Consumer Health Informatics

Chapman & Hall/CRC Healthcare Informatics Series

Consumer Health Informatics
Enabling Digital Health for Everyone
Catherine Arnott Smith, Alla Keselman

Process Modeling and Management for Healthcare
Carlo Combi, Giuseppe Pozzi, Pierangelo Veltri

For more information on this series please visit: https://www.routledge.com/
Chapman--HallCRC-Healthcare-Informatics-Series/book-series/HEALTHINF

Consumer Health Informatics

Enabling Digital Health for Everyone

Catherine Arnott Smith
University of Wisconsin-Madison

Alla Keselman
National Library of Medicine

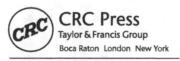

CRC Press
Taylor & Francis Group
Boca Raton London New York

CRC Press is an imprint of the
Taylor & Francis Group, an **informa** business

A CHAPMAN & HALL BOOK

First Edition published 2020
by CRC Press
6000 Broken Sound Parkway NW, Suite 300, Boca Raton, FL 33487-2742

and by CRC Press
2 Park Square, Milton Park, Abingdon, Oxon, OX14 4RN

Library of Congress Cataloging-in-Publication Data
Names: Smith, Catherine Arnott, author. | Keselman, Alla, author.
Title: Consumer health informatics : enabling digital health for everyone /
Catherine Arnott Smith, University of Wisconsin-Madison, Alla
Keselman, National Library of Medicine.
Description: First edition. | Boca Raton : CRC Press, 2021. | Series:
Chapman & Hall/CRC healthcare informatics series | Includes
bibliographical references and index.
Identifiers: LCCN 2020037236 | ISBN 9781138337459 (hardback) | ISBN
9780429442377 (ebook)
Subjects: LCSH: Medical informatics. | Telecommunication in medicine.
Classification: LCC R858 .S563 2021 | DDC 610.285--dc23
LC record available at https://lccn.loc.gov/2020037236

ISBN: 978-1-138-33745-9 (hbk)
ISBN: 978-0-429-44237-7 (ebk)

Typeset in Minion Pro
by SPi Global, India

Contents

I

Foundations

Individuals' Opportunities and Challenges in the Era of Participatory Healthcare

Alla Keselman

THIS CHAPTER DISCUSSES opportunities and challenges created by the growing societal conviction that individuals should be active participants in their healthcare. It opens with a history of the relationship between medical care and its recipients as it shifts from "doctor knows best" to recognition of individuals' right to exercise control over their bodies and lives. The chapter discusses the role of the internet in democratizing health information access and its impact on patient empowerment. It also addresses the role of informatics, precision medicine, and pharmacogenomics in the rise of patient-driven data platforms enabling user-driven information exchange, research, and communication. The chapter provides examples of people's involvement in their care, biomedical and healthcare research (defining priorities, proposing hypotheses, initiating studies, crowdsourcing data collection), and medical technology development. In one of these examples, a patient guides a team of engineers and doctors collaborating on developing a modification for a surgical procedure. In another, a group of concerned parents of children with diabetes builds a successful grassroots community that develops an effective approach for diabetes-related data sharing and integration. The chapter also discusses how patients' self-experimentation, shared and propagated via patient platforms or online communities, can both lead to new clinical trials and give rise to ethical concerns. There is also an overview of participatory medicine societies and conferences and a discussion of participatory medicine's impact on individuals' health outcome and healthcare cost. Lastly, the chapter discusses challenges to people's effective participation in healthcare, such as persistent medical paternalism and limited individuals' health literacy. At the closing, it turns to how consumer health informatics can support people by providing tools that help overcome the barriers.

1.1 FROM PATERNALISTIC ROOTS TO ETHICAL PATIENT ENGAGEMENT

Before the germ theory of disease gained acceptance in the late 19th century (Bantock, 1899), medicine was not exactly science-based (science itself was very different then). Doctors were not held in very high regard, and people sought care from a variety of sources, including experienced family and community members and traditional healers (Roberts, 1999). There was no sharp delineation between "professional" and non-professional healing-related knowledge. However, as 19th-century discoveries in science and technology came into medicine, knowledge gaps between doctors and the lay public grew, and so did the respect and authority afforded to the medical profession. On the one hand, it was customary to assume that, since the doctor knew best, the patient did not need to know. On the other hand, when patients did want to know more, the medical establishment attempted to guard medical information and restrict lay access to it, out of fear that it would be misused in incorrect self-diagnosis and inappropriate self-treatment. Before the internet, professional medical information was principally found in medical libraries, and many medical libraries restricted the public's access to their stacks. In an overview of "Medical information for the consumer before the World Wide Web", Catherine Arnott Smith quotes from a 1934 *Bulletin of the Medical Library Association* article, published by Mildred Farrow, a medical librarian at the San Diego Medical Society (Arnott Smith, 2015). In the article, Ms. Farrow calls for closing the medical library to the public. She points out that the lay patrons "read on subjects of which they had not the slightest knowledge", so one "can but marvel why … this problem was not solved long ago" (Farrow, 1934).

The position on the public's rights to medical information started changing in the 1970s. At that point, the impetus was ethical, rather than utilitarian. Civil rights movements of the 1960s and 1970s stressed the ethical imperative of supporting empowerment of a growing number of disadvantaged groups. In the context of those societal changes, it suddenly became quite reasonable to suggest that individuals have the right to information and should be involved in decisions that affect their lives and well-being. This was aided by the realization of the need to protect participants in biomedical research, the urgency of which came to light in the case of the infamous 1932–1972 US Public Health Service Tuskegee Syphilis Study. The study, which recruited poor rural Black sharecroppers diagnosed with syphilis, studied the natural progression of the disease. When the study began, there was no effective treatment for syphilis, so observation without treatment did not deviate from the established standard of care. However, when penicillin became the standard treatment in 1947, participants were kept in the dark about it and prevented from seeking care outside the study. Eventually, leaks to the press and the ensuing public outrage led to very significant changes in federal legislature regulating research with human subjects (Centers for Disease Control, 2020).

The movements of the 1970s led to calls for patient empowerment and shared decision-making. Throughout the 1990s, as attracting and retaining patients by provider networks became more competitive, healthcare increased its focus on "patient-centeredness" (Roberts, 1999). These social and healthcare developments stressed the importance of gaining patients' perspectives and priorities and engaging patients in decision-making.

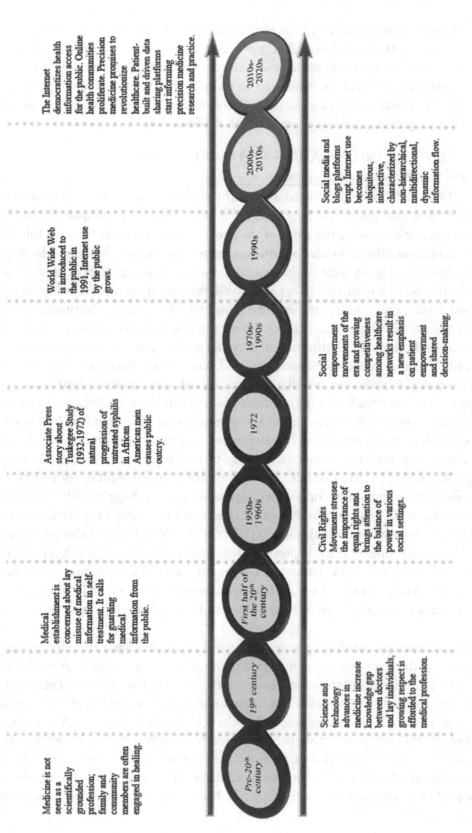

FIGURE 1.1 Brief historical timeline of the patient–healthcare establishment relationship.

A growing number of initiatives within the healthcare industry emphasized the importance of helping patients understand relative risks and benefits of various treatment approaches, as well as the trade-off between effective treatments and quality of life. The advent of managed care and its reimbursement model that rewarded lower per-patient expenditure also prompted an emphasis on wellness and public health initiatives devoted to increasing the public's understanding of health determinants.

1.2 21ST-CENTURY INFORMATION TECHNOLOGY AS GAME-CHANGER

While the 1970s–1990s changed attitudes about the public's rights and engagement, it was the technological changes of the 21st century that propelled the participatory medicine movement, greatly expanding the scope of the public's engagement with health information and healthcare. The rationale for patient engagement shifted, from an ethical discourse on people's rights to their bodies to a utilitarian discourse on improved safety and quality of care and cost reduction. Two particular developments merit discussion here.

The first development is the internet and its role in democratizing health information access for the public. The internet changed both the ease with which people can reach information and the kinds of information they can access. The era when well-meaning medical librarians or health professionals could serve as gatekeepers of information, barring the public from access, is well behind us. Health information websites and apps proliferate, with new ones becoming available daily. While their quality varies and navigating to high-quality information is not always easy (as we will see in Part I: Chapter 4; Part II: Chapter 8), many authoritative government, academic, non-profit, and for-profit organizations now provide accurate, reliable, up-to-date information, written in simple language. According to many sources, Americans are taking advantage of this access, with the majority going online for health information (Fox & Duggan, 2013). In emerging economies, in 2018 as many as 70% of Mexicans and Jordanians reported accessing health information on their mobile phones (Silver et al., 2019). Patients also join forums and platforms that connect them to powerful information networks. This has given rise to a new kind of patient. These patients are knowledgeable, skilled at consumer health information seeking, connected with others, empowered, and ready to be vital collaborators on issues extending beyond their values and lifestyle preferences (deBronkart, 2015).

The second development shifting patient participation in healthcare from the ethical to the pragmatic is the changing face of medicine in the 21st century. 21st-century medicine is more and more informed by pharmacogenomics: the study of how a person's genes affect his or her susceptibility to diseases or conditions and response to treatments. This revolutionary model, termed "precision medicine", is changing biomedical research and clinical care. From the research perspective, precision medicine studies require large datasets of genetic, clinical, and behavioral data. Such data are not routinely collected in a doctor's office and can only be obtained from actively collaborating participants. From a clinical care perspective, treatments are matched not to a disease, but to a patient's genetic profile.

While the resulting treatments are tailored to subgroups rather than individual patients, precision medicine increases the emphasis on the individuals and their response. The development of precision medicine occurs via initiatives that encourage patient engagement and collaboration between researchers, patients, and clinicians. Some of these initiatives are patient-driven. For example, PatientsLikeMe is an online data sharing platform that was founded in 2004 by family members of a young man living with Amyotrophic Lateral Sclerosis (ALS; see also Part II: Chapter 10). The platform enables its members to enter longitudinal information on various aspects of their conditions and functioning, with the goal of discovering what treatments proved effective for those with similar profiles (PatientsLikeMe, 2019). At the time of writing of this chapter, in July of 2020, PatientsLikeMe provides a platform to members sharing data on over 2800 conditions, including COVID-19, currently in its active pandemic phase. PatientsLikeMe data have also been used by the platform's research team and its commercial and academic collaborators in order to conduct research and advance treatment development. Another effort to accelerate precision medicine research is the NIH *All of Us* Research Program that aims to collect genetic, clinical, lifestyle, and environmental data from more than one million individuals in the US. *All of Us* recruits program participants via an active engagement and education campaign. Jointly, the democratization of consumer health information access and the precision medicine revolution in healthcare make active patient engagement in healthcare not only ethical, but also practical, and likely conducive to better outcomes.

1.3 INFORMATION SOURCES FOR FACILITATING PATIENTS' AND THE PUBLIC'S ENGAGEMENT WITH HEALTHCARE

Throughout this book, you will see chapters dedicated to various specific online information sources and types of tools that support engaged consumer health functioning. This section is just a brief overview of their universe. Of these tools and resources, the oldest, most similar to traditional print sources, but more easily accessible, are traditional information websites. While they do not provide interactivity or connection to a community, at their best, they deliver authoritative quality information. An example of such a site is medlineplus.gov from the National Library of Medicine that provides free quality information about diseases, conditions, treatments, and wellness issues.

Later generations of information sources include more dynamic, interactive tools such as blogs, social media forums, and patient platforms like PatientsLikeMe (patientslikeme.com). Traditionally, most information that patients could obtain about diseases and treatments was written from the provider's perspective. Topics included symptoms, available treatments, and survival curves, but little space was devoted to managing the impact of a disease on lifestyles, relationships, friendships, work, and sense of self. The internet changed that. Consider the case of Jeri Burtchell. Burtchell was diagnosed with multiple sclerosis (MS) in 1999, enrolled in a clinical trial of an investigational drug for her condition in 2007, and searched for information about what it felt like to be a participant (Burtchell, 2016). When, to her surprise, she could not find such information written from a patient perspective, she started a blog documenting her clinical trial experience. Today Jeri is a health activist and a blogger who writes and delivers talks about different aspects of living with MS. Another blogger and pioneer of internet-enabled patient engagement is Dave deBronkart, or e-Patient Dave. In 2007, Dave was diagnosed with Stage 4 renal cell carcinoma and given a median survival prognosis of 24 weeks. After Dave received experimental treatment in a clinical trial – a trial that he identified with the help of his primary care physician-recommended online patient community – his cancer went into remission (deBronkart, 2018). Dave and his oncologist also credit Dave's pre-clinical online information gathering with his readiness and ability to tolerate the trial medication's serious side effects. Following his remission, Dave deBronkart became a vocal advocate of the patient engagement movement, giving speeches and writing books, articles, and blog posts. He also co-founded the Society for Participatory Medicine, a non-profit organization that publishes the peer-reviewed *Journal of Participatory Medicine*, and became a frequent contributor to the Society's blog. While Jeri and Dave's blogs are unusually broad and multi-faceted in their coverage of health-related issues, they exemplify a growing genre giving voice to patients who want to share their stories – and help those looking for such stories to become informed and inspired.

A blog is a voice of a single individual. Online forums and listservs are examples of platforms that support community discussions and exchange of opinions. These communities vary in their coverage, membership, and degree of moderation, ranging from grassroots unmoderated Google and Yahoo groups and social media accounts (e.g., Twitter, Facebook) to moderated communities maintained by hospitals and healthcare organizations (e.g., Mayo Clinic Connect; see Part II: Chapter 10). When Web-based communities first arose, there was concern among health professionals about their potential to spread misinformation along with support. Spread of health misinformation in online networks is, indeed, a justified concern. Yet, it appears that, in the case of Web-based communities of patients and families, the concern was not well-founded, as the kind of information patients seek from one another (emotional and lifestyle support) is often different from the information they seek from healthcare providers. The most sophisticated level of patient communities are platforms like PatientsLikeMe, mentioned above, which not only enable and facilitate conversations among patients, but allow structured data entry, aggregation, visualization, and analysis, supporting citizen science and traditional research.

Tools that connect patients with one another and support knowledge sharing and generation are extremely important. So are tools that support wellness and disease management and access to individual information recorded and analyzed by providers. Promoters of participatory medicine thus actively advocate for patients' access to their medical records. The model of such access is exemplified by the growing OpenNotes initiative that calls for providers to adopt technological solutions that enable their patients to read their records (https://www.opennotes.org/). Studies suggest that, despite the initial worry among some providers, opening notes to patients does not increase providers' workload and positively affects patients' sense of control and empowerment, without leaving them frightened or confused; it also improves patient adherence to medication (DesRoches et al., 2019). In addition to using their patient portals to access their individual data entered by providers, patients can maintain and share their own records using online tools and apps dedicated to various aspects of health information management, from appointment scheduling to setting medication reminders. Part II of this book is dedicated to specific tools enabling patient and consumer health empowerment.

1.4 PARTICIPATORY HEALTHCARE SOCIETIES AND CONFERENCES

A number of membership organizations, publications, and conferences are dedicated to promoting the participatory model in healthcare and supporting patients seeking greater involvement in their care. For example, The Institute for Patient- and Family-Centered Care (IPFCC), a non-profit organization founded in 1992, aims to "[provide] essential leadership to advance the understanding and practice of patient- and family centered care" (Institute for Patient- and Family-Centered Care, n.d.). It provides consulting and guidance to healthcare organizations that would like to increase their engagement with patients and families. One real-world result: the development of PFACS, or Patient and Family Advisory Councils. A recent survey of 6700 family physicians found that 24% of respondents engaged with patients using a PFAC structure (Sharma et al., 2018). The previously mentioned Society for Participatory Medicine, formed in 2009, unites "patients, physicians, nurses, caregivers, policy makers, consultants, and others who are part of the healthcare system" in "dozens of countries around the world" (https://participatorymedicine. org/memberships/). The Society publishes a peer-reviewed journal, organizes an annual conference, conducts free webinars, and maintains a blog. Patient advocacy organizations such as the American Cancer Society and American Heart Association provide patient education and support, and engage in research funding and health policy work. European Cancer Patient Coalition (ECPC) advocates for patient-centered government policies and better alignment between cancer patients' needs and EU cancer research priorities. It also promotes patient engagement in research design and active data gathering (http://www. ecpc.org/).

Another relatively new phenomenon, related to the e-patient movement, is patient conferences. For example, Kathi Apostilidis, President of ECPC, organizes a yearly Patient Power conference in Greece (deBronkart, 2015). Another patient activist, Imogen Cheese, created an annual melanoma patient conference in the UK (Cheese, 2017). The Neuroendocrine Tumor Research Foundation, faced with an 80% rate of misdiagnosis of this incurable cancer, began holding free educational conferences in 2009 to increase awareness, and in 2019 reported that more than 3000 people had attended (NETRF, 2020). The Los Angeles NET Society features not only an annual conference, but a videotaped Speaker Series posted on YouTube. The objective of such conferences is to bring together patients, caregivers, patient advocates, and health professionals to network, learn, and discuss treatment, research, and policy priorities. As we are writing this chapter at the height of the COVID-19 pandemic, we would be amiss not to mention the pandemic's canceling impact on opportunities for face-to-face conferences. Yet, we hope that technology, including conferencing technologies, will help participatory healthcare societies find innovative alternative ways to connect patients, families, advocates, and providers.

1.5 PATIENT PARTICIPATION IN DIFFERENT ASPECTS OF MEDICAL CARE, RESEARCH, AND DEVELOPMENT

As suggested above, patient participation in healthcare can take many forms. This section provides examples and case studies of patient participation in their personal care, biomedical research, and treatment development.

1.5.1 Patient Participation in Their Care

Shared decision-making – the process when doctors and patients discuss various treatment options and jointly choose the optimal course of treatment based on the patient's priorities – represents an early model of patient engagement. By discussing their values and priorities with their providers, patients can give input into therapeutic goal-setting and treatment selection. This may involve a decision, for example, about submitting to more aggressive treatment, given the possible side effects, or choosing which medication options best fit into the individual's lifestyle. Making treatment and disease management decisions often involves processing large amounts of complex information. As the appreciation of the patients' role in decision-making grows, so does the understanding that patients need support dealing with this complex information. Patient Decision Aids help individuals make treatment decisions (Agin et al., 2018). They exist in a variety of formats, from print charts to electronic apps. They have been developed and studied in a range of conditions and patient groups, from cancer care to pregnancy. Studies suggest that, when well designed, decision aids lead to increased knowledge, decreased inner conflict around making the decision, and the alignment between stated lifestyle preferences and chosen decision options (McAlpine et al., 2018). While technology can provide valuable assistance, it does not replace human interaction. The process of shared decision-making should include true collaboration between the patient and the health professional, during which the patient has the opportunity to ask questions and express concerns without being rushed, with the provider helping with both the cognitive and the emotional burden of the process.

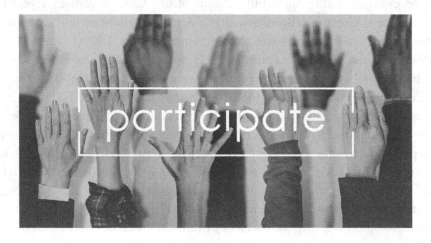

Other examples of patient engagement in care are situations when patients, connecting with others and reviewing information, discover a new diagnostic hypothesis or treatment option that was not suggested to them by the physician. This is highly controversial: lay individuals certainly do not have the training and expertize that providers use in their decisions. Yet, in the digital universe, what individuals often have is the time and motivation to crowdsource questions; they can spend much more time searching for information pertaining to their case than any provider can afford. Providers are understandably wary of this shift in power, and yet, in the world of today's rapidly developing medical knowledge, patients may discover valuable information that their provider does not know. Through sites like PatientsLikeMe, they can also compare themselves to others with similar conditions and clinical and demographic profiles. For example, Todd Small was a man living with MS whose symptoms were not alleviated by the muscle relaxant medication he was taking. After registering for PatientsLikeMe, Small was able to look at self-reported medication dosages for about 200 other site members taking the same medication. After doing so, Small saw that, despite his impression that he was taking the maximum recommended dose of the drug, his dose was actually on the low end. He asked his neurologist to increase the dose, which led to significant alleviation of the symptoms. While Small did not have his neurologist's knowledge of the pathophysiology and pharmacology involved in this decision, he did have access to a large dataset of cases that provided him with a perspective his doctor did not have (Goetz, 2011).

Doctors' reaction to patients bringing in suggestions they found during online networking and research varies tremendously. deBronkart (2018) points out that a doctor's objection to patients' googling information is equivalent to saying "If I don't already know something, it can't add value to the case". He then adds that, on the other hand, expecting the doctor to know everything puts an unfair burden on the doctor, concluding: "Let patients help". deBronkart' s doctor concurs, commenting: "I don't know if you could have tolerated enough medicine if you hadn't been so well prepared" (deBronkart, 2013). Ultimately, when providers are justifiably concerned about the quality of information brought to them for discussion by patients, explaining this in a respectful conversation, rather than dismissing it outright, is likely to be better and the relationship.

1.5.2 Patients as Influencers and Promoters of Biomedical Research

Much innovation is happening in patients' contribution to research. The collective force of information technology-enabled patient communities drives this innovation. Such communities can propose research questions and participate in determining biomedical research priorities. As seen in the section on patient conferences, patient advocacy organizations see influencing decisions about research priorities and funding as one of their key functions. IPFCC-run PFACS, along with their other functions, provide platforms for clinicians or researchers to generate ideas and obtain members' input and feedback. In addition, online patient communities like PatientsLikeMe, where patients contribute their data to repositories, can demand a voice in how their data are used in research. As participatory medicine is becoming the norm, invitations to patients to contribute to defining research agendas may come from unusual places. For example, 23andMe, a direct-to-consumer commercial genetic testing service company, encourages its customers, who are not necessarily patients, to propose new research questions and submit project ideas (Prainsack, 2014). While a single individual is not likely to impact the research agenda of a biomedical field, unless she or he is a celebrity, vocal engaged communities can affect science policy and funding.

PatientsLikeMe and 23andMe community members participate in a large number of studies, organized by these companies with collaboration from industry and academic researchers. Participants generally feel comfortable sharing their data via these platforms (Wicks et al., 2010), as they are able to contribute to the discourse about research priorities. Much of the research conducted with PatientsLikeMe participants consists of observational studies that help researchers understand how diseases progress and affect participants. These data have been used to inform improving questionnaires for assessing patients' functioning (e.g., in ALS patients) (Swan, 2012). Another significant research area is tracking patients' response to off-label use of treatments. Off-label use, both legal and common, occurs when a medication is prescribed for diagnoses or in doses different from those defined in its FDA approval (Food and Drug Administration, 2018). For example, a drug that causes an undesirable side effect (e.g., jitters and insomnia) may be used for a disease where that side effect would be welcome (e.g., MS-induced fatigue). Wicks points out that prescribing physicians often do not treat enough patients with the condition to assess the effectiveness of such off-label use and describes several cases when PatientsLikeMe provided positive data that encouraged further investigation in traditional research.

Engaged patients can also help the research community with promoting studies and recruiting participants into them – a practice called crowdsourced recruitment – as well as promoting the importance of research in general. For example, Kantor et al. (2018) point out that patient community websites, such as http://mymsteam.com Multiple Sclerosis support community, promote information about clinical trials. Organizations and companies like PatientsLikeMe and 23andMe use their extensive networks to recruit participants for researcher-organized studies (Swan, 2012).

1.5.3 Patient Communities as Participant-Organized Crowdsourcing Networks

In a revolutionary departure from the previous biomedical research models, online patient communities can use the power of their aggregate data to conduct their own studies. Swan (2012) points to a number of social network communities that conduct participant-organized studies. These include PatientsLikeMe and Quantified Self, the networks that support self-tracking and communication, as well as DIY Genomics that is specifically dedicated to conducting research via crowdsourcing.

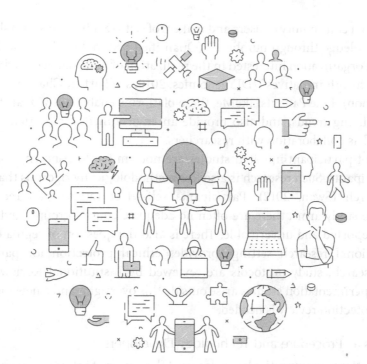

Some of these studies emerged out of self-experimentation by individuals living with serious incurable diseases and unwilling to put up with the slow traditional research and drug approval process. For example, a 2008 *New York Times* article describes how, several months prior to publication, the ALS community became energized with the buzz that Italian researchers had found that lithium significantly slowed down ALS progression. Although this information did not come from published research, a group of PatientsLikeMe members with ALS obtained lithium prescriptions from their doctors and self-organized into a spontaneous patients-run clinical trial, aggregating their data via the platform (Goetz, 2008). Eventually, the impact of lithium on ALS progression was studied by PatientsLikeMe-associated researchers, and then in traditional clinical studies. Researchers ultimately concluded that while lithium did not slow ALS progression, the drug presented no safety concern (UKMND-LiCALS Study Group et al., 2013).

The lithium story illustrates both the potential benefits and the potential serious pitfalls of patient-run crowdsourced research. On the one hand, such self-organized clinical trials by patients may provide fast-track confirmatory or disconfirmatory data for traditional research, facilitating its progress. On the other hand, the processes that slow down traditional research and drug approval are patient safety measures. Patients pressuring their doctors into off-label prescription of approved medications, designed for different conditions, on the basis of early/inconclusive research, could be inviting dangerous consequences.

Despite and alongside the concerns, participants-organized medical research is growing, with new online platforms emerging for that purpose. For example, Quantified Self is "an international community of users and makers of self-tracking tools who share an interest in 'self-knowledge through numbers'" (Quantified Self, n.d.). DYIgenomics is "a nonprofit research organization interested in the realization of personalized medicine through crowdsourced health initiatives" (DIYgenomics, 2019; see Part II, Chapter 11 for more on this phenomenon). Like PatientsLikeMe, these platforms enable individuals to input their data for visualizing trends, and also provide an environment for participant-organized studies, as well as collaboration with researchers.

Criticisms of participant-initiated studies are not limited to concerns about potential harm to participants. Such research is also less methodologically rigorous than traditional medical research (Swan, 2012). Participants self-select rather than receive random assignments to study arms, there are often no adequate control groups, and much of the data are self-reported and unverifiable. There is also the question of regulatory oversight that in traditional research settings provides ethical protection for participants. In traditional research, study protocols are reviewed by Institutional Review Boards, but ad-hoc self-experimentation studies arise outside this oversight, and a new model of safety and ethical protection review is needed.

1.5.4 Patients as Procedure and Technology Developers

Patients and patient communities have also used the power of information access and connectivity, afforded by modern information technologies, to contribute to developing and improving medical devices and procedures. The Smart Homes chapter of this book describes the #WeAreNotWaiting grassroots diabetes community movement, started by tech-savvy parents of children with Type 1 Diabetes. The movement, which sprang out of parents' concern about lack of interoperability standards in glucose monitoring technology, gave rise to several open-access DIY technology projects. One of these projects is Nightscout, described in the Smart Homes chapter (Part II: Chapter 9). It supports continuous upload of blood glucose measures from wearable monitors to the cloud, enabling parents and family members to monitor their children's glucose values remotely, at any time of day, using a range of devices. The technology, of course, is useful beyond pediatric settings (Nightscout, 2020).

Another project that grew out of the #WeAreNotWaiting movement is #OpenAPS, a patient community dedicated to building open-access Artificial Pancreas System (APS) technology. "Artificial pancreas" refers to technology that automatically monitors and adjusts blood glucose levels via an insulin pump. Insulin is a hormone that metabolizes glucose (sugar). A certain minimum level of insulin in the blood is required at all times to maintain normal blood glucose level. That minimum level fluctuates somewhat depending on factors such as activity level. In addition, a greater infusion of insulin is required at mealtimes. Traditionally, patients or family members computed these insulin doses using mathematical formulas, with some trial-and-error tweaking. The OpenAPS community developed Autotune, an automated tool for determining relevant insulin dosing variables on the basis of the data obtained from continuous glucose monitoring devices (Lewis & Leibrand, 2017). The technology relies on open-source software and, according to deBronkart (2015), "a $35 pocket computer".

Another noteworthy example of medical technology developed via participatory medicine involves a collaboration not among a group of patients, but between a patient and a multidisciplinary team of engineers, physicians, and scientists (deBronkart, 2015). Tal Golesworthy, a UK patient with Marfan syndrome, faced very serious surgery on his aorta, the main artery that carries oxygenated blood from the heart to the rest of the circulatory system. Stretching, or enlargement, of the aorta is a common complication of Marfan syndrome. It is very dangerous and may be life-threatening because it may lead to leaking or bursting of the aorta. The standard treatment involves surgery in which the enlarged segment of the aorta is replaced. This type of surgery – detaching and re-attaching the aorta – requires using extreme cooling to induce hypothermia, dropping patient's body temperature to about 64.4F, stopping the patient's heart, and transferring the heart and lungs function to a machine. After the surgery, the patient needs to be on a continuous regimen of blood-thinning medications. Not surprisingly, Tal was very motivated to find an alternative treatment for his condition. An R&D process engineer, Tal set out to solve what he described as "just a plumbing problem" to develop a mesh that could be used to wrap and, thus, contain, the bulging section of the aorta. He was able to obtain funding for the project and assemble a multidisciplinary team that, among others, involved engineers, cardiac specialists, a radiologist, and a chemist. The team collected multiple MRI and CT scan images of Tal's aorta. The scans were used to create a plastic, and then mesh, model of the bulging section of his aorta. The tailored mesh was then used to wrap that aorta section. The resulting surgery was a much shorter process than the traditional procedure and did not require artificial heart and lungs machine and body cooling. In explaining his investment in the project, Tal said in his TED talk, "The great advantage of an external support, for me, was that I could retain all of my own bits, all of my own endothelium and valves, and not need any anticoagulation therapy" (Golesworthy, 2011). The method developed by Tal has since been used for a number of patients with aortic dilation.

1.6 IMPACT OF PARTICIPATORY MEDICINE ON HEALTH OUTCOMES AND THE COST OF CARE

Proponents of participatory medicine believe that this approach has the potential to improve health outcomes and reduce costs. For example, in the *Observations* section of BMJ, one of the world's most authoritative medical journals, its patient partnership editor and patient advocate Tessa Richards argues: "[patient empowerment is] not just a nice thing to do but a cost effective intervention that can be implemented widely" (Richards, 2011). Building empirical evidence for this claim is not straightforward because there is no agreed-upon definition of participatory medicine. To study a concept, researchers need a universal definition of it that can be translated into specific measures. Participatory medicine, as we have seen, comprises a range of things, from shared decision-making about treatment to patients-organized research using patients-aggregated data.

There are, however, studies that look into how different characteristics of healthcare that are associated with participatory medicine affect health outcomes and costs. One well-studied characteristic is patient-centeredness of care. Patient-centeredness refers to the extent to which physicians view their patients' health in the larger context of their lives, inquire about patients' understanding of their disease and their priorities, and develop decision-making partnership. The hypothesis that patient-centeredness increases the effectiveness and efficiency of care seems intuitive. Its advocates propose that it gives the patient a sense of empowerment and leads to greater and more effective engagement with the healthcare system. If patient-centeredness and the resulting patient engagement lead to better understanding and, thus, utilization of preventive and routine care, as well as better adherence to treatment and lifestyle measures (Bauman et al., 2003), this is likely to lead to better outcomes and reduced costs.

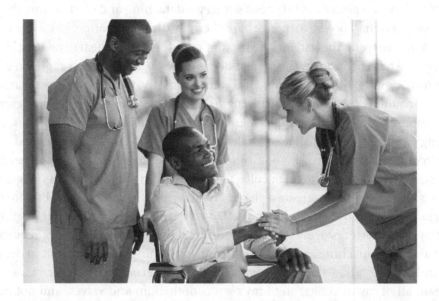

The data support the hypothesis. In a study of 599 patients, Bertakis and Azari (2011) found that patient-centered care style by family physicians and general internists was related to fewer hospitalizations, fewer visits to specialists, fewer diagnostic and lab tests, and reduced overall cost of care. The authors assessed patient-centeredness via Davis Observation Code developed and validated by their team (Callahan & Bertakis, 1991). This instrument identifies patient-centered interactions in six different patient care clusters (e.g., technical cluster that focuses on physical examination and treatment planning, preventive services cluster, etc.). This allows representation of patient-centeredness as a multidimensional concept that involves different physician-initiated topics and behaviors. Examples of these topics and behaviors include discussing social history and family functioning, asking and inviting questions about exercise and nutrition, and assessing patient's beliefs and health and disease. The study design did not allow determination of the mechanism by which greater patient-centeredness may lead to reduced number of hospitalizations and specialist visits. The authors hypothesized, however, that such care may reduce patients' anxiety, increase their trust in their primary care doctors, and, thus, reduce requests for referrals to specialists (Bertakis & Azari, 2011). It is also possible that such care improves patients' health practices and home medication schedule, making their health more stable and reducing the need for hospitalization and specialist care, usually utilized in acute situations. In healthcare, the frequency of hospitalizations and emergency services utilization is often used as a proxy for health status. More research is needed to connect models of care with outcomes and cost reduction.

As this chapter demonstrates, a frequently discussed component of patient engagement is online patient networks. Of their various purposes, the most studied component is their support group function. There is evidence suggesting that participating in online support groups has positive impact on disease management, health behaviors, and health outcomes (e.g., Griffiths et al., 2012; Laranjo et al., 2015; Mo & Coulson, 2013). For more information on the impact of patient communities on patients' lives, see Part II: Chapter 10 of this book.

More research is needed to assess the impact of various aspects of participatory medicine on individuals' health outcomes and cost of care. In order for such research to be meaningful, we need a meaningful definition of participatory care. Perhaps, following Bertakis and Azari's (2011) work, the concept of participatory medicine can be represented as a set of patient behaviors and patient-system interactions within clusters of individuals' relationships with healthcare: for example, individual care, biomedical research, R&D. Then the impact of the behaviors on health outcomes can be studied both jointly and separately. It is also important to remember that participatory care is a property of a system, rather than a patient or a provider. A highly engaged patient may, nevertheless, be unsuccessful in initiating participatory care if his provider does not welcome this model or if the healthcare organization erects barriers to the information essential for the collaboration (e.g., page charges for medical records). By the same token, no matter how patient-centered the provider, the care will not be participatory if the patient prefers a paternalistic model, in which she relies on the doctor's recommendations without asking probing questions (e.g., as a way to manage anxiety of living with a disease). Lastly, it is important to collect evidence, so that we can answer the question "Under what circumstances does participatory medicine lead to better health outcomes?" Different factors can serve as barriers and enablers with regard to the impact on outcomes. One likely barrier to the effectiveness of participatory medicine, as will be discussed further, is patients' limited health literacy. In such cases, we hope that informatics tools can provide needed supports, helping achieve the desired outcome despite the barriers. Such possible enablers will be briefly discussed further in this chapter, and later, in great detail, throughout the book.

1.7 SYSTEMIC BARRIERS AND CHALLENGES TO PATIENT ENGAGEMENT

This chapter is full of examples of striking successes of collaborative care approaches between patients and their healthcare providers. Yet, while such collaborations are becoming more common, providers vary greatly in their openness to them. Doctors' and other health professionals' resistance to participatory medicine is a significant barrier slowing the cultural change. In their e-patient advocacy talks and publications, deBronkart and Tessa Richards (deBronkart, 2011, 2015; Richards, 2014) give example of physicians' very different responses to patients' attempts to ask for decision-making partnership. For example, Richards describes doing extensive online research for a patient with drug-resistant rheumatoid arthritis. Her research suggested that biologics are potentially helpful, yet, prescribed inconsistently. The patient's doctor, however, refused to prescribe biologics and did not welcome the discussion. The patient changed the provider, and the new doctor immediately agreed that biologics were indicated.

Many doctors are weary of patients coming to their office with the information they found on the internet, asking questions about alternative treatments and procedures. In considering their attitude, we must remember that the internet is full of inaccurate, incomplete, and misleading information, some of it placed there intentionally, by unscrupulous snake oil salesmen praying on people's despair. Yet, it is also important to remember that a patient's stake in a healthcare interaction is their health and their life; denying them decision-making power is ethically unjustifiable. Moreover, if the decision they would like to make is based on incorrect or incomplete information, simply dismissing their search for alternatives is likely to have dismal results.

The famous, or rather, infamous, UK case of a five-year-old patient Ashya King illustrates this point. In 2014, Ashya underwent a brain tumor removal surgery in Southampton General Hospital. His doctors felt that the appropriate follow-up treatment was conventional radiotherapy, while his parents wanted Ashya to receive proton beam therapy, which at the time was not routinely provided by NHS, the UK national healthcare system. Ashya's parents requested that the procedure be performed abroad, but his doctors did not support their decision and, according to Ashya's father, threatened to involve the court in resolving the disagreement. This led to Ashya's parents leaving the hospital with the boy and taking him to Spain without informing hospital staff. The hospital appealed to court, which issued a European arrest warrant. Ashya's parents were arrested and put in prison in Spain, and Ashya made a ward of the court. As a result of the ensuing international backlash, Ashya was finally allowed to receive proton beam treatment in a Prague clinic (Dyer, 2014). His UK doctors maintain that proton beam therapy was suboptimal treatment for Ashya's case. Today Ashya is alive and cancer-free (ITV, 2019). Doctors may be justified in involving the courts in pediatric cases when they believe that the parents are preventing the child from receiving life-saving treatment. But a situation like Ashya's illustrates another danger: of communication breakdown between the doctors and the patients and families, with the two parties coming to see each other as adversaries, rather than collaborators.

Paternalism and attempts to discourage patients and families from active participation in decision-making may come not only from individual providers, but from entire healthcare systems. Frequently, this manifests in barring information access to medical records and other types of patient data, or making such access difficult. In the US, patient access to their medical records is guaranteed by the Health Information Portability and Accountability Act (HIPAA; The Health Insurance Portability and Accountability Act, 1996). This does not mean there are no barriers to obtaining records; besides technological difficulties transferring information between healthcare systems, providers can charge individuals "reasonable costs" to copy and mail the records. There are also unique challenges inherent is some special cases. For example, "records" consisting of data emitted by medical devices remain a complicated medicolegal problem, on which the FDA – which has the responsibility for devices – has issued guidance (Center for Devices and Radiological

Health, 2017). Hugo Campos is a patient advocate who lives with an implanted cardiac defibrillator. His experience of attempting to access the data generated by his defibrillator made Hugo a campaigner for patients' rights to the data collected by their implanted medical devices (Campos, 2012; Gurkan, 2019). Hugo felt that monitoring his data would help him understand what triggers his arrhythmia and avoid those triggers. While implantable device makers send these data to doctors, they are extremely reluctant to share them with patients in whose bodies the devices are implanted. This means, among other things, that patients without health insurance have to pay very high fees for data analysis via a specialist office visit. Hugo Campos' advocacy involved meeting with FDA regulators and device manufacturers, resulting in much positive press coverage and earning him White House Champion of Change for Precision Medicine honor. Yet, patient access to implanted device data remains a challenge, and systemic change in healthcare that would welcome patient engagement and make it easy is far from completed.

1.8 THE CHALLENGE OF HEALTH LITERACY AND DIGITAL LITERACY REQUIREMENTS FOR PARTICIPATION

For patients and consumers, effectively dealing with health information requires a number of competencies. These competencies, which constitute capacity to "obtain, process, and understand basic health information" are often referred to as "health literacy" (Ratzan & Parker, 2000, p. vi). Dealing with health information in the digital domain presents additional requirements (e-Health literacy).

The concepts of health literacy and e-Health literacy are complex and have no single agreed-upon definition, issues discussed at length in Part I: Chapter 3. Yet, if we think about them as a set of skills, they involve, among others, traditional reading ability and numeracy, understanding how to search and evaluate information, background science knowledge, and the ability to use computers and the internet.

Studies suggest that the level of health literacy in the US population is disconcertingly low. According to the most comprehensive 2003 US National Assessment of Adult Literacy (NAAL) (https://nces.ed.gov/naal/), only 12% of US adults have a "proficient" level of health literacy, while 14% are at the "below basic" level. NAAL's methods of assessing health literacy are not perfect, and there is no corresponding national study on e-health literacy (more on that in Part I: Chapter 3). Yet, the list of skills and the statistics jointly show that entering the field of medical decision-making is not an easy task. Individuals like Tal Golesworthy, possessing the knowledge and skills to lead teams of engineers and physicians in medical discovery tailored to their specific medical requirements, are extremely rare and few people would dream of attempting such a collaboration. But even much simpler participatory medicine tasks, such as choosing between two treatment regimens, involve a lot of complexity.

Imagine a family faced with the situation in which Ashya King's parents found themselves: dealing with multiple information streams and evaluating the pros and cons of conventional radiotherapy and proton beam therapy for their five-year-old. The information involved is complex and highly technical, with much specialized terminology and statistical data. There is uncertainty and disagreement among experts and among healthcare systems of different countries. In addition, the situation is emotionally charged, and the stakes are enormous. While we view participation in her or his healthcare as a patient's right, the exercising of which has many benefits for the patient, it is also a burden and a challenge. People's underlying competencies vary, and those who are in the greatest need (older adults, individuals with low socioeconomic and less than high school level of education, those in poor health) may have the greatest difficulty navigating and using health information. Understanding this, doctors and healthcare systems should not only welcome collaboration, but see it as their task to provide needed supports.

1.9 PATIENT ENGAGEMENT: RIGHT VERSUS RESPONSIBILITY

From the perspective of this book's authors, as well as from the perspective of patients wishing to choose treatment options or seeking access to their data, participatory medicine is a patients' right, and so is the access to information needed to exercise that right. Paradoxically, advocacy for supporting those rights harbors a potential ethical pitfall of presenting the right as a responsibility. deBronkart points out that becoming an e-patient is not a choice that everybody wants to make. Some people find the task of becoming experts in disease mechanisms and treatment procedures too anxiety-provoking. They would like to protect themselves from the mental and physical burden of being constantly engaged in reading, tracking information, and thinking about their disease. Additionally, the repertoire of tasks, described in this chapter as illustrating patient participation, is broad and far-reaching. While all people are experts in their quality of life preferences and disease experience, very many lack requisite skills for distinguishing between more and less reliable information and interpreting data trends. Even fewer are able to lead teams of doctors and engineers in designing medical procedures tailored to their unique needs. Given this reality, it is somewhat disconcerting to read about patient engagement as a tool for lessening doctors' professional burden. While the healthcare system is right to embrace the appearance of empowered digital patient networks that provide advice and data for comparison searching, we should also recognize that their emergence is evidence of deficiencies in the "official" healthcare system. After all, many of these entrepreneurial initiatives grew out of patients' dissatisfaction with what their providers were able to offer them. Greater attention to medical informatics and information science in medical education, producing e-doctors with data analytics skills to match those of savvy e-patients, may reduce the participatory "workload" burden of the patient.

It is also important to remember that, ideally, participatory healthcare is about collaboration, rather than about division of responsibilities. Networks like PatientsLikeMe aggregate invaluable data. However, reviewing trends that emerge from these datasets, like looking at medication dosages prescribed to patients' with specified diagnoses and characteristics, does not have to be a patient's task. In an ideal world, these data platforms would be integrated with patients' electronic medical records, and doctors would be spending some billable hours reviewing the data as the context for caring for their patients.

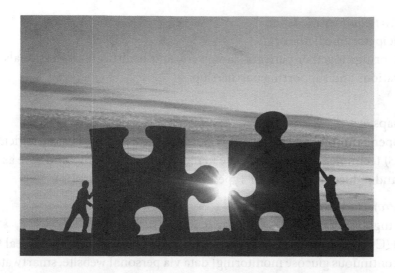

1.10 ROLE OF CONSUMER HEALTH INFORMATICS TOOLS IN SUPPORTING PARTICIPATORY HEALTHCARE

This chapter makes a case for how information technology and consumer health informatics – the research field concerned with IT in healthcare (see Part I: Chapter 2) – have been instrumental in bringing the participatory medicine model to the forefront of healthcare, presenting patient participation as not just an ethical imperative, but also a way to decrease cost and improve outcomes. There is a lot the field can do toward turning this model into a universal standard of care. This means continuing to build platforms, resources, and tools that connect people to health information – including the information produced by their own bodies – and health professionals to one another. Most importantly, informatics should continue striving to make these platforms, tools, and resources tailored to users' needs, effective, easy to understand, and easy to use. The tools should embed information authority and accuracy checks, lowering health and e-health literacy demands of information tasks, and, thus, making participation easier. The remaining chapters of this book discuss how this can be accomplished by different types of information tools, developed to support different tasks and optimized for different population groups.

WEB RESOURCES

All of Us Research Program
https://allofus.nih.gov/
This National Institutes of Health (NIH) program aims to create a very large (one million participants) and diverse database of individuals' health, behavioral, and genomic data for biomedical research and discovery. It thus relies on the participation and support of patients and consumers.

PatientsLikeMe
https://www.patientslikeme.com/
PatientsLikeMe is a very large patients' data sharing platform that supports patients' trend discovery, networking and communication, and research.

Society for Participatory Medicine
https://participatorymedicine.org/
This Society brings together patients, caregivers, and healthcare professionals, encouraging collaborations and supporting partnership.

#OpenAPS
https://openaps.org/
This is an open community project "to make safe and effective basic Artificial Pancreas System (APS) technology widely available to more quickly improve and save as many lives as possible and reduce the burden of Type 1 diabetes".

Nightscout Project #WeAreNotWaiting
http://www.nightscout.info/
"Nightscout (CGM in the Cloud) is an open source, DIY project that allows real time access to a CGM [continuous glucose monitoring] data via personal website, smartwatch viewers, or apps and widgets available for smartphones".

e-Patient Dave's (David deBronkart's) TED Talk
https://www.ted.com/speakers/dave_debronkart
In this TED talk, cancer survivor and patient advocate Dave deBronkart talks about how patients can participate in their care, stressing the importance of personal data ownership and connection with other patients.

Tal Golesworthy's TED Talk
https://www.ted.com/talks/tal_golesworthy_how_i_repaired_my_own_heart#t-129,209
In this TED talk, Tal Golesworthy, an engineer with Marfan syndrome, talks about his experience leading a team of engineers and doctors in developing a medical device that made his required heart surgery less invasive.

REFERENCES

Agin, F., Madhani, Z., Zahmatkeshan Khorasani, A., Zehtab, H., & Aslani. A. (2018). Patient Decision Aid systems: An overview. *Studies in Health Technology and Informatics*, 249:208–211.

Bantock, G. G. (1899). The modern doctrine of bacteriology, or the germ theory of disease. *British Medical Journal*, 1, 846–848. doi:10.1136/bmj.1.1997.846

Bauman, A. E., Fardy, H. J., & Harris, P. G. (2003). Getting it right: Why bother with patient-centred care? *The Medical Journal of Australia*, 179(5), 253–256.

Bertakis, K. D., & Azari, R. (2011). Patient-centered care is associated with decreased health care utilization. *Journal of the American Board of Family Medicine*, 3, 229–239. doi:10.3122/jabfm.2011.03.100170

deBronkart, D. (2011, April). *Meet e-patient Dave. [video]* https://www.ted.com/speakers/dave_debronkart

deBronkart, D. (2013). How the e-patient community helped save my life: an essay by Dave deBronkart. *BMJ*, 346:f1990.

deBronkart, D. (2015). From patient centered to people powered: autonomy on the rise. *BMJ* 350:h148 doi: 10.1136/bmj.h148

deBronkart, D. (2018). The patient's voice in the emerging era of participatory medicine. *International Journal of Psychiatry in Medicine*, 53(5–6) 350–360.

Burtchell, J. (2016). *About me.* http://jeriburtchell.com/blog/about-me/

Callahan, E. J., & Bertakis, K. D. (1991). Development and validation of the Davis observation code. *Family Medicine,* 23(1), 19–24.

Campos, H. (2012, Jan. 19) *Fighting for the right to open his heart data: Hugo Campos at TEDxCambridge 2011.* https://www.youtube.com/watch?v=oro19-l5M8k

Center for Devices and Radiological Health, Food and Drug Administration, U.S. Department of Health and Human Services. (2017, Oct. 30). *Manufacturers sharing patient-specific information from medical devices with patients upon request: Guidance for industry and Food and Drug Administration staff.* https://www.fda.gov/media/98519/download

Centers for Disease Control. (2020, March 2) *The Tuskegee timeline.* https://www.cdc.gov/tuskegee/timeline.htm

Cheese, I. (2017). Patient perspective: life in the melanoma patient community and the emergence of the melanoma patient conference. *Melanoma Management,* 4(2):89–93.

DesRoches, C. M., Bell, S. K., Dong, Z., Elmore, J., Fernandez, L., Fitzgerald, P., … Walker, J. (2019). Patients managing medications and reading their visit notes: A survey of OpenNotes participants. *Annals of Internal Medicine,* 171(1), 69–71. doi:10.7326/m18-3197

DIYgenomics (2019, January 2). *About DIYgenomics.* https://www.diygenomics.org/about.php

Dyer, C. (2014). Judge rules that boy with brain cancer can be treated in Prague. *BMJ,* 349, g5570. doi:10.1136/bmj.g5570

Farrow, M. (1934). Closed to the public. *Bulletin of the Medical Library Association,* 22 (4): 225–227.

Food & Drug Administration. (2018, Feb. 5). *Understanding unapproved use of approved drugs "off label".* https://www.fda.gov/patients/learn-about-expanded-access-and-other-treatment-options/understanding-unapproved-use-approved-drugs-label

Fox, S., & Duggan, M (2013). *Health Online 2013.* https://www.pewresearch.org/internet/2013/01/15/health-online-2013/

Goetz, T. (2008, Mar. 23). Practicing patients. *New York Times.*

Goetz, T. (2011). *The decision tree: How to make better choices and take control of your health.* Rodale.

Golesworthy, T. (2011). *How I repaired my own heart.* [video]. https://www.ted.com/talks/tal_golesworthy_how_i_repaired_my_own_heart#t-129,209

Griffiths, K. M., Mackinnon, A. J., Crisp, D. A., Christensen, H., Bennett, K., & Farrer, L. (2012). The effectiveness of an online support group for members of the community with depression: A randomized controlled trial. *PLoS One,* 7(12), e53244. doi:10.1371/journal.pone.0053244

Gurkan, A. (2019, Sept. 12). Hugo Campos has waged a decade-long battle for access to his heart implant. *Economist.*

HIPAA (1996), *The Health Insurance Portability and Accountability Act of 1996. Pub. L. 104–191. Stat. 1936.*

Institute for Patient- and Family-Centered Care. (n.d.) *About us.* https://www.ipfcc.org/about/index.html

ITV. (2019, August 19). *Proton beam therapy facility opens in Reading.* https://www.itv.com/news/meridian/2019-08-19/proton-beam-therapy-facility-opens-in-reading/

Kantor, D., Bright, J. R., & Burtchell, J. (2018). Perspectives from the Patient and the Healthcare Professional in Multiple Sclerosis: Social Media and Participatory Medicine. *Neurology and therapy,* 7(1), 37–49. https://doi.org/10.1007/s40120-017-0088-2

Laranjo, L., Arguel, A., Neves, A. L., Gallagher, A. M., Kaplan, R., Mortimer, N., … Lau, A. Y. (2015). The influence of social networking sites on health behavior change: A systematic review and meta-analysis. *Journal of the American Medical Informatics Association,* 22 (1), 243–256. doi:10.1136/amiajnl-2014-002841

Lewis, D.M., & Leibrand, S. (2017) *Automatic estimation of basals, ISF, and carb ratio for sensor-augmented pump and hybrid closed-loop therapy.* Poster presented at American Diabetes Association's 77th Scientific Sessions. San Diego, CA, June 9–13, 2017.

McAlpine, K., Lewis, K. B., Trevena, L. J., & Stacey, D. (2018). What is the effectiveness of patient decision aids for cancer-related decisions? A systematic review subanalysis. *JCO Clinical Cancer Informatics*, 2, 1–13. doi:10.1200/cci.17.00148

Mo, P. K., & Coulson, N. S. (2013). Online support group use and psychological health for individuals living with HIV/AIDS. *Patient Education and Counseling*, 93(3), 426–432. doi:10.1016/j. pec.2013.04.004

Morrison, K. E., Dhariwal, S., Hornabrook, R., Savage, L., Burn, D. J., Khoo, T. K., … Majid, T. (2013). Lithium in patients with amyotrophic lateral sclerosis (LICALS): A phase 3 multicentre, randomized, double-blind, placebo-controlled trial. *Lancet Neurology*, 12(4), 339–345. doi:10.1016/ s1474-4422(13)70037-1

NETRF, Neuroendocrine Tumor Research Foundation. (2020). *Patient and caregiver conferences*. https://netrf.org/events/patient-and-caregiver-conferences/

Neuroendocrine Tumor Research Foundation. (2019). *Patient and caregiver conferences*. https:// netrf.org/events/patient-and-caregiver-conferences/

Nightscout (2020). *Welcome to Nightscout*. http://www.nightscout.info/

PatientsLikeMe. (2020). *About us*. Available online: https://www.patientslikeme.com/about.

Prainsack, B. (2014). The powers of participatory medicine. *PLoS Biology* 12(4): e1001837.

Quantified Self (n.d.). *What is Quantified Self?* https://quantifiedself.com/about/what-is-quantified-self/

Ratzan, S. C., & Parker, R. M. (2000). Introduction. In C. R. Selden, M. Zorn, S. C. Ratzan, & R. M. Parker (Eds.), *National Library of Medicine current bibliographies in medicine: Health Literacy*. NLM Publishing No. CBL 2000-1. Bethesda, MD: National Institutes of Health, U.S. Department of Health and Human Services.

Richards, T. (2011). Enlist the patients' help. *BMJ*, 343, d5827. doi:10.1136/bmj.d5827

Richards, T. (2014, Sept. 4). *When doctors and patients disagree*. https://blogs.bmj.com/ bmj/2014/09/04/tessa-richards-when-doctors-and-patients-disagree/

Roberts, K. J. (1999). Patient empowerment in the United States: A critical commentary. *Health Expectations*, 2(2), 82–92. doi:10.1046/j.1369-6513.1999.00048.x

Sharma, A. E., Knox, M., Peterson, L. E., Willard-Grace, R., Grumbach, K., & Potter, M. B. (2018). How is family medicine engaging patients at the practice-level?: A national sample of family physicians. *Journal of the American Board of Family Medicine*, 31(5), 733–742. doi:10.3122/ jabfm.2018.05.170418

Silver, L., Huang, K., & Taylor, K. (2019). *In Emerging Economies, Smartphone and Social Media Users Have Broader Social Networks*. Pew Research Center. https://www.pewresearch.org/internet/wp-content/uploads/sites/9/2019/08/PI-PG_2019-08-22_social-networks-emerging-economies_FINAL.pdf

Smith, C. (2015). Medical information for the consumer before the World Wide Web. In C. Arnott Smith and A. Keselman (Eds.), *Meeting health information needs outside of health care: Opportunities and challenges* (pp 41–73). Chandos.

Swan, M. (2012). Crowdsourced health research studies: An important emerging complement to clinical trials in the public health research ecosystem. *Journal of Medical Internet Research*, 14(2), e46. doi:10.2196/jmir.1988

UKMND-LiCALS Study Group, Morrison, K. E., Dhariwal, S., Hornabrook, R., Savage, L., Burn, D. J., Khoo, T. K., Kelly, J., Murphy, C. L., Al-Chalabi, A., Dougherty, A., Leigh, P. N., Wijesekera, L., Thornhill, M., Ellis, C. M., O'Hanlon, K., Panicker, J., Pate, L., Ray, P., Wyatt, L., … Majid, T. (2013). Lithium in patients with amyotrophic lateral sclerosis (LiCALS): a phase 3 multicentre, randomised, double-blind, placebo-controlled trial. *The Lancet. Neurology*, 12(4), 339–345. https://doi.org/10.1016/S1474-4422(13)70037-1

Wicks, P., Massagli, M., Frost, J., Brownstein, C., Okun, S., Vaughan, T., … Heywood, J. (2010). Sharing health data for better outcomes on PatientsLikeMe. *Journal of Medical Internet Research*, 12(2), e19. doi:10.2196/jmir.1549

CHAPTER 2

Consumer Health Informatics as a Field

Catherine Arnott Smith

THIS CHAPTER INTRODUCES the reader to consumer health informatics as an interdisciplinary field in which academia, healthcare practice, the health IT industry, and the federal government are principal players and stakeholders.

2.1 WHAT IS CONSUMER HEALTH INFORMATICS?

Consumer health informatics is a subset of a larger field called *Medical informatics*, which is itself a subset of an even larger field called *Informatics*. The term *Informatics* originated in a German publication in 1957 (Steinbuch, 1957) and spread across Western Europe. In various European languages, the term means "computer science" or "computing science"; in English, it has a sense of "information science." While both information and computer science involve the use of computers, the difference between the two is that computer science "may or may not involve the existence of information" (LIMSwiki.org, 2015). Informatics students, educators, and researchers are focused on information.

Various professional associations have been attempting to formulate lists of desirable skill sets for students at the intersection of healthcare and computer sciences since at least 1978, when the ACM (Association for Computing Machinery) proposed a computer science curriculum for "health computing." The types of students identified as *needing* such a curriculum give a sense of the diversity of the field: students of medicine (by the Association of American Medical Colleges, 1998); nursing (by the American Nursing Association, 2001); dentistry (by the AMIA Dental Informatics Working Group, 2006); medical librarianship (by the Medical Library Association, 2006); and public health (Public Health Informatics Competencies Working Group, funded by the Centers for Disease Control and Prevention) (Kulikowski et al., 2012). Today, the umbrella term *biomedical informatics* is often used to denote the intersection of health with computing.

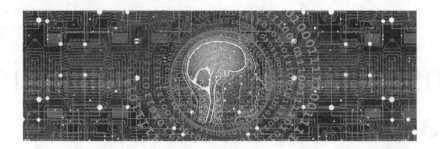

Medical informatics has been defined as "the field that is concerned with the optimal use of information, often aided by the use of technology, to improve individual health, health care, public health, and biomedical research." It was identified as a core competency for all healthcare professionals by the Institute of Medicine in 2003. The Institute defined it as: the ability to "communicate, manage knowledge, mitigate error, and support decisionmaking using information technology. [boldface mine; CAS]" (Greiner & Knebel, 2003). The other four competencies were "Provide patient-centered care"; "Work in interdisciplinary teams"; "Employ evidence-based practice"; and "Apply quality improvement." These were all identified as *core* competencies because the skills involved are not specific to any one clinical area of practice or type of professional, but are instead required of professionals across the healthcare system.

There are numerous subfields and variant fields within and including health informatics, a situation which has been referred to as "our adjective problem" (Hersh, 2009, para 8). These adjectives may define how informatics is applied, where the informatics work takes place, or the particular kind of people who do that work. Charles Friedman, a leader in biomedical informatics education, proposed a "fundamental theorem" for the field: That "a person working in partnership with an information resource is 'better' than that same person unassisted'" (Friedman, 2009, p. 169).

Other subfields within health informatics include *bioinformatics* (informatics in cellular and molecular biology); *imaging informatics* (the informatics of clinical imaging, such as the retrieval, delivery, and display of CT or PET scans); and *nursing, dental, pathology, oncology, pediatric informatics* (all informatics practiced by particular biomedical disciplines); as well as *public health informatics* (informatics in a public health context) (see Figure 2.1 from Hersh, 2009).

"Consumer health informatics", or CHI, is a term for the subfield of informatics that focuses on consumer and patient perspectives, simultaneously as users and beneficiaries of information systems that empower them to manage their own health.

Note that *consumer* is not identical with *patient*. One commonly used definition from the Agency for Healthcare Quality and Research is: "anyone who seeks or uses health care information for nonprofessional work" (p. 13) (Gibbons et al., 2009). This includes people who are living with a diagnosis (e.g., Type 2 diabetes) as well as people who are not (e.g., teachers of a child living with Type 2 diabetes).

From this perspective, consumers are active agents who both use and are affected by information technology. The American Medical Informatics Association is the principal

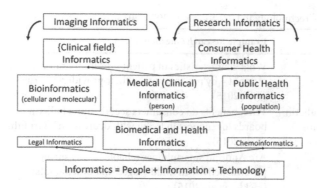

FIGURE 2.1 Subcategories of "informatics". From Hersh (2009).

professional organization for practitioners and researchers in biomedical informatics. Its definition for CHI states that "The focus is on information structures and processes that empower consumers to manage their own health – for example, health information literacy, consumer-friendly language, personal health records, and Internet-based strategies and resources." (American Medical Informatics Association, 2019). The International Medical Informatics Association, which holds a triennial conference in different countries, is the international organization aggregating AMIA and its sister associations all over the world.

2.2 SCOPE OF THE CHI FIELD

In this very broad field, any space in which consumers and patients interact with information and information systems is included. This includes the design and deployment of decision support tools, information management tools, communication tools (patient-to-patient, or clinician-to-patient), and therapies that enhance interpersonal relationships – for example, smartphone-based meditation apps. It also includes attention to health information sources themselves, for example, the quality of health information exchanged in online patient communities or made available on the Web. Finally, CHI tools' effects on the larger society in which health information is exchanged are also subjects of research in consumer health informatics. For example: What is the impact of the digital divide on access to CHI tools and consumer health information? How do different demographic variables (majority/minority race/ethnicity; spoken language; literacy) relate to uptake and usage of CHI tools in different populations?

Smith et al.'s scoping review of CHI research studies published in the literature of computer science, information science, and engineering between 2008 and 2015 (2020) found these topics to be particularly popular (Table 2.1).

2.3 WHO DOES CONSUMER HEALTH INFORMATICS?

The same systematic review by Smith et al. (2020) examined the literatures in which CHI research was published. The 271 studies published between 2008 and 2015 appeared in no

TABLE 2.1   Classes of Technology in CHI Research, 2008–2015

Class of Technology	Example Research Question	Number of Studies
Personal health records, patient portals	What characteristics of patient portals are rated highly – or not – by patients and by their providers? (Kruse et al., 2015)	60
Online communities/bulletin boards/discussion forums	What benefits do consumers see in online bulletin boards for support in living with depression? (Griffiths et al., 2015)	55
Self-tracking apps	Are Android smartphones reliable in measuring physical activity in middle-aged and older adults? (Hekler et al., 2015)	44
Social media	What is the evidence for social media health interventions in the indigenous population of Australia? (Brusse et al., 2014)	38
Communication, interaction with providers	How useful is asynchronous communication between patients and providers in the context of chronic illness? (de Jong et al., 2014)	21
Text messaging	Is a text-based intervention feasible for consumers seeking to maintain their weight? (Shaw et al., 2013)	19
Web-based applications	Can Internet-based self-management programs benefit caregivers of dementia patients? (Boots et al., 2016)	17
Search engines	How do women use technology to acquire information when they are pregnant? (Kraschnewski et al., 2014)	16
Sensors	Can ubiquitous sensors be used to capture information about consumers' activities of daily life (ADL) in the home? (Lee & Dey, 2015)	14
Web-based information resources	Can a website created to target a Hispanic/Latino population increase knowledge about organ transplants? (Gordon et al., 2016)	13

less than 63 different journals and 22 different conference proceedings. The top five fields and representative journals are listed in Table 2.2.

Figure 2.2 illustrates the career trajectories of people who receive training in biomedical informatics, from undergraduate degrees through employment in sectors including healthcare and other industries besides academic and government settings.

Consumer health informatics stands at the crossroads of other disciplines. This field is both multi- and interdisciplinary; on the technical side, biomedical engineers, computer scientists, data scientists, and information scientists are contributors to the work. They collaborate with healthcare practitioners and researchers as well as information providers and educators such as medical librarians, nutritionists, and patient educators. They also collaborate increasingly with patients and the consumers who act as the caregivers and advocates for patients (see Chapter 1). This textbook is for undergraduate students thinking about future careers in any or all of these professional fields.

TABLE 2.2   Fields and Journals in CHI Research, 2008–2015

Field	Example Journal	Studies
Health informatics	Journal of Medical Internet Research	65%
Information science/Library & information science	Journal of the American Society for Information Science and Technology	15%
Computer Science	Soft Computing	10%
Medicine	Journal of Adolescent Health	4%
Engineering	IEEE Journal of Biomedical and Health Informatics	2%

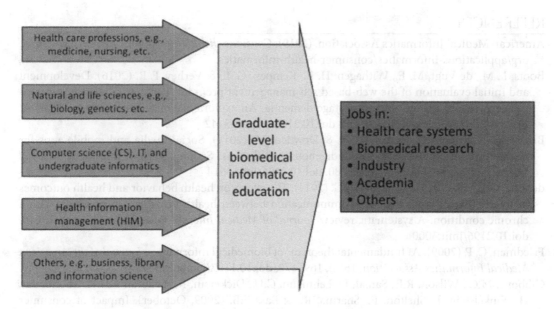

FIGURE 2.2 Career pathways in biomedical and health informatics (Hersh, 2009).

WEB RESOURCES

American Medical Informatics Association
The principal professional organization for biomedical informatics, including the subspecialty of consumer health informatics. Web presence for working groups for students and other interest and affinity collectives.
www.amia.org

>   Student Working Group
>   https://www.amia.org/programs/working-groups/student

Consumer Health Informatics Working Group
https://www.amia.org/programs/working-groups/consumer-and-pervasive-health-informatics

Medical Library Association
Principal professional organization for health sciences librarianship in the US and Canada.
https://www.mlanet.org/

International Medical Informatics Association
International nongovernmental organization (NGO) serving as bridge organization "across professional and geographical boundaries."
https://imia-medinfo.org/wp/

REFERENCES

American Medical Informatics Association. (2019). *Consumer health informatics.* https://www.amia.org/applications-informatics/consumer-health-informatics.

Boots, L. M., de Vugt, M. E., Withagen, H. E., Kempen, G. I., & Verhey, F. R. (2016). Development and initial evaluation of the web-based self-management program "partner in balance" for family caregivers of people with early stage dementia: An exploratory mixed-methods study. *JMIR Research Protocols*, 5(1), Article e33. doi:10.2196/resprot.5142

Brusse, C., Gardner, K., McAullay, D., & Dowden, M. (2014). Social media and mobile apps for health promotion in Australian indigenous populations: Scoping review. *Journal of Medical Internet Research*, 16(12), Article e280. doi:10.2196/jmir.3614

de Jong, C. C., Ros, W. J., & Schrijvers, G. (2014). The effects on health behavior and health outcomes of internet-based asynchronous communication between health providers and patients with a chronic condition: A systematic review. *Journal of Medical Internet Research*, 16(1), Article e19. doi:10.2196/jmir.3000

Friedman, C. P. (2009). A "fundamental theorem" of biomedical informatics. *Journal of the American Medical Informatics Association*, 16(2), 169–170. doi:10.1197/jamia.M3092

Gibbons, M.C., Wilson, R.F., Samal, L., Lehmann, C.U., Dickersin, K., Lehmann, H.P., Aboumatar, H., Finkelstein, J., Shelton, E., Sharma, R., & Bass E.B. (2009, October). Impact of consumer health informatics applications. *Evidence Report/Technology Assessment No. 188*. (Prepared by Johns Hopkins University Evidence-based Practice Center under contract No. HHSA 290–2007-10061-I). AHRQ Publication No. 09(10)-E019. https://www.ahrq.gov/downloads/pub/evidence/pdf/chiapp/impactchia.pdf

Gordon, E. J., Feinglass, J., Carney, P., Vera, K., Olivero, M., Black, A., O'Connor, K.G., Baumgart, J.M., & Caicedo, J. C. (2016). A website intervention to increase knowledge about living kidney donation and transplantation among Hispanic/Latino dialysis patients. *Progress in Transplantation*, 26(1), 82–91. doi:10.1177/1526924816632124

Greiner, A.C., & Knebel, E. (Eds.) (2003). *Health professions education: A bridge to quality*. Washington (DC): National Academies Press. https://www.ncbi.nlm.nih.gov/books/NBK221519/#ddd00052.

Griffiths, K. M., Reynolds, J., & Vassallo, S. (2015). An online, moderated peer-to-peer support bulletin board for depression: User-perceived advantages and disadvantages. *JMIR Mental Health*, 2(2), Article e14. doi:10.2196/mental.4266

Hekler, E. B., Buman, M. P., Grieco, L., Rosenberger, M., Winter, S. J., Haskell, W., & King, A. C. (2015). Validation of physical activity tracking via android smartphones compared to Actigraph accelerometer: Laboratory-based and free-living validation studies. *JMIR Mhealth Uhealth*, 3(2), Article e36. doi:10.2196/mhealth.3505

Hersh, W. (2009). A stimulus to define informatics and health information technology. *BMC Medical Informatics & Decisionmaking*, 9. http://www.ncbi.nlm.nih.gov/pmc/articles/PMC2695439/?tool=pubmed.

Kraschnewski, J. L., Chuang, C. H., Poole, E. S., Peyton, T., Blubaugh, I., Pauli, J., & Reddy, M. (2014). Paging "Dr. Google": Does technology fill the gap created by the prenatal care visit structure? Qualitative focus group study with pregnant women. *Journal of Medical Internet Research*, 16(6), Article e147. doi:10.2196/jmir.3385

Kruse, C. S., Argueta, D. A., Lopez, L., & Nair, A. (2015). Patient and provider attitudes toward the use of patient portals for the management of chronic disease: A systematic review. *Journal of Medical Internet Research*, 17(2), Article e40. doi:10.2196/jmir.3703

Kulikowski, C. A., Shortliffe, E. H., Currie, L. M., Elkin, P. L., Hunter, L. E., Johnson, T. R., ... Williamson, J. J. (2012). AMIA board white paper: Definition of biomedical informatics and specification of core competencies for graduate education in the discipline. *Journal of the American Medical Informatics Association*, 19(6), 931–938. doi:10.1136/amiajnl-2012-001053

Lee, M. L., & Dey, A. K. (2015). Sensor-based observations of daily living for aging in place. *Personal Ubiquitous Computing*, 19(1), 27–43. doi:10.1007/s00779-014-0810-3

LIMSwiki.org. (2015, Mar. 21). *Informatics (academic field)*. https://www.limswiki.org/index.php/Informatics_(academic_field)#cite_note-3.

Shaw, R. J., Bosworth, H. B., Hess, J. C., Silva, S. G., Lipkus, I. M., Davis, L. L., & Johnson, C. M. (2013). Development of a theoretically driven mhealth text messaging application for sustaining recent weight loss. *JMIR Mhealth Uhealth*, 1(1), Article e5. doi:10.2196/mhealth.2343

Smith, C.A., Yu, D., Maestre, J.F., Backonja, U., Boyd, A.D., Buis, L.R., Chaudry, B.M., Huh-Yoo, J., Hussain, S.A., Jones, L.M., Lai, A.M., Senteio, C.R., Siek, K.A., & Veinot, T.C. (2020). *Consumer health informatics research: A scoping review of informatics, information science and engineering literature*. [Unpublished manuscript submitted for publication.]

Steinbuch, K. (1957). *Informatik: Automatische informationsverarbeitung [Informatics: Automatic information processing]*. Berlin: SEG-Nachrichten.

CHAPTER 3

Health Literacy and Other Competencies

The Skills Consumers Need in Order to Be Effective in the Digital Health Information Environment

Alla Keselman

M ANAGING ONE'S HEALTH and effectively participating in one's care is not only a right; it is also a challenge that requires knowledge and a number of information-related skills. This chapter discusses health literacy and other competencies that people need to have in order to interact with consumer health information and consumer health information technology effectively. It includes several definitions of health literacy, explaining their history, coverage, and benefits and challenges they present for research and practice. The chapter also discusses health literacy assessment instruments and their relationship with the definitions. It describes levels of health literacy in the population, which present a public health concern (only about 12% of Americans are "Proficient") and reviews research on how health literacy may be associated with health behaviors and outcomes. The chapter then introduces the concept of e-health literacy (Norman & Skinner, 2006), positioning health literacy in a broader framework of e-health information competencies that also include traditional literacy, information literacy, media literacy, computer literacy, and scientific literacy. Finally, the chapter discusses how consumer health informatics can support each of these competencies, ameliorating problems and helping individuals deal with health information effectively.

3.1 HEALTH LITERACY

No matter what background and goals bring you to this book, there is a good chance that you have heard of the concept of "health literacy" as a prerequisite for successfully navigating the health domain as a patient or consumer. What, exactly, is health literacy, and why is it important? One of several influential definitions describes it as the "degree to which individuals have the capacity to obtain, process, and understand basic health information and services needed to make appropriate health decisions" (Ratzan & Parker, 2000, p. vi). Clearly, the capacity to "obtain, process, and understand basic health information" is an essential competency for health functioning. However, you may notice that the concept is defined in a way that makes it difficult to measure, or, indeed, fully grasp. Saying that the "capacity to obtain, process, and understand basic health information" is essential for navigating health information is somewhat circular. So, what is it exactly? While the concept is important, the answer is not as easy as we would like it to be.

3.1.1 The Concept's Beginnings

We believe that a useful way to understand health literacy is by following the evolution of the concept. "Health literacy" grew out of the field of adult literacy. It has long been known that general literacy, or the ability to read and comprehend written text, affected one's ability to deal with health information effectively. This is unsurprising, because, after all, reading and comprehending a health-related text is just a specific case of engaging general reading comprehension competency. Yet, around the late 1980s and 1990s, leading health educators, communicators, and researchers started noticing that general adult reading test scores were not as strong predictors of individuals' ability to deal with health information as were their health-domain-specific reading skills (Doak & Doak, 1987; Doak et al., 1996; Logan, 2015). Moreover, the two kinds of literacies seemed to constitute separate constructs; general vocabulary breadth and reading scores were not necessarily closely connected with medical terminology knowledge and ability to understand health information.

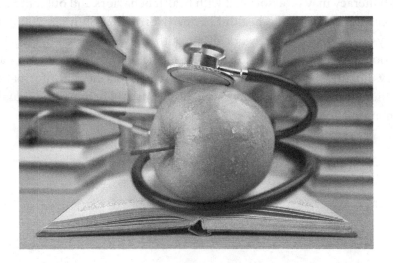

3.1.2 Early Assessment of Health Literacy

Around the same time, researchers started developing tests for measuring health literacy in research and clinical practice. Having widely agreed-upon instruments for measuring health literacy is important for several reasons. First, this allows investigators to estimate health literacy competency in the general population as well as different subgroups of that population (e.g., older adults). Second, this enables researchers to conduct research studies into the relationship between health literacy (as measured by the instruments) and health behaviors and outcomes. After all, limited health literacy is only a problem if it is associated with poor health outcomes. Third, it allows researchers and health educators to create and evaluate programs and activities directed at improving health literacy.

Two early and still widely used instruments are Rapid Estimate of Adult Literacy in Medicine (REALM) and Test of Functional Health Literacy in Adults (TOFHLA) (Davis et al., 1991; Parker et al., 1995). REALM presents individuals with a list of 66 health-related words of varying complexity to read aloud (e.g., flu, pill, eye, kidney, nutrition, menopause, hemorrhoids). Based on the number of correctly pronounced words, the results are assigned to one of the four reading levels, corresponding to (1) third grade and below, (2) fourth to sixth grades, (3) seventh to eighth grades, and (4) high school. Each correctly pronounced word earns a point. Only participants at the highest level are expected to be able to read and understand most patient education materials.

TOFHLA consists of 17 numeracy questions and 50 reading comprehension questions (Parker et al., 1995). Numeracy questions require participants to interpret specific directions and perform necessary computations. For example, participants read prescription instructions and determine the time to take the second and third daily doses if the first one was taken at 8 a.m.; or determine whether a specified monthly household income would qualify a family with three children for free care at a clinic with particular income requirements. Reading comprehension section uses what is called a Cloze test (the word is an abbreviation of the word "closure") (Taylor, 1953). Cloze tests exist in hundreds of domains; they are passages of text with some words removed. Responders choose from several multiple-choice options to fill in the blanks. For example, in the TOFHLA, it might read: "I agree to give correct information to _____ if I can receive Medicaid"; "hair," "salt," "see," and "ache" as possible answer choices) (Institute of Medicine [IOM], 2004, p. 306).

Both the REALM and TOFHLA tests, as short as they are, have even briefer versions that have been shown to correlate well with the longer ones. Moreover, they are very easy to administer and do not require much training. For these reasons, even though, as you will see, the concept of health literacy has evolved greatly since its inception, these older tests are still the ones most widely used.

3.1.3 Health Literacy Levels in the Population

Having a concept and instruments to measure it allowed assessment of levels of health literacy in the general population. For example, the development of TOFHLA involved giving the test to 200 English-speaking and 203 Spanish-speaking patients who visited a large public hospital in Atlanta, Georgia, for acute and emergency care. Spanish speakers were given a Spanish-language version of the test. The results were troubling. Only "half of the

English-speaking and less than a third of the Spanish-speaking patients completed 80% of or more of items correctly" (Parker et al., 1995). These individuals – actual patients visiting a hospital for acute care – had trouble with TOFHLA tasks that were directly relevant to their care, such as correctly interpreting medication instructions.

An important milestone for formalizing the concept of health literacy was the 2003 US National Assessment of Adult Literacy (NAAL), which is "the nation's most comprehensive measure of adult literacy" (U.S Department of Education, n.d., What is NAAL? Section, para. 1). The 2003 NAAL assessed health literacy separately from general literacy, which is defined, similarly to REALM and TOFHLA, as "the ability to understand medical terms and information" (Logan, 2015 p. 22). The test provided the most comprehensive assessment of health literacy in the US, concluding that only 12% of American adults had Proficient level of health literacy, while 14% had a level of proficiency that was "Below Basic" (U.S. Department of Education, 2006, Introduction section, p. v). Low levels of health literacy are the most prevalent among older adults, representatives of racial and ethnic minorities, individuals with less than high school level of education, those with low socioeconomic status, non-native English speakers, and individuals with poor health status.

3.2 ASSOCIATION WITH HEALTH BEHAVIORS AND OUTCOMES

Poor health literacy is only a problem if it leads to negative health outcomes. By now, the knowledge we have about health behaviors and outcomes associated with different levels of health literacy is quite extensive. An article by Berkman et al. (2011) provides a systematic review of this research. The review is a synthesis of 96 studies of good or fair quality, reported in 111 published articles: 98 focusing on health literacy and 22 on health numeracy. Studies typically measured health literacy via versions of REALM or TOFHLA, and numeracy via general math tests not specifically designed for the health-related context. The big picture created by the systematic review suggests that lower health literacy is associated with several poor outcomes. For a number of health conditions (asthma, congestive heart failure) and populations groups (elderly, inner-city patients), it is associated with higher rate of ER visits and hospital admissions, which suggests poorer disease management and more complications (Baker et al., 2004; Cho et al., 2008; Hope et al., 2004). Lower health literacy is also associated with underuse of important preventive services such as mammography screening and flu vaccination (Guerra et al., 2005; White et al., 2008). Individuals with lower health literacy also have more difficulty interpreting medications and nutritional labels and taking medications as directed (Davis et al., 2006; Kripalani et al., 2006). They also have more trouble interpreting health messages (Davis et al., 2006). Studies also suggest that, for the elderly, lower health literacy may be related to overall poorer health (Cho et al., 2008; Lee et al., 2009) and higher mortality (Baker et al., 2017; Baker et al., 2008; Sudore et al., 2006).

For a number of other outcomes (e.g., access to care, various specific health behaviors), the evidence of association with health literacy was deemed insufficient because of poor methodology of studies or inconsistent results. The relationship between numeracy and health outcomes was similarly judged as presently inconclusive because of insufficient or inconsistent findings. This means that there are some studies pointing at such associations, but it is too early to make a conclusive statement about it. As more research evidence is accumulated and methodology is refined, this evidence may emerge with stronger support.

3.3 IS THE RELATIONSHIP BETWEEN HEALTH LITERACY AND OUTCOMES CAUSAL?

You will have noticed that the previous section, as well as research studies cited in it, talk about limited health literacy being "associated" with poor health outcomes. The studies reviewed by Berkman, Sheridan, Donahue, Halpern, and Crotty (2011) find that individuals with low health literacy tend to have poorer outcomes, even when other factors that usually correlate with low health literacy – for example, lower general literacy, education, and income level – are taken into consideration. However, demonstrating an association between two phenomena is not the same as demonstrating causality. In research studies, causality is typically demonstrated in experiments. For example, individuals with different levels of the variable of interest might be randomly assigned to different groups, and then the groups are compared with regard to the outcome of interest. However, in some cases, setting up experiments is unethical or methodologically impossible, and health literacy presents one of those cases. We cannot randomly appoint people to low or high levels of health literacy conditions, as their health literacy is a function of their life experience. Even if we could, such experimentation would not be ethical.

When experimentation is impossible, two things can provide indirect evidence of the causal nature of the relationship. The first is a plausible mechanism, supported by evidence that relates the variables. The second is evidence that health literacy interventions improve health outcomes for those at risk.

Paasche-Orlow and Wolf (2007) propose a model of "causal pathways between limited health literacy and health outcomes." In this model, health literacy, which is a function of many social, cultural, demographic, cognitive, and health status factors (e.g., age, education, income, language, culture, memory, reasoning, hearing, vision), influences three areas of health functioning:

1) Access and utilization of health care,

2) Provider-patient interaction, and

3) Self-care.

Health literacy affects care access and utilization because limited health literacy creates personal and systemic barriers to obtaining care. On a personal level, individuals with lower health literacy are less likely to understand prevention and recognize early symptoms of disease. On a systemic level, they may find it more difficult to navigate the complexities of US healthcare with its referrals, pre-authorizations, and for-profit insurance. As a result, people with lower health literacy are likely to have fewer preventive and routine visits and encounter the healthcare system when they are sicker and need more intensive services. With regard to provider-patient interactions, patients with limited health literacy may avoid asking questions out of shame; they may not know which questions to ask; or they may not understand doctors' explanations because they do not know the terminology and may not have the requisite background knowledge. Self-care is also likely to be affected if people have difficulty understanding labels and instructions (as shown in the discussion of "Early Assessment" above), which then may affect their level of knowledge and their skills related to health management. The three areas, considered jointly, negatively impact health outcomes.

This model, which is necessarily complex, is still a simplification of even more complex reality and does not lend itself to predictions. While its components are plausible, and many are supported by empirical evidence, it is only one of multiple proposed mechanisms that provide a framework for thinking about the impact of health literacy on health outcomes.

Analyzing this impact is made tricky by the complexity of the concept, which is related to knowledge of medical terminology, comprehension in context, numeracy, and, as we will soon see, a web of other skills, the exact composition and nature of which are still being debated by experts. Under these circumstances, it is impossible to specify what, exactly, should constitute a "health literacy intervention." Additionally, health literacy is something likely to develop over years, shaped by many life experiences, so it is very unlikely to be changed by several presentations or workshops. However, interventions may aim to provide knowledge and information skills in a specific domain (e.g., to improve self-management of a specific chronic illness). Interventions may also attempt to mitigate gaps between individuals' health literacy levels and literacy or numeracy requirements of specific documents (e.g., by lowering readability level of a hospital discharge summary).

Another comprehensive systematic review by Berkman et al., (2011) focused on intervention studies aiming to mitigate effects of low health literacy on various outcomes. The review found evidence that studies that included mixed intervention strategies, targeting several competencies related to health literacy, had a positive impact on several health-related outcomes. For example, there was moderately strong evidence that "intensive self-management and adherence interventions appear to be effective in reducing emergency room visits and hospitalizations" (p. ES-7). Also, educational interventions about cancer prevention and early detection via screening increased participation in colorectal and prostate cancer screening. There was also moderately strong evidence that disease management programs improved self-management of diseases targeted by the interventions. For a number of other variables, including self-efficacy, medication adherence, quality of life, and cost of healthcare, results were insufficient or inconclusive. However, as the field is rapidly developing, an updated investigation may provide additional insight about them.

Investigators have tried specific strategies to improve outcomes by mitigating readability or numeracy requirements of documents, and by providing visual aids (e.g., graphs, charts, diagrams). Berkman et al., (2011) noted some promising strategies that improved comprehension for low-literacy participants in a small number of studies as meriting further investigation. Examples of such strategies include presenting most important information first; presenting it by itself; lowering readability levels; and including illustrations with text. Yet, the summative strength of evidence of these single-strategy interventions on supporting low-health-literacy individuals was low, largely due to diversity in the studies' design and the difficulty in generalizing across them. This does not mean that the relationship does not exist, but suggests that it has not been studied sufficiently, systematically, and via enough well-designed studies to warrant an evidence-based conclusion with a high level of certainty.

Overall, the conclusion that low health literacy contributes to poor health outcomes seems reasonable, even though exact pathways and ways to impact the relationship need to be studied further. The field proposes models with plausible mechanism of action, and interventions produce improvements in outcomes. Given the complexity of health literacy as a concept, it is not surprising that mixed multi-faceted interventions may be more impactful than single-strategy ones. At the same time, it remains essential to know more about the potential effectiveness of specific strategies.

3.4 NEWER DEFINITIONS AND MEASURES OF HEALTH LITERACY

Let's think back to the definition of health literacy as the "capacity to obtain, process, and understand basic health information and services" (Ratzan & Parker, 2000, p. vi). Clearly, this definition is much broader than its original driver: the observation that literacy in a health-related context is somewhat different from overall functional literacy. Indeed, while adult literacy was the impetus that drew attention to the issue, researchers and policymakers realized that capacity to interact with health information and services effectively included a broad range of cognitive, social, and motivational factors. For example, the World Health Organization (WHO) defined health literacy as "the cognitive and social skills which determine the motivation and ability of individuals to gain access to, understand, and use information in ways which promote and maintain good health" (World Health Organization [WHO], 2009). Nutbeam (2008) pointed out that the US model of improving health literacy centered on remediating deficits in individuals' health-related knowledge and reading, writing, numeracy, and oral communication skills; but the WHO definition stressed the importance of bolstering people's sense of empowerment. Others pointed out that early definitions presented health literacy as a competency residing solely with the individual, while in reality, one's capacity to navigate health information is influenced by the interaction between that individual, the healthcare system, and the larger society (D. W. Baker, 2006).

These definitional discussions may seem abstract and removed from the world of design and patient and consumer engagement. But they have direct impact on the efforts we undertake in consumer health informatics to support individuals in their health functioning. For example, if we define health literacy primarily as the ability to comprehend complex health texts, we may then have concerns about the potential benefit of consumer health tools, such as apps and patient portals, that provide complex information characterized by uncertainty. At the same time, conceiving health literacy as part of an individual's sense of empowerment would prompt viewing CHI tools as health literacy interventions strengthening individuals' capacity to function in the world of health information by inviting their full participation. Of course, as the process of navigating health information effectively is very complex, different conceptions of health literacy will draw our attention to its different prerequisite and component skills, all of which are important.

As the concept of health literacy evolved, the health literacy research community real-ized the need for assessment instruments that would reflect its multidimensional complex-ity. However, attempts to design measures that reflected the evolving concept resulted in instruments that were impractically lengthy and difficult to validate. At the time this chap-ter is being written, REALM and TOFHLA are still the most prevalent instruments used in the clinical and research settings. However, the movement to capture the complexity of health literacy in assessment continues. Osborne, Batterham, Elsworth, Hawkins, and Buchbinder (2013) developed the Health Literacy Questionnaire that assesses nine scales of health literacy. These scales encompass multiple dimensions, from *cognitive* (e.g., Appraisal of health information, Ability to find good health information, Understanding health information well enough to know what to do), to *social* (e.g., Social support for health) and *emotional* (Feeling understood and supported by healthcare providers) dimensions. The tool was developed via a careful multi-phase process involving several rounds of psycho-metric analysis and revision and validated in several settings. Assessment along each scale consists of four to five multiple-choice questions or statements with which respondents agree or disagree (e.g., "I have at least one person who can come to medical appointments with me" and "I ask healthcare providers about the quality of the health information I find"). The Health Literacy Tool Shed, a free online database of health literacy measures developed by researchers at Boston University, Communicate Health, and RTI International, provides more information about the Health Literacy Questionnaire and 197 other instru-ments; find it at https://healthliteracytoolshed.bu.edu.

Researchers working in the field of health literacy today recognize that it is comprised of many dimensions. However, the absence of a single agreed-upon definition is detrimental

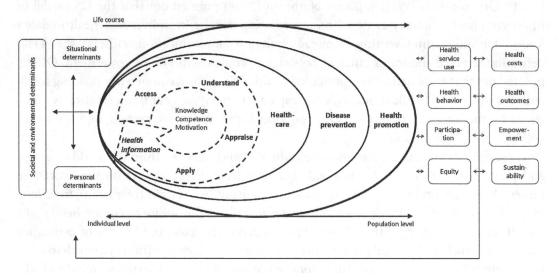

FIGURE 3.1   An integrated cumulative health literacy model, from a systematic analysis from Sørensen et al. (2012). [*NOTE.* Adapted from "Health literacy and public health: A systematic review and integration of definitions and models," by K. Sørensen, S. Van den Broucke, J. Fullam, G. Doyle, J. Pelikan, Z. Seolnska, H. Brand, and (HLS-EU) Consortium Health Literacy Project European, 2012, *BMC Public Health, 12*(80). (https://doi.org/10.1186/1471-2458-12-80). Copyright 2012 by Sørensen et al.; BioMed Central Ltd. CC BY 2.0]

to the field (Logan, 2015). It complicates development of assessment measures and interventions research, and negatively impacts the field's credibility. Sørensen et al. (2012) conducted a systematic analysis of 12 conceptual models and 17 definitions of health literacy (Figure 3.1). From these, they developed an integrated conceptual model of health literacy. This model takes into account personal, societal, and environmental determinants of health and acknowledges cognitive and social/emotional/motivational factors as central to health literacy. It also presents exercising health literacy as a process involving accessing, understanding, appraising, and applying information. Successful execution of each step in the process may require different cognitive competencies and be helped or hindered by different characteristics of health information, tools, organizations, and relationships.

3.5 FROM HEALTH LITERACY TO E-HEALTH LITERACY: OTHER RELEVANT COMPETENCIES

As if the list of health literacy competencies was not long enough, transition of much of health information functioning into the digital arena adds a new set of requisite component skills with which to contend. This reality is reflected in the concept of e-health literacy. In an influential article, Norman and Skinner (2006) define e-health literacy as "the ability to seek, find, understand, and appraise health information from electronic sources and apply the knowledge gained to addressing or solving a health problem" (p. 2). They also present a model in which e-health literacy is comprised of six component literacies:

1) **Traditional literacy**, or the ability to read and understand, as well as write, texts. Traditional literacy is important to dealing with e-health resources because at present, much of electronic information is text based.

2) **Information literacy**, or understanding "how knowledge is organized, how to find information, and how to use information in such a way that others can learn from them" (American Library Association, 1989). This definition, adopted by Norman and Skinner, was put forward in 1989 by the American Library Association Presidential Committee on Information Literacy.

3) **Media literacy**, or the ability to take media content and context into consideration when interpreting health information. This involves considering the larger social context of messages, such as market drivers and audience relations. While media literacy is important in all informational contexts, the internet removes many print publication process steps that traditionally ensured some quality control.

4) **Health literacy**, as defined previously in the chapter.

5) **Computer literacy**, or the ability to use computers effectively.

6) **Science literacy**, or the ability to understand goals, methods, limitations, and the larger social context of scientific studies. This competence helps one understand the scientific foundation of health information.

The six dimensions outlined by Norman and Skinner (2006) are not the only way to conceptualize competence in dealing with health information in the digital age. For example, when discussing health literacy, Norman and Skinner cite the 1999 American Medical Association definition that is closely tied to traditional literacy and numeracy and does not discuss the background knowledge or social and motivational issues (American Medical Association [AMA], Ad Hoc Committee on Health Literacy for the Council on Scientific Affairs, 1999). Similarly, their definition of science literacy focuses on the understanding of the nature of science (the how and why science is done) as opposed to knowledge of specific scientific content. Science education research, the field that focuses on lay science competency with a more fine-grained view, distinguishes among *conceptual scientific knowledge*, *knowledge about science* (similar to science literacy as defined by Norman and Skinner), and *attitudes toward science* (Bybee et al., 2009; Organization for Economic Co-operation and Development [OECD], 2016). All three competencies are likely to be important for navigating health information effectively.

Norman and Skinner also make a choice to present the six competencies of their model as non-hierarchical. Building an alternative representation, one can make a case for traditional literacy, media literacy, information literacy, and science literacy as subdomains of health literacy. *Information literacy* and *traditional literacy* roughly correspond to the cognitive health literacy dimensions (Osborne et al., 2013), described in the previous section. However, ultimately, the issue of just how the distinct components of e-health literacy (or health literacy) relate to one another is not of critical importance. Norman and Skinner's model draws attention to the ever-expanding set of competencies that are needed for dealing with health information in the digital age.

3.6 PRACTICAL CONSIDERATIONS FOR DESIGNERS AND PROMOTERS OF CONSUMER HEALTH INFORMATION TOOLS

What are we to take from the almost three decades of research into health literacy competencies, as well as recent e-health literacy work? We believe that valuing individuals' right to play an active role in their healthcare is an ethical imperative, rather than a function of its empirical utility testing. Because of our position, we will always focus on using technology to help people participate, rather than on debating whether the public has the competencies to benefit (e.g., from access to their health records).

That said, viewing health literacy in terms of its more recent, public-health-oriented definitions that emphasize the role of social and motivational factors in effective dealing with health information, we see technology as an important facilitator of health literacy. The very existence and the spread of consumer health information tools create a social environment that empowers individuals, sending them a strong invitation to participate. Patient portals, health-oriented online forums, lifestyle support and disease management apps all aim to ease information delivery and support interactions with healthcare. Consumer health informatics tools can also provide social and emotional supports for health by enabling their users to stay in touch with remote caregivers (e.g., their family members at work), share data (e.g., by having it shared with physicians via at-home monitoring devices, such as glucose meters), and communicate with healthcare providers (e.g., via electronic messages). In Part II: Chapter 9, we will also visit the world of emotional support robots.

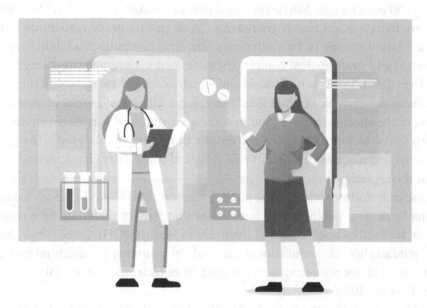

At the same time, technology's ability to facilitate, rather than complicate information use, depends on its usability and fit to user needs. Reading this book, you will see that while consumer health information resources proliferate exponentially, only a subset of these resources is characterized by high quality.

Also in line with the newer definitions of health literacy, we see health literacy competency as a function of the match between an individual and a resource. Rather than discussing the level of reading skills, knowledge, etc., needed for people to be considered sufficiently "health literate," we would like to focus on ways technology can lower these entry requirements. Unfortunately, to-date research on health literacy interventions has not been sufficiently rigorous and systematic to provide strong evidence for what health literacy mitigation strategies (e.g., lowering readability, adding visual aids and multimedia) work in what circumstances (Berkman et al., 2011). What we know is that when different mitigation strategies are tried together, it leads to better information use experience and health outcomes (Berkman et al., 2011). What we present here is based on the state of knowledge we have today, with the hope that the next decade will increase the precision of the recommendations.

The rest of this section addresses common ways to support various e-health-related competencies, as well as ways in which technology can be used to lower the bar of competency requirements. The structure of the presentation roughly follows Norman and Skinner's e-health literacy model, without subscribing to the model's representation of the relationships between various competencies.

3.6.1 Reading Competency Problems

The field of health literacy (and subsequently, e-health literacy) grew out of the concern of the mismatch between the public's reading competency and complexity of typical patient education materials, instruction, and other health-related content. Text complexity is often expressed in terms of grade levels. You are probably aware of readability formulas built into text editing software such as Microsoft Word that can assign a grade level to a text. What does it mean, to have a text that is graded at a 7th or an 11th grade readability level? Most formulas are based on one of two principles. The first computes readability level on the basis of lexical and grammatical complexity, estimated via average word length and sentence length in a text. The Flesch–Kincaid and Flesch Reading Ease tests built into Microsoft Word products are examples of this (Microsoft, n.d.). The second looks at how frequently words used in the specific text are used in some gold-standard corpus (from the Latin for "body," this is the technical term for the dataset of text being analyzed). The grade level assigned to the text suggests that results reflect typical complexity characteristic of texts for students in those grades.

Many research studies evaluated the public's reading skills (NAAL), which led to recommendations by several public health authorities that patient materials be written at the 6th-8th grade readability level (National Institutes of Health [NIH], 2016; Weiss, 2007). Yet, numerous studies show that educational materials in a number of health-related fields are written at a level above the recommended guidelines (Aaronson et al., 2018; Baker et al., 2017; Fajardo et al., 2019).

Readability formulas were originally developed to evaluate complexity of materials for school children. For this reason, their use with reading materials for adults, and specifically in the health domain, is not without controversy. While formulas are often based on word length, there are many short medical terms that are less familiar to a typical lay reader than certain longer terms (e.g., "angina" vs. "hospitalization"). Also, artificial simplification of texts by breaking longer complex sentences into shorter simple sentences may actually make texts more difficult to understand by removing relationships between clauses.

Still, criticisms aside, writing consumer-oriented text in simple, jargon-free language is essential for good consumer health applications. In authoring such materials, being aware of the readability level and aiming for the 6th-8th grade level range is an important first step. However, with the aid of technology, consumer health information tools can deliver much more. In the last decade, consumer health informatics researchers dedicated much time mapping lay health terms (i.e., health-related language used by regular people in conversations, such as "heart attack") to professional medical terminologies (or language used by doctors, such as "myocardial infarction"). Like many professions, medicine has its own language, which serves a useful purpose by enabling quick, effective communication among health professionals. At the same time, it often creates a language barrier between doctors and patients, especially when patients access medical documents not written specifically for them, such as their medical records. An average lay reader may or may not know that "neoplasm" may be another way of saying "cancer." She is less likely to know that "paresthesia" stands for a strange skin sensation such as burning or what she might call "pins and needles." In addition to making comprehension more difficult, different vocabularies complicate searching: will my search for "pins and needles" produce lower-quality, less authoritative results than a search for "paresthesia"?

Consumer health informatics can help address this issue by using a consumer health vocabulary to translate terms found in documents and search queries. For example, the National Library of Medicine maintains the Unified Medical Language System (UMLS), a free service that coordinates many health and biomedical vocabularies, including Consumer Health Vocabulary (CHV). The UMLS is running behind the scenes at PubMed database of biomedical and life sciences literature, meaning that a searcher who uses a lay term for a health concept – or a professional medical, nursing, dental, etc. term for a health concept – retrieves journal articles that use the technical term. Using the UMLS can allow developers to map consumer health terms onto terms commonly used in medical systems (e.g., the International Classification of Diseases, used to identify diagnoses and procedures for billing purposes). It can thus facilitate both translation and comprehension.

In addition to lowering readability levels, designers can also follow guidelines for creating useful, usable, easily readable content, such as those put forward in federal Plain Language Guidelines (https://www.plainlanguage.gov/guidelines/). These guidelines, consistent with cognitive psychology principles of text comprehension, emphasize that texts need to be concise, state the most important information first, chunk information into short passages, and utilize subheadings and bullet lists.

Simplifying texts and linking terminologies, however, is only one way of ameliorating the readability requirement. One of the advantages of information technology is its ability to present information via a variety of modalities including audios, videos, and interactive animations.

Cognitive psychology, public health communication, and informatics make numerous research-based recommendations for making information easier to comprehend. Yet, while following them, we should remember that, at present, we do not have conclusive data linking these measures to more optimal health behaviors and outcomes. This stresses the need for designers and developers to be humble, employing user-centered design with iterative rounds of feedback.

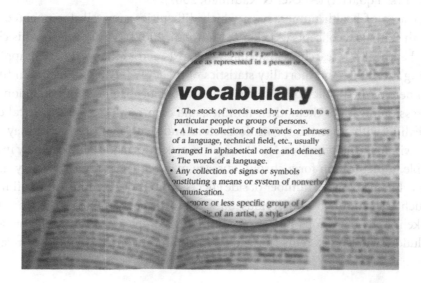

3.6.2 Numeracy Problems

Definitions of health literacy usually combine numeracy with traditional literacy without delving into greater depth. Yet, some authors produce a unique, nuanced definition of health numeracy, insisting that the potential impact of numeracy on individual and public health requires greater and more focused attention. For example, Golbeck et al. (2005) define health numeracy as "the degree to which individuals have the capacity to access, process, interpret, communicate, and act on numerical, quantitative, graphical, biostatistical, and probabilistic health information needed to make effective health decisions" (p. 375).

Examples of health-related tasks drawing on numeracy competence are interpreting instructions for taking medications; reading food values; understanding test results and other numbers in doctors' records; evaluating consumer health information that refers to risks and prevalence; making treatment course decisions on the basis of known statistical risks; and interpreting visuals like tables and graphs. Ancker and Kaufman (2007) identify three categories of numeracy skills that are important in health contexts:

1) Basic quantitative skills such as computation, estimation, and understanding statistical concepts (e.g., uncertainty, randomization);

2) Ability to use information artifacts such as tables, charts, and graphs; and

3) Ability to communicate quantitative information to providers (e.g., explain adherence to medication regimens).

Studying lay performance on tasks that require health numeracy, researchers documented many difficulties. National surveys such as NAAL showed that individuals with low levels of numeracy have difficulty performing the calculations to compute medication dose as a function of body weight, or calculating nutritional values for different portion sizes. People also have trouble recognizing equivalence between different numerical formats (e.g., 1/4 vs. 0.25 vs. 25% vs. a quarter) (Ancker & Kaufman, 2007).

Another area of health numeracy in which difficulties are well documented involves dealing with statistical concepts (Ancker & Kaufman, 2007). We are writing this chapter at the time when health researchers and epidemiologists across the world are grappling with determining morbidity and mortality statistics of the COVID-19 pandemic. In the meantime, members of the public contemplate what various probabilities of contagion and disease progression mean for them, their families, and communities. Most medical decisions involve dealing with uncertainty; while doctors and drug manufacturers may offer the odds, they will make no promises. For this reason, risk information is extremely important. For example, a medication for a chronic disease may reduce the severity of symptoms of that disease, but also cause a number of side effects, from more common and mildly annoying to much less common and serious ones. Unfortunately, quantitative variables that express likelihoods of various outcomes are highly complex. For example, prescriptions often include various risk reduction data. A commonly used statistic is relative risk reduction, RRR, which is the difference between the number of events (e.g., hospitalizations, side effects) in the control and treatment groups divided by the number of events in the control group (BMJ Best Practice, n.d.). If you are not sure that you grasped the meaning of this formula, you can peruse the BMJ Best Practice Evidence Based Medicine (EBM) Toolkit page on how to calculate risk (https://bestpractice.bmj.com/info/us/toolkit/learn-ebm/how-to-calculate-risk/) or other similar tools. Our objective here is to simply show that the task is not a trivial one. For a detailed primer on communicating risk in decision support aids, see Trevena et al. (2013).

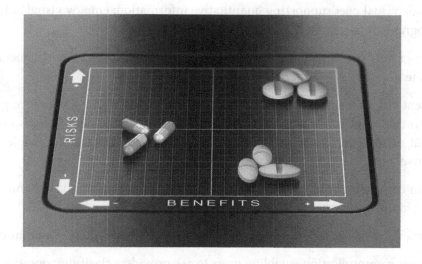

Risk information is so complex, in fact, that researchers have investigated the effectiveness of descriptive labels as an alternative; for example, discussing things that happen "frequently" or "rarely" instead of assigning a number. However, these studies have shown that people preferred more precise numeric information, and that numeric information produced more accurate understanding (West et al., 2013). Individuals with low numeracy skills had more difficulty interpreting the numbers and were aided to a greater degree by pictographs and simple graphics. Several studies also pointed to the benefit of combining quantitative and narrative information.

We have previously suggested that lay ability to deal with health information is a function of both lay knowledge/skills and the packaging, content, and delivery of the said information. Ancker and Kaufman (2007) review studies that focus on patients' ability to deal with quantitative health information in different information materials as related to design characteristics of those materials. They note that individuals, especially those with lower health literacy, often have difficulty locating the essential while excluding extraneous information, dealing with information in multiple formats, and reading tables and graphs. They give an example of patients in a diabetes telemedicine study who had no trouble reading their systolic and diastolic blood pressure on the display of their blood pressure meter, but did not recognize the same values in a table of an online patient portal.

What design features are likely to alleviate demands on health numeracy and improve understanding? Ancker and Kaufman (2007) and Trevena et al. (2013) make the following suggestions (refer to the papers for complete lists):

- Do not include extraneous information, but do reduce the need for computation (e.g., include dosages for different weight ranges rather than require computation; include caloric values for the whole food packet rather than some arbitrary portion)

- Include multiple representational formats or allow switching between representations

- Include visual cues supporting quantitative information; employ visual aids such as pictographs, charts, and diagrams

- Keep graphs simple (employ user testing to verify simplicity), supplement graphs with text

- Present risk of a single event with a denominator, specifying a reference group for which the event is relevant; keep the denominator simple, with a basis of 10 (e.g., "5 out of 100 people who test positive" is better than "1 out of 20 people who test positive")

- When comparing risks or probabilities, use the same format and the same denominator for all events that are being compared

- Whenever possible, tailor information and presentation to the user's situation

- Support communication, enabling users to ask providers clarifying questions

As with literacy supports, user engagement and iterative design are essential for effective implementation of these recommendations. Remember that understanding statistical information characterized by uncertainty (e.g., comparative probabilistic outcomes of different treatments, expected change over time) is, perhaps, the most cognitively challenging of health numeracy tasks. Human interpretation of risk statistics and willingness to assume risks is heavily influenced by presentation of information. While an in-depth guide on health risk communication is outside the scope of this book, it is important that developers and communicators be aware of the complexity of the problem and the need for a careful, deliberate approach to risk communication (for a greater discussion of risk, refer to Part II: Chapter 11).

3.6.3 Supporting Media and Information Literacy

Searching for health information online has been compared to drinking water from a firehose, and users need help distinguishing between the credible and the problematic. A number of organizations and projects attempted to help the public by developing evaluation criteria for online information. Two most established criteria-based tools are HONcode and DISCERN.

HON, or Health on the Net Code, is run by a nonprofit foundation that awards criterion-based certification to health-related websites that apply for it. Certification suggests that a site meets the following eight criteria:

- Authoritative – authors have satisfactory qualification in the subject matter

- Complementarity – information intends to support, rather than replace relationship with healthcare providers

- Privacy – the site respects privacy and confidentiality of users' personal data

- Attribution – sources of information are clearly cited

- Justifiability – claims about benefits of treatments are backed by evidence

- Transparency – the site is easy to comprehend and includes accurate contact information

- Financial disclosure – the site's funding sources are clearly stated

- Advertising policy – advertisement is clearly differentiated from the rest of the content

HON Foundation website includes a specialized search engine that allows queries of HON-certified sites. In June 2019, the foundation counted over 7,300 websites from 102 countries among recipients of its certificate (Health on the Net Foundation [HON], 2019).

Unlike HON, DISCERN [http://www.discern.org.uk/], developed as a collaborative project between the UK National Health Service and the British Library in 1996-97, comprises a set of criteria for evaluating consumer health information. Its original purpose was to help individuals evaluate information about medical treatments, though it has since been applied to a broader range of documents. Unlike HON, DISCERN does not certify documents, but rather, helps users decide whether those documents fit specific quality criteria. Users evaluate whether the publication is reliable and whether the treatment information it presents is of high quality. Reliability criterion considers factors such as clear aims, relevance, clarity of sources, absence of bias, and statement of uncertainty. Information quality criterion considers whether treatment mechanism and risks and benefits are discussed, whether alternative treatment options are described, and whether the document supports shared decision-making with health professionals and family members. Ultimately, the user rates the document on a scale from 1 (serious or extensive shortcomings) to 5 (minimal shortcomings).

While DISCERN supports more in-depth analysis of a document's quality, it leaves the judgment to subjective analysis by the user. In addition, it was developed for print documents and may not constitute the best fit for the contemporary digital information ecosystem that includes videos and social media posts (Keselman, Arnott Smith, Murcko, & Kaufman, 2019). Consumer health informatics can help by developing information quality evaluation criteria tailored to web media and by creating algorithms for evaluating information quality. In the meantime, developers can help users by following HON and DISCERN recommended criteria, by being aware of HON and other emergent certification systems, and by considering obtaining these certifications (for more discussion about the evaluation of health information and the role of tools like these, refer to Part I: Chapter 5).

3.6.4 Supporting Computer Literacy

Computer literacy, or the ability to use computers effectively, can refer to a number of skills, from basic (turning on a computer, using a mouse) to very advanced (writing computer algorithms in a programming language). Computer tasks relevant to consumer health information technology include knowing how to: turn computers, phones, and tablets on and off; operate a mouse and a touch screen; open a browser and access applications; access and navigate websites; read and send email; and use apps. They also involve updating applications and operating systems and downloading software.

Populations differ in how easy, on average, their members find these tasks. Much has been written about the digital divide and its relationship to age (on average, older adults have more limited computer skills), income, health status, and other demographic variables (Hong & Cho, 2017; Reiners et al., 2019; see also Part I: Chapter 6 of this book). Physical access to technology– getting a computer or internet-enabled device – is the first-level digital divide; having the skills to get information online is the second-level; and using that access to receive real benefit from that connectivity is the third-level (van Deursen & van Dijk, 2019). Some aspects of the divide are narrowing with spread of information technology in society. More and more people have computers with internet access and smartphones. The number of seniors owning a smartphone more than doubled between 2013 and 2017 (Anderson & Perrin, 2017). Internet and smartphone use is also growing among lower-income Americans (Anderson & Kumar, 2019). Yet, in other ways, the divide is persisting. Younger and wealthier Americans use technology differently. They are more likely to own multiple devices, have access to large-screen devices (lower-income individuals are more likely to use smartphones as their sole device) (Anderson & Kumar, 2019), and download sophisticated apps. Younger, wealthier individuals are also more likely to have the skills to enable technology to function smoothly and effectively (e.g., connecting devices into a network) (for more on the digital divide, refer to Part II: Chapter 7).

As with the other competencies discussed in this chapter, enabling successful functioning is in part accomplished by embedding an understanding of that functioning in information design. Everyone benefits from better usability (and thus from usability testing); but users with less sophisticated computer skills benefit from simpler designs. Designing for lowering computer literacy requirements involves ensuring that designs work well on different devices and in different browsers, for example, by employing responsive design. While designers can be drawn to cutting-edge technologies, they should remember that users may not have the optimal hardware to run software making heavy demands on computer memory. These users may also not have the latest browser versions and operating systems. In addition, special guidelines make detailed design recommendations for users living with disability or age-related mobility, vision, and hearing impairments.

In addition to being mindful of computer literacy demands posed by various technologies, the information professionals who select and introduce them can support users via education and training. If you are reading this book, you are probably a very savvy computer user. It is, therefore, very important for you to get to know the computer skills of your users or clients, as they may be very different from what you consciously or unconsciously view as the default. In one striking example, a colleague of the authors – who is another consumer health informatics researcher – once pointed to a link on a computer screen and asked a user with low computer literacy to "please, click here." The user lifted the mouse up to the place on the monitor that the researcher was touching. While this took place around 2001 and one can expect such experiences to be becoming less and less common in the US, it is a cautionary anecdote: nothing replaces getting to know your users.

3.6.5 Supporting Science Literacy

Science literacy is defined by the ability to understand scientific basis of health information. This literacy generally develops through school science instruction, as well as in informal science contexts (e.g., via reading science-related books and magazines, going to science museums, etc.). Unfortunately, these experiences are often insufficient. In the 2015 leading global educational assessment project, US 15- and 16-year-olds ranked 19th out of the 35 Organization for Economic Co-operation and Development (OECD) participating member countries on their science learning (31st in math), falling behind many countries with a comparable level of development (Organization for Economic Co-operation and Development [OECD], 2016). In addition, although the standard school science curriculum in the US includes biology, it is rarely taught in the context of health and disease management and healthcare (Keselman, 2017). Instead, schools usually teach health as a separate subject, focused on wellness and health promotion, and taught without in-depth analysis of biological mechanisms or the nuances of the scientific method.

This situation is particularly disconcerting because of the spread of inaccurate online health information that tries simultaneously to discredit established science and to present itself as grounded in science (Keselman et al., 2019). In fact, health literacy and science literacy are intertwined challenges. In a study of web pages about natural treatments for type 2 diabetes, we found that most pages promised or strongly implied definitive cures (Keselman et al., 2019). This is noteworthy because, according to authoritative evidence-based medical science, type 2 diabetes can be put into remission, but generally not cured or reversed. In spite of this scientific consensus, most of the webpages we explored, from informational texts to YouTube videos, made references to and provided descriptions of biological mechanisms behind their proposed treatments and mentioned scientific studies. Often, their descriptions of mechanisms were very complex, so that judging their accuracy was a task likely exceeding the competency of a typical layperson, regardless of how much attention that person paid in a high school biology classroom. The authors of these webpages, however, also made statements that could raise suspicion in someone with reasonably good understanding of how science works. For example, some sites claimed breakthrough discoveries by unspecified teams of scientists that contradicted mainstream science. But while science develops through debates, and disagreements among scientists are possible, science is rather conspiracy-proof. It is highly unlikely that a breakthrough treatment for a disease that constitutes a major public health threat would exist without such findings appearing in authoritative journals and entering prominent mainstream media. Problematic webpages with promises of a cure also often exaggerate or misrepresent results of scientific studies, or point to studies characterized by poor methodologies and published in low-authority publications. Recognizing these characteristics and viewing them as a signal of potentially problematic information requires a rather high level of science literacy that many users don't have. Combine that with the common and desperate hope for a cure and the power of today's information technology to spread misinformation, and you will see why sites promoting various unconfirmed remedies are doing quite well.

What can information designers, consumer health informatics researchers, and other information professional do? Given the complexity of science literacy, it may be wise to focus on supporting media and information literacy (see Part I: Chapter 5 for more information), and helping users recognize reliable and authoritative information sources. After all, if my preferred source of information for advances in type 2 diabetes treatments is the American Diabetes Association, I am not likely to encounter there a promise that an ancient herb will help me get rid of my diabetes in 14 days. Consumer health informatics researchers can also develop machine algorithms for detecting misinformation and inaccurate health information. Such algorithms can rely on rule-based and machine-learning (probabilistic) approaches, identifying linguistic and conceptual features of inaccurate information. Unfortunately, while such research is potentially promising, it is currently uncommon. Finally, another potentially fruitful direction is contributing to raising the public's science literacy as it relates to health education through outreach events and workshops, as well as by pointing out important characteristics of scientific evidence behind quality health information content.

3.7 CONCLUSIONS

In summary, individuals' ability to successfully locate, evaluate, understand, and use health information is grounded in a number of cognitive, social, emotional, and motivational factors. In health, these competencies are most often discussed under the umbrella of the concept of health literacy. Extensive research has recorded insufficient levels of health literacy in the population as well as the relationship between poor health literacy, suboptimal health behaviors, and poor outcomes. While the concept of health literacy is useful, it is characterized by a diversity of definitions and component skills ascribed to it. Assessments of health literacy used in studies are generally easy-to-administer proxies that test health vocabulary knowledge and reading ability in health contexts. At the same time, researchers and professionals understand that health literacy is much more complex than vocabulary and paragraph comprehension. Another concept that has been studied in the context of digital health information is e-health literacy. Research literature also mentions health numeracy, information literacy, computer literacy, and science literacy.

In discussing these literacies, one can visualize different hierarchical relationships among them. The most important thing to remember is that there are multiple cognitive competencies that underlie dealing with online health information. These competencies include reading ability, knowledge of health terminology, ability to operate with numbers and understand health statistics and different representations of health data, ability to use computers efficiently, knowledge of characteristics of quality health information and information sources, some knowledge of the underlying science, and understanding of the scientific method and its value. Add to this written and oral communication skills and motivation to pursue information that is tied to cultural, social, and emotional factors, and you will understand why the issue is so immensely complex.

Fortunately, competency requirements are not static requirements of the user; rather, they arise from the interaction between the user's skills/knowledge/background and characteristics of information technology. This means that you, as a current or future professional involved in designing, developing, selecting, or promoting health information technology or conducting research around it, can help the public in navigating this complexity.

WEB RESOURCES

Health Literacy Tool Shed
http://healthliteracytoolshed.bu.edu
This site is "an online database of health literacy measures," maintained by Boston University.

Plain Language Guidelines
https://www.plainlanguage.gov/guidelines/
Federal plain languages guidelines for US federal agencies, aiming to support and promote clear communication to the public.

Unified Medical Language System (UMLS)
https://www.nlm.nih.gov/research/umls/index.html
This is "a set of files and software that brings together many health and biomedical vocabularies and standards to enable interoperability between computer systems"; it includes Consumer Health Vocabulary (CHV).

BMJ Best Practice: How to Calculate Risk
https://bestpractice.bmj.com/info/us/toolkit/learn-ebm/how-to-calculate-risk/
This page includes definitions and formulas for various risk-related concepts that may be discussed in health information resources.

REFERENCES

Aaronson, N. L., Joshua, C. L., & Boss, E. F. (2018). Health literacy in pediatric otolaryngology: A scoping review. *International Journal of Pediatric Otorhinolaryngology*, 113, 252–259. https://doi.org/10.1016/j.ijporl.2018.08.013

American Library Association. (1989). Presidential committee on information literacy: Final report. http://www.ala.org/acrl/publications/whitepapers/presidential

American Medical Association [AMA], Ad Hoc Committee on Health Literacy for the Council on Scientific Affairs. (1999). Health literacy: Report of the council on scientific affairs. *Journal of the American Medical Association*, 281(6), 552–557. https://doi.org/10.1001/jama.281.6.552

Ancker, J. S., & Kaufman, D. (2007). Rethinking health numeracy: A multidisciplinary literature review. *Journal of the American Medical Informatics Association*, 14(6), 713–721. https://doi.org/10.1197/jamia.M2464

Anderson, M., & Kumar, M. (2019). *Digital divide persists even as lower-income Americans make gains in tech adoption.* Pew Research Center. Retrieved February 29, 2020, from https://www.pewresearch.org/fact-tank/2019/05/07/digital-divide-persists-even-as-lower-income-americans-make-gains-in-tech-adoption/

Anderson, M., & Perrin, A. (2017). *Technology use among seniors.* Pew Research Center. Retrieved February 29, 2020, from https://www.pewresearch.org/internet/2017/05/17/technology-use-among-seniors/

Baker, D. M., Marshall, J. H., Lee, M. J., Jones, G. L., Brown, S. R., & Lobo, A. J. (2017). A systematic review of internet decision-making resources for patients considering surgery for ulcerative colitis. *Inflammatory Bowel Diseases, 23*(8), 1293–1300. https://doi.org/10.1097/MIB.0000000000001198

Baker, D. W. (2006). The meaning and measure of health literacy. *Journal of General Internal Medicine, 21*(8), 878–883.

Baker, D. W., Gazmararian, J. A., Williams, M. V., Scott, T., Parker, R. M., Green, D., Ren, J., & Peel, J. (2004). Health literacy and use of outpatient physician services by Medicare managed care enrollees. *Journal of General Internal Medicine, 19*(3), 215–220. https://doi.org/10.1111/j.1525-1497.2004.21130.x

Baker, D. W., Wolf, M. S., Feinglass, J., & Thompson, J. A. (2008). Health literacy, cognitive abilities, and mortality among elderly persons. *Journal of General Internal Medicine, 23*(6), 723–726.

Baker, D. W., Wolf, M. S., Feinglass, J., Thompson, J. A., Gazmararian, J. A., & Huang, J. (2007). Health literacy and mortality among elderly persons. *Archives of Internal Medicine, 167*(14), 1503–1509.

Berkman, N. D., Sheridan, S. L., Donahue, K. E., Halpern, D. J., & Crotty, K. (2011). Low health literacy and health outcomes: An updated systematic review. *Annals of Internal Medicine, 155*(2), 97–107. https://doi.org/10.7326/0003-4819-155-2-201107190-00005

Berkman, N. D., Sheridan, S. L., Donahue, K. E. , Halpern, D. J., Viera, A., Crotty, K., Holland, A., Brausure, M., Lohr, K. N., Harden, E., Tant, E., Wallace, I., & Viswanathan, M. (2011). Health literacy interventions and outcomes: An updated systematic review. *Evidence Report/Technology Assessment, 199,* 1–941. Agency of Healthcare Research and Quality Publication No. 11-E006.

BMJ Best Practice. (n.d.). *EMB toolkit: How to calculate risk.* BMJ Publishing Group Limited. https://bestpractice.bmj.com/info/us/toolkit/learn-ebm/how-to-calculate-risk/

Bybee, R., McCrae, B., & Laurie, R. (2009). PISA 2006: An assessment of scientific literacy. *Journal of Research in Science Teaching, 46*(8), 865–883. https://doi.org/10.1002/tea.20333

Charnock, D., & Shepperd, S. (n.d.). DISCERN: Quality criteria for consumer health information. *Radcliffe Online.* Retrieved February 29, 2020, from http://www.discern.org.uk/

Cho, Y. I., Lee, S.-Y. D., Arozullah, A. M., & Crittenden, K. S. (2008). Effects of health literacy on health status and health service utilization amongst the elderly. *Social Science & Medicine, 66*(8), 1809–1816.

Davis, T. C., Crouch, M. A., Long, S. W., Jackson, R. H., Bates, P., George, R. B., & Bairnsfather, L. E. (1991). Rapid assessment of literacy levels of adult primary care patients. *Family Medicine, 23*(6), 433–435.

Davis, T. C., Wolf, M. S., Bass, P. F. 3rd, Thompson, J. A., Tilson, H. H., Neuberger, M., & Parker, R. M. (2006). Literacy and misunderstanding prescription drug labels. *Annals of Internal Medicine, 145*(12), 887–894.

van Deursen, A. J., & van Dijk, J. A. (2019). The first-level digital divide shifts from inequalities in physical access to inequalities in material access. *New Media & Society, 21*(2), 354–375. https://doi.org/10.1177/1461444818797082

Doak, C. C., Doak, L. G., & Root, J. H. (1996). *Teaching patients with low literacy skills* (2nd ed.). Lippincott.

Doak, L. G., & Doak, C. C. (1987). Lowering the silent barriers for patients with low health literacy skills. *Promoting Health, 8*(4), 6–8.

Fajardo, M. A., Weir, K. R., Bonner, C., Gnjidic, D., & Jansen, J. (2019). Availability and readability of patient education materials for deprescribing: An environmental scan. *British Journal of Clinical Pharmacology, 85*(7), 1396–1406. https://doi.org/10.1111/bcp.13912

Golbeck, A. L., Ahlers-Schmidt, C. R., Paschal, A. M., & Dismuke, S. E. (2005). A definition and operational framework for health numeracy. *American Journal of Preventative Medicine, 29*(4), 375–376. https://doi.org/10.1016/j.amepre.2005.06.012

Guerra, C. E., Krumholz, M., & Shea, J. A. (2005). Literacy and knowledge, attitudes and behavior about mammography in Latinas. *Journal of Health Care for Poor and Underserved, 16*(1), 152–166. https://doi.org/10.1353/hpu.2005.0012

Health on the Net Foundation [HON]. (2019). *HONcode certification.* Retrieved February 29, 2020, from https://www.hon.ch/en/

Hong, Y. A., & Cho, J. (2017). Has the digital health divide widened? Trends of health-related internet use among older adults from 2003 to 2011. *Journals of Gerontology: Series B, 72*(5), 856–863. https://doi.org/10.1093/geronb/gbw100

Hope, C. J., Wu, J., Tu, W., Young, J., & Murray, M. D. (2004). Association of medication adherence, knowledge, and skills with emergency department visits by adults 50 years or older with congestive heart failure. *American Journal of Health-System Pharmacists, 61*(19), 2043–2049.

Institute of Medicine [IOM]. (2004). *Health literacy: A prescription to end confusion* (L. Nielsen-Bohlman, A. M. Panzer, D. A. Kindig, Eds.). The National Academies Press. https://doi.org/10.17226/10883

Keselman, A. (2017). Health information literacy as a tool for addressing adolescent behaviors, knowledge, skills, and academic trajectories. In V. Patel, J. F. Arocha, & J. S. Ancker (Eds.), *Cognitive informatics in health and biomedicine: Understanding and modeling health behaviors* (pp. 119–136). Springer. https://doi.org/10.1007/978-3-319-51732-2_6

Keselman, A., Arnott Smith, C., Murcko, A. C., & Kaufman, D. R. (2019). Evaluating the quality of health information in a changing digital ecosystem. *Journal of Medical Internet Research, 21*(2), e11129. https://doi.org/10.2196/11129

Kripalani, S., Henderson, L. E., Chiu, E. Y., Robertson, R., Kolm, P., & Jacobson, T. A. (2006). Predictors of medication self-management skill in a low-literacy population. *Journal of General Internal Medicine, 21*(8), 852–856. https://doi.org/10.1111/j.1525-1497.2006.00536.x

Lee, S.-Y., Arozullah, A. M., Cho, Y. I., Crittenden, K., & Vicencio, D. (2009). Health literacy, social support, and health status among older adults. *Educational Gerontology, 35*(3), 191–201. https://doi.org/10.1080/03601270802466629

Logan, R. A. (2015). Health literacy research's growth, challenges and frontiers. In C. A. Smith and A. Keselman (Eds.), *Meeting health information needs outside of healthcare* (pp. 19–38). Chandos. https://doi.org/10.1016/C2014-0-03754-9

Microsoft. (n.d.). *Get your document's readability and level statistics.* Retrieved February 29, 2020, from https://support.office.com/en-us/article/get-your-document-s-readability-and-level-statistics-85b4969e-e80a-4777-8dd3-f7fc3c8b3fd2

National Institutes of Health [NIH]. (2016). *Clear & Simple: What is clear & simple? NIH Office of Communications and Public Liaison.* Retrieved February 29, 2020, from https://www.nih.gov/institutes-nih/nih-office-director/office-communications-public-liaison/clear-communication/clear-simple

Norman, C. D., & Skinner, H. A. (2006). eHEALS: The eHealth literacy scale. *Journal of Medical Internet Research, 8*(4), e27. https://doi.org/10.2196/jmir.8.4.e27

Nutbeam, D. (2008). The evolving concept of health literacy. *Social Science & Medicine, 67*(12), 2072–2078. https://doi.org/10.1016/j.socscimed.2008.09.050

Organization for Economic Co-operation and Development [OECD]. (2016). *Country notes: Key findings from PISA 2015 for the United States* (pp. 1–76). OECD Publishing. Retrieved February 29, 2020, from https://www.oecd.org/pisa/PISA-2015-United-States.pdf

Osborne, R. H., Batterham, R. W., Elsworth, G. R., Hawkins, M., & Buchbinder, R. (2013). The grounded psychometric development and initial validation of the Health Literacy Questionnaire (HLQ). *BMC Public Health*, 13, 658.

Paasche-Orlow, M. K., & Wolf, M. S. (2007). The causal pathways linking health literacy to health outcomes. *American Journal of Health Behavior*, 31(Suppl. 1), S19–S26.

Parker, R. M., Baker, D. W., Williams, M. V., & Nurss, J. R. (1995). The test of functional health literacy in adults: A new instrument for measuring patients' literacy skills. *Journal of General Internal Medicine*, 10(10), 537–541. https://doi.org/10.1007/bf02640361

Ratzan, S. C., & Parker, R. M. (2000). Introduction. In C. R. Selden, M. Zorn, S. C. Ratzan & R. M. Parker (Eds.), *National Library of Medicine current bibliographies in medicine: Health Literacy*. NLM Publishing No. CBL 2000-1. Bethesda, MD: National Institutes of Health, U.S. Department of Health and Human Services.

Reiners, F., Sturm, J., Bouw, L. J. W., & Wouters. E. J. M. (2019). Sociodemographic factors influencing the use of eHealth in people with chronic diseases. *International Journal of Environmental Research and Public Health*, 16(4), 645. https://doi.org/10.3390/ijerph16040645

Sørensen, K., Van den Broucke, S., Fullam, J., Doyle, G., Pelikan, J., Solnska, Z., Brand, H., & (HLS-EU) Consortium Health Literacy Project European. (2012). Health literacy and public health: A systematic review and integration of definitions and models. *BMC Public Health*, 12(80). http+s://doi.org/10.1186/1471-2458-12-80

Sudore, R. L., Yaffe, K., Satterfield, S., Harris, T. B., Mehta, K. M., Simonsick, E. M., Newman, A. B., Rosano, C., Rooks, R., Rubin, S. M., Ayonayon, H. N., & Schillinger, D. (2006). Limited literacy and mortality in the elderly: The health, aging, and body composition study. *Journal of General Internal Medicine*, 21(8), 806–812.

Taylor, W. L. (1953). "Cloze procedure": A new tool for measuring readability. *Journalism Quarterly*, 30(4), 415–433. https://doi.org/10.1177/107769905303000401

Trevena, L. J., Zikmund-Fisher, B. J., Edwards, A., Gaissmaier, W., Galesic, M., Han, P. K., King, J., Lawson, M. L., Linder, S. K., Lipkus, I., Ozanne, E., Peters, E., Timmermans, D., & Woloskin, S. (2013). Presenting quantitative information about decision outcomes: A risk communication primer for patient decision aid developers. *BMC Medical Informatics and Decisionmaking*, 13(Supplement 2), S2–S7. https://doi.org/10.1186/1472-6947-13-S2-S7

U.S Department of Education. (n.d.). *National assessment of adult literacy (NAAL)*. Institute of Education Sciences, National Center for Education Statistics. Retrieved February 29, 2020, from https://nces.ed.gov/naal/

U.S. Department of Education. (2006). *the health literacy of America's adults: Results from the 2003 national assessment of adult literacy (NAAL)*. Institute of Education Sciences, National Center for Education Statistics. https://nces.ed.gov/pubs2006/2006483.pdf

Weiss, B. D. (2007). *Health literacy and patient safety: Help patients understand: A manual for Clinicians* (2nd ed., pp. 1–62). Chicago, IL: American Medical Association Foundation and American Medical Association & AMA Foundation.

West, S. L., Squiers, L. B., McCormack, L., Southwell, B. G., Brouwer, E. S., Ashok, M., Lux, L., Boudewyns, V., O'Donoghue, A., & Sullivan, H. W. (2013). Communicating quantitative risks and benefits in promotional prescription drug labeling or print advertising. *Pharmacoepidemiology and Drug Safety*, 22(5), 447–458. https://doi.org/10.1002/pds.3416

White, S., Chen, J., & Atchison, R. (2008). Relationship of preventive health practices and health literacy: A national study. *American Journal of Health Behavior*, 32(3), 227–242. https://doi.org/10.5993/AJHB.32.3.1

World Health Organization [WHO]. (2009). *Track 2: Health literacy and health behavior. 7th global conference on health promotion*, Nairobi, Kenya. https://www.who.int/healthpromotion/conferences/7gchp/track2/en/

CHAPTER 4

Online Databases to Support Consumer Health Informatics

Catherine Arnott Smith

T<small>HIS CHAPTER DISCUSSES</small> high-quality digital information resources which can meet the needs of CHI students, researchers, and practitioners alike. Examples of licensed commercial databases include the ACM Digital Library, IEEE Xplore, CINAHL, Health and Psychosocial Instruments (HaPI), and PsycINFO. Free high-quality health information resources from the federal government, such as PubMed MEDLINE, as well as citation products Web of Science, Scopus, and Google Scholar, are also explored.

4.1 HEALTH INFORMATION ONLINE: AN INTRODUCTION

The most important thing to understand about health information online is that there is a vast amount of it. Google's virtual monopoly on market share – 92% overall in the United States, and 95% on mobile devices, as of December 2019 (Merkle, 2019) – together with the ease of use of this particular product has led to the misconception that everything digital can be found using a search engine. While search engines are extremely useful agents for presenting and organizing information, their prominence and ease of use means that they also function as mass media channels "broadcasting" information in response to a specific query (Segev, 2010). What many users don't realize is that search engines (1) aren't searching the entire Web, but only that portion of the Web which has been indexed by the engine and (2) use multiple dimensions of user profiling to tailor results not just to a specific query, but to a specific user on a specific computer. This means that users of search engines don't know what results they're missing. Author Eli Pariser's TED talk – and book – *The Filter Bubble* explains why this matters:

> In a broadcast society – this is how the founding mythology goes .. there were these gatekeepers, the editors, and they controlled the flows of information. And along came the Internet and it swept them out of the way, and it allowed all of us to connect together, and it was awesome. But that's not actually what's happening right

now. What we're seeing is more of a passing of the torch from human gatekeepers to algorithmic ones. With these kinds of algorithmic filters, these personalized filters .. because they're mainly looking at what you click on first .. You don't decide what gets in. And more importantly, you don't actually see what gets edited out.

(Pariser, 2011)

Health information is, of course, high need in human society and high risk as well, so the ability to understand how search engines work can be literally a matter of life and death. Chinese student Wei Zexi, a cancer patient, used Google to discover that he'd been misled by advertising online:

> [Wei] was treated for a rare form of cancer with radiation and chemotherapy; when these did not work, he looked online for other options. He found a hospital in Beijing that claimed to have an experimental treatment for his condition, but after traveling to the hospital and taking the expensive treatment, he found it was neither effective nor experimental. In a widely circulated post before his death, Mr. Wei blamed China's largest search engine, Baidu, for directing him to the hospital by providing him with paid advertisements that masqueraded as objective information. "Baidu, a top-ranked hospital … everything must be legitimate," CNN reported him writing, "A Chinese student in the United States helped me Google relevant information. Only then did we find out that American hospitals had long stopped using the technology (used in the treatment) due to poor results in clinical trials."

(Yom-Tov, 2016)

Research takes place at all stages of study of consumer health informatics – whether for health information seeking, website or app design, analysis of results, or a term paper. Research means finding high-quality sources of published information, authored by experts, and processed in a way that guarantees "editorial oversight" (Markey, 2019). How, in the era defined by the World Wide Web, do we find this information? The answer is that we need to look in the right places. This chapter focuses on two important places: bibliographic databases and websites.

4.2 BIBLIOGRAPHIC DATABASES

What is a database and why should you use one? A database is a kind of collection: a collection of digital resources (such as full-text articles or conference papers) or of digital pointers to digital resources (such as physical books held by libraries). A bibliographic database may contain citations to published articles, conference proceedings, book chapters, and other scholarly works in a particular field. Because the database has been curated, quality control has been achieved at several different points, each of which increases a searcher's chance of finding good published information.

For example, MEDLINE (discussed below) is a key database for healthcare and health informatics students and professionals, produced by the US National Library of Medicine but available and widely used internationally. In medicine (as well as nursing and other related health fields) the dominant unit of communication is the journal, not books or conference proceedings. Specific journals accept submissions from authors, send potentially publishable articles out for review by people in the same field as the authors, and make decisions based on the opinion of reviewers and editors who are selected for journals' editorial boards because of their own relevant experience and qualifications. This is quality control at the *article* level. A similar process occurs for other publication venues such as conference proceedings.

There is also quality control occurring at the *journal* level. Journals are submitted for consideration for indexing and inclusion, for example, in the MEDLINE database (for details, see National Library of Medicine, 2019a). "Indexing" means that individual articles in the journals are read and tagged, using a standardized process, by human beings and computers, working together. The metadata used in indexing makes the article content accessible on the article level.

The process by which journals are selected for indexing is publicly available, and so are the criteria used for selection (see National Library of Medicine, 2019b). The complete list of journals indexed is also publicly available in its own searchable database (see https://www.nlm.nih.gov/lstrc/j_sel_faq.html). Databases also have specific audiences in mind. To understand a database, consider the kind of journals indexed by that database. Some journals are aiming at a practitioner readership (industry professionals, physicians, nurses), and some at students (computer or data science undergraduate majors). By inspecting the nature of journals indexed by a database, users can assess for themselves whether the editorial criteria used by that database conform with their own personal or professional values as well as their purpose for needing the information. For example, a student interested in researching alternative medicine will have *some* of their needs met by MEDLINE, but a different database, Consumer Health Complete, may be a better choice (see below).

Why use a database and not a search engine? For research purposes, it is necessary, in the 21st century, to use both. But databases are still necessary: in part because of the built-in content quality filter that any database provides when compared to any search engine. Another reason: the Invisible Web, defined as:

> Text pages, files, or other often high-quality authoritative information available via the worldwide web that general-purpose search engines cannot, due to technical limitations, or will not, due to deliberate choice, add to their indices of web pages.
>
> (Sherman & Price, 2001)

Much online content remains "invisible," or hidden from search engines, because it is of one of two types: either it is password-protected *or* it appears on page 42 of a 500-page result list. This content is not available to web crawlers for indexing and so it will not be seen by the searcher.

Table 4.1 presents other significant differences between search engines and databases in terms of functions and content.

The access question is important. Because many (but not all) databases are commercial products and can cost many thousands of dollars a year for access, it is typical for libraries

TABLE 4.1 Databases versus Search Engines

Function	Database	Search Engine
Collects content through…	Submission process based on journal editorial board, peer review, etc.	Web crawler
Indexing happens by…	Access points created to article-level metadata ("author," "subject", etc.)	N/A
Retrieval happens when…	Information stored in database record and/or full text of article is searched by internal search engine	Information stored in document matches keywords submitted by searcher
Results are displayed in …	Order specified by the searcher; default is often "relevance ranking" but other choices include publication date (oldest or newest first), alphabetical order by author, etc.	"Relevance ranking"
Characteristics		
Scope of the content retrieved is …	Typically organized with a particular purpose, subject OR audience in mind. All records retrieved have something in common according to purpose, subject, or audience	Anything and everything based on keyword matching
Content retrieved consists of …	Depends on nature of database; can be full-text, can be citations or abstracts only	Depends on what content owner has decided to make available; can be full-text, can be citations or abstracts only
Authority of the content is determined by …	For peer-reviewed publications: The editorial process (review might be single-blind – reviewer knows who wrote it, but the author doesn't know who's reviewing it; or double-blind: neither reviewer nor author knows who the other person is). In all publications: The publisher of the journal or other publication venue; editors and editorial boards	N/A
Content is updated by …	Database publisher determines how frequently updates will happen	Crawler specifications determine frequency of update
Cost	Incredible variability, from free to hundreds of thousands of dollars. Factors include: cost of production; licensing agreements between journal publishers and database publishers; subsidizing of access by user's company, library, university, etc.	Incredible variability, from free to hundreds of thousands of dollars, depending on what the publisher has made available for *legal* access
Access	Depends on cost. Public, university, and corporate libraries and knowledge management centers make databases available to different kinds of users. See also discussion below.	Anywhere online

(*Continued*)

TABLE 4.1 (*Continued*) Databases versus Search Engines

Function	Database	Search Engine
Full-text	Depends. The availability of full-text documents in commercial *or* free databases depends on the licensing agreements in place at the university library in which these sometimes very expensive products can be found. If libraries have subscriptions to digital full-text, a technology called a "link resolver" makes that full text accessible to searchers at the touch of a button. If libraries do not, interlibrary loan services can be used to acquire full text copies at cheap or no cost, depending on the level of funding of the academic or public library.	Depends. See "Cost" above.

in different settings to subscribe to specific databases so that their individual users do not have to. Academic libraries (serving students, faculty and staff in settings from vocational schools to four-year research universities) provide access to databases that serve their particular user community's needs. In industry settings, libraries and knowledge centers open only to employees of the corporation can fulfill that same function. Even public libraries have databases available to the general public. In the sections that follow, we provide brief descriptions of key databases that are valuable for CHI. To find out what databases you have access to yourself, we recommend that you investigate your university library.

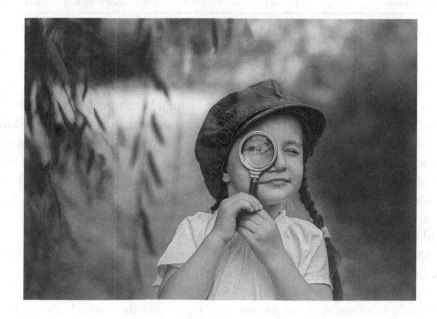

4.3 DATABASES AND LITERATURE FOR CHI

It is important to understand literature for CHI from both a research and a practice angle. Key information resources in CHI provide access to high-quality literature that supports the whole life cycle of CHI research and practice – from studying systems, to building systems, to using systems, and back again. This literature communicates CHI research to scholars and students as well as practitioners.

Note: Full-text databases aimed at a general audience, such as Academic Search, ProQuest Research, and JSTOR are generally not sufficient for academic or industry research of any breadth and depth. JSTOR in particular has a "rolling embargo" that restricts most content to no more recent a date than three to five years ago, which makes it less useful for health-related research (JSTOR, 2020). However, these databases can provide content that points you to the key people, institutions, organizations, and ideas you're looking for. You can then use more focused, specialized databases, such as those listed below, to do more in-depth research.

To find high-quality literature in CHI, you need to search the bibliographic databases that index the published literature of that domain. Researchers and writers who contribute content to the authoritative published literature of health information technology occupy four principal domains (see Table 4.2), and sometimes several at the same time:

Domain of Practice	Typical Bibliographic Databases
Healthcare: Medicine	*Healthcare:* PubMed; MEDLINE; PsycINFO
Healthcare: Nursing	Cumulative Index to Nursing and Allied Health Literature (CINAHL)
Healthcare: Consumer-facing	Consumer Health Complete
Engineering	*Engineering:* Engineering Village (Compendex; INSPEC); IEEE Xplore
Computer Science	ACM Digital Library
Information Science	Library & Information Science & Technology Abstracts (LISTA)

4.3.1 Healthcare: Medicine

4.3.1.1 PubMed and MEDLINE

The United States has five national libraries: The National Transportation Library, focused on transportation information and the transportation community; the National Library of Education, for all education information; The National Library of Agriculture, for materials related to agriculture; the National Library of Medicine, for materials related to medicine; and the Library of Congress, for everything else. The National Library of Medicine, or NLM, began its institutional life in 1836 as the Library of the Surgeon General's Office. One of its most important products today, the MEDLINE database, began as a printed index – the first bibliographic index of biomedical literature in the entire world – in 1879.

MEDLINE may be "the best-known IR [information retrieval] application in all of health or biomedicine" (Hersh, 2009, p. 121). Research supports this statement: one study of healthcare providers in 56 hospitals in 2017 found the MEDLINE database was the second most frequently used resource for patient care, right after the journals themselves (both print and digital) (Dunn, Marshall, Wells, & Backus, 2017). It is the principal international database of biomedical literature, including the literature of medical computing and health information technology. That literature is largely made up of scholarly journals, but there are newspapers, magazines, and newsletters included as well. Its intended audience is people in the health professions: "researchers, practitioners, educators, administrators, and students" – although this database is also used by consumers and patients, and NLM cautions: "Health consumers are encouraged to discuss search results with their health care provider" (National Library of Medicine, 2019c). Publishers submit journals for consideration for indexing by an NLM committee; this committee meets three times a year and makes selections based on criteria such as scope/coverage and quality of content, editorial work, and production. During the fiscal year 2017, 3.3 billion searches were done in MEDLINE; and 5150 unique journal titles were indexed for the database (National Library of Medicine, 2018). As a print index (*Index Medicus*), MEDLINE dates from 1879. As a digital product (first known as MEDLARS), it dates from 1964. Just six years later, 24,000 MEDLINE searches were being done annually from only ten computers nationwide. It was renamed MEDLINE in 1972. After the dawn of the World Wide Web, in July 1997, MEDLINE became free via the PubMed service, an event announced by Vice President Al Gore. To underscore the importance of PubMed and MEDLINE: Google™ has been scraping PubMed citations for results for Google searches since at least 2005 (Nahin, 2005).

PubMed is the name for the search engine for the MEDLINE database, described below, but also an access portal for dozens of other databases containing content from books to genomes. While it is common in healthcare to hear references to "PubMed" and "MEDLINE" interchangeably, in fact they are two different things; for more information, see NLM's FactSheet (National Library of Medicine, 2019d).

While the core MEDLINE database consisting of bibliographic citations – author, title, publication information, and an abstract – is free, and has been since 1997, the data are also available as a licensed product from commercial database vendors with value-added features such as enhanced metadata searching capabilities. Commercial vendors selling MEDLINE to libraries integrate the database with licensed full-text content; while much of this full-text content is available for free online via PubMed Central after a period of time has elapsed, commercial vendors make some of the same full-text content – and more – available much faster.

4.3.1.2 PsycINFO

PsycINFO is the principal database concentrating on the literature of psychology and its related fields. (It is important to note: psychology, not psychiatry; psychiatry requires an MD degree to practice and so is better represented in MEDLINE.) It is a product of the American Psychological Association and indexes more than 2500 journals identified as "psychologically relevant, archival, scholarly, peer-reviewed, and regularly published." Its target audience is "students, researchers, educators, and practitioners" (PsycINFO, 2019). This classic and valuable product is very widely found in college and university libraries in North America.

4.3.2 Healthcare: Nursing

4.3.2.1 CINAHL

The Cumulative Index to Nursing and Allied Health Literature, or CINAHL, is the principal database serving the needs of nursing and allied health professions. In addition to more than 50 specialties within nursing, the allied health professions whose literature is covered here include emergency services, nutrition/dietetics, audiology, physical therapy, and surgical technology. Like most databases, this commercial product began as a print index. In 1977, "allied health" was added to the scope of coverage and the title, and CINAHL launched as a digital product in 1984. Its indexed content includes not only academic journals and practitioner-oriented magazines, but consumer-oriented magazines and newsletters like Vegetarian Times, evidence-based care sheets to support nursing practice; overviews of specific diseases and conditions; and research instruments, such as psychology questionnaires. Its target audience is "students, faculty, and practitioners in the nursing and allied health fields" (Ebsco Health, 2020). This database is so key to nursing education that it can be found wherever nursing students can be found: in libraries from community colleges through research universities. Larger public libraries offer access to this commercial database as well.

4.3.2.2 HaPI

Health and Psychosocial Instruments, or HaPI, indexes the published literature of healthcare (medicine, nursing, public health, psychology) and the social sciences (social work, communication, sociology). HaPI's content is articles, but they are all articles that relate to *instruments* – that is, the tools of and for data collection, such as surveys, tests, indexing schemes, checklists, rating scales, and scenarios. Records in this database provide the searcher with, at minimum, information about who has published research using the instrument. Some records contain sample items from the instrument and more detailed information. This commercial database is found in academic libraries.

4.3.3 Healthcare: Consumer-Facing

4.3.3.1 Consumer Health Complete

The commercial database Consumer Health Complete and similar consumer-facing products assume a consumer- and patient-facing audience as opposed to a health professional audience. CHC indexes publications likely to be useful to the general public. This database features magazines as well as journals (e.g., *Fit Pregnancy*), patient education pamphlets from publishers including NIH and Harvard Health, health reference books and encyclopedias, animations with audio narration, and medical images. This makes this database an ideal source not only to obtain a general understanding of health topics and how content might be tailored to the public, but to appreciate the consumer and patient *perspective* on health topics. Consumer Health Complete is a good source for complementary and alternative medicine information as well as pharmaceutical information. This product is found in academic libraries but also public libraries.

4.3.4 Computer and Information Science

4.3.4.1 ACM Digital Library

The Association for Computing Machinery is the largest professional association for computing sciences, and it is also a major publisher of journals, books, and conference papers presented at its numerous conferences. Just as ACM conferences attract both academics and industry researchers, so do their publications represent both audiences. The ACM Digital Library is thus the most efficient place to find high-quality publications from this association publisher. In February 2020, the Library incorporates 1405 journals and magazines, 26,251 conference proceedings, and 181,692 books, in addition to 74,545 student theses and 25,462 technical reports (Association for Computing Machinery, 2020). However, ACM Digital Library is not a good place to look for content that did *not* originate in an ACM conference or journal. This database is common in academic libraries serving computer science students and faculty.

4.3.5 Library and Information Science

The field of library and information science includes research areas relevant to consumer health informatics, such as health information-seeking behaviors (what health information do people look for? And why?) and information retrieval (the science of search; database and search engine construction and functions). Two particular databases in this subject area have different strengths and foci.

4.3.5.1 LISTA (Library, Information Science & Technology Abstracts)

Library, Information Science & Technology Abstracts (LISTA) is an online database available for free to the entire world from its commercial vendor, Ebsco. While the full text of articles that are indexed and abstracted is not necessarily free, users who have citations from LISTA – or any other commercial database discussed in this chapter – can request the full text from their university or public library. LISTA indexes more than 600 periodicals, plus books, research reports, and proceedings. The target audience is library and information science professionals and student professionals, but because of the technology aspect, data science, IT, and computer science students will find content here to interest them as well.

4.3.5.2 LISA (Library and Information Science Abstracts)

LISA is a different product, a commercial database that covers >400 periodicals including conference proceedings as well as academic journals, published in more than 68 countries and more than 20 different languages. The principal difference between LISA and LISTA is that LISA has more international coverage of countries such as Australia and the African continent. Like LISTA, the target audience is in library and information science, but the possible users are a much bigger group of professions and students of professions.

4.3.6 Engineering

4.3.6.1 IEEE Xplore

The Institute of Electrical and Electronics Engineers, or IEEE, describes itself as "the world's largest technical professional association dedicated to advancing technology for the benefit of humanity" (IEEE, 2019). "Technology" covers everything from consumer electronics to cloud computing; for this reason, if an engineering perspective on consumer health informatics is required, the IEEE Xplore Digital Library is the best place to look for IEEE publications: journals, conference proceedings, technical standards, and books. The IEEE Digital Library is found in academic libraries that serve engineering students.

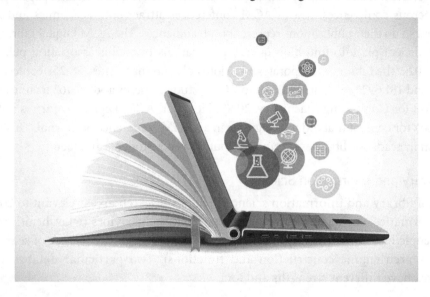

4.3.6.2 INSPEC

This commercial database published by the Institution of Engineering and Technology features over 18 million records (journals and conference papers) (Institution of Engineering and Technology, 2020) in the fields of physics, computer science, electrical engineering, information technology, and related disciplines. Researchers go to INSPEC because it indexes more than IEEE content, so if a wider net is required for your search, INSPEC would be the preferred choice; seekers of IEEE content alone would be best served with IEEE Xplore. Like Xplore, INSPEC is a staple of academic libraries serving undergraduate through faculty engineering-oriented users.

4.3.7 IT Industry

To stay current with industry trends and news reports, the best source is your appropriate professional organization (see Part I, Chapter 2, for key organizations in consumer health informatics). Professional associations typically maintain a resource library of focused, relevant content, including unpublished content such as research reports and surveys, that is open to members and supported by membership dues. The American Medical Informatics Association (AMIA), for example, releases a daily news bulletin relating to medical informatics as a benefit to its members.

Follow the various free newsfeeds available at major organization websites such as HIMSS' Health IT Pulse (https://www.himss.org/news).

Two databases are of particular use not only to follow industry trends, but to better understand industries. The technical term for content like this is "market research."

Although databases of this type are among the most expensive in existence, these databases can be found in academic libraries serving the needs of business faculty and students.

4.3.7.1 IBISWorld

This business intelligence product features original content, instead of indexed material published somewhere else: current Industry Market Research reports that provide overviews of industries including health IT. These overviews feature definitions, key statistics, major companies involved, the supply chain, operating conditions such as regulatory environments, and a helpful list of jargon used in the industry. For example, a search for the keyword "medicine" in this database produces reports on industries from allergy medicine and cough and cold manufacturing, through sports medicine practitioners.

4.3.7.2 BCC Research

BCC Research features original research reviews that spotlight global markets in industries including both information technology and healthcare, for example, smart home technologies (see Part II, Chapter 3, of this book) and wearable medical devices. The research reviews include information on factors affecting the market as well as historical background, exemplar products, company profiles, acronyms, and more.

4.4 CITATION DATABASES

Citation databases were developed to serve as double discovery tools. Searchers can use them to identify high-impact research in a particular academic field. Then, they can find out what other authors have cited those specific works, so the searcher can build a network of authors doing work in that field. All three of these key citation database products discussed below include citations and abstracts only. For full text of articles and conference papers, refer to Table 4.1.

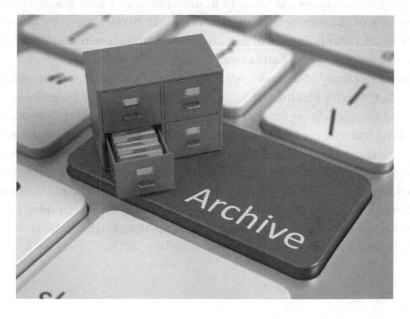

4.4.1 Web of Science

Web of Science is a long-running commercial product from Clarivate Analytics. It provides 1.7 billion citations from over 34,000 "high-impact" journals, 205,000 conference proceedings, and over 104,000 books. Despite the name, this database is multidisciplinary, covering literature of the humanities, social sciences, and sciences – all of which can be relevant to consumer health informatics (Clarivate, 2020). This database is so key to research in the 21st century that it can be found in any research-intensive university's academic library.

4.4.2 Scopus

Scopus, another commercial product developed to compete with Web of Science, advertises that it is "the largest" curated citation database, with over 75 million records including citations to over 24,600 peer-reviewed journals and 194,000 books, and 740 book series, over 9 million conference papers and more than 300 trade publications (Elsevier, 2020). Like its competition, Web of Science, it is multidisciplinary: 25% health sciences, 27% physical sciences, 16% life sciences, and 32% social sciences. A newer product, it is not quite as widely available as Web of Science, but is catching up, and targets the same users: research-intensive students through faculty at universities.

4.4.3 Google Scholar

Google Scholar, a free Google product, was also developed to compete with Web of Science, but Scholar was the brainchild of a Google developer (Levy, 2014). Like the other two citation databases, Scholar links to full-text content where available, but it also points to commercial document delivery services. These help searchers who lack credentials to access through a university or public library and do not know about interlibrary loan services that are cheaper (see Table 4.1). In the 16 years since its launch, Google Scholar has received much attention by researchers anxious to understand why a user would choose Google Scholar over one of the commercial alternatives. Since many university libraries link to Google Scholar and offer licensed full-text content to searchers with university affiliations, this is a topic of interest to librarians as well.

A comprehensive study of Google Scholar content across disciplines has been difficult to accomplish, but Martín-Martín, Orduna-Malea, Thelwall, and Delgado López-Cózar (2018) assessed Google Scholar for citations from 252 different subject categories – including the medical sciences, computer sciences, electrical engineering, and information science. Forty-seven percent of all citations they investigated were found by all three citation products. Google Scholar has been found to include more unique content than Web of Science; in addition to the usual journal articles, it includes "many publication types … doctoral theses, conference proceedings, anthology articles, monographs, regional and online journals, publication outlets in other languages than English, and research reports from policy-oriented think tanks" (Andersen & Nielsen, 2018).

4.5 DATABASES VERSUS SEARCH ENGINES: A COMPARISON

Here is a graphic example of how much difference a database can make to a research question. Imagine that you are a computer science student, part of a group tasked with developing an app designed for people living with Type I diabetes, which is a disease caused by the failure of the pancreas to make insulin. Patients living with Type 1 diabetes are dependent on insulin for their entire lives. Type 1 diabetes is an autoimmune disorder that is not preventable (National Library of Medicine, 2020), unlike Type 2 diabetes, which is caused by excessive blood sugar levels (National Library of Medicine, MEDLINEPlus, 2020b) and can be treated through lifestyle changes such as diet and exercise (National Library of Medicine, MEDLINEPlus, 2020c). So the distinction between Type 1 and Type 2 diabetes is important as a research question, a product development question, an academic question, and – ultimately – a consumer health question.

Your team has designated you to be the researcher on the project. Your task: Find out what elements of a person's diet are important for that person to track if they are living with Type 1 diabetes. Your team is only interested in results from the last five years, published in English.

Table 4.2 displays some possible search strategies for this research question and results from three very different sources: PubMed MEDLINE, Google, and Google Scholar.

TABLE 4.2 Type 1 Diabetes Question: Database versus Search Engines*

MEDLINE	Results	Google	Results	Google Scholar	Results
"Diabetes Mellitus, Type 1/diet therapy"[Majr] AND ("2015/03/02"[PDat]: "2020/02/28"[PDat] AND English[lang])**	84	diet type 1 diabetes	449,000,000 Top five sources by relevance: Medicinenet.com WebMD.com Healthline.com Health.usnews.com Diabetes.org.uk	diet type 1 diabetes	272,000 First five sources sorted by date: *Pediatrics* *Nutrition Journal* *Asia Pacific Journal of Clinical Nutrition* *PLoS One* *Nutrition Research*
		Type 1 diabetes diet	570,000,000 results Top five sources by relevance: Medicinenet.com WebMD.com Healthline.com Health.usnews.com UIchildrens.org	Type 1 diabetes diet	324,000 results First five sources sorted by date: *Pediatrics* *Nutrition Journal* *International Journal of Case Report Images* *Asia Pacific Journal of Clinical Nutrition* *Clinical Immunology*

* Searches run Feb. 28, 2020.
** Wondering how I did this? Visit this PubMed tutorial page: https://www.nlm.nih.gov/oet/ed/pubmed/quicktours/topic_how_it_works/index.html

One of these search processes is much more efficient than the other two and returns information already vetted to be of high quality. All 84 records returned by the PubMed search could be skimmed, and the most relevant of the articles read in their entirety. The same could not be said of Google or Google Scholar's performance. However, of the results briefly noted in Table 4.2, both PubMed MEDLINE and Google Scholar return results that could, in theory, be useful to the team building this app from a *scientific* point of view. The Google results would provide a consumer-readable perspective on the same question. In the end, for consumer health informatics, multiple sources of information and multiple frames of reference are required. The trick is to know when to use which sources.

WEB RESOURCES

Eli Pariser TED Talk on "filter bubbles"
Classic, but unfortunately timeless, 5-minute talk, delivered to key players in the search and information industries about the dangers of social media and siloed news.
https://www.ted.com/talks/eli_pariser_beware_online_filter_bubbles/transcript?language=en

National Library of Medicine
World's largest medical library and key website for numerous information resources in the domain of health information and informatics, from PubMed MEDLINE to grant funding to scholarships to a consumer-facing medical encyclopedia.
> Literature Resources
> https://www.ncbi.nlm.nih.gov/guide/literature/
> Journals referenced in the NCBI databases
> https://www.ncbi.nlm.nih.gov/nlmcatalog/journals
> Fact Sheet: MEDLINE journal selection
> https://www.nlm.nih.gov/lstrc/jsel.html
> MEDLINE, PubMed, and PMC (PubMed Central): How are they different?
> https://www.nlm.nih.gov/bsd/difference.html
> Online tutorials, videos, and other NLM instructional materials
> https://learn.nlm.nih.gov/

University of Wisconsin-Madison
How do I find scholarly articles?
https://www.library.wisc.edu/college/research-help/how-do-i/how-do-i-find-scholarly-articles/
How do I know if a source is good?
https://www.library.wisc.edu/college/research-help/how-do-i/how-do-i-know-if-a-source-is-good/

Your University Library
For resources specific to you and your needs – ask a librarian!

REFERENCES

Andersen, J. P., & Nielsen, M. W. (2018). Google Scholar and Web of Science: Examining gender differences in citation coverage across five scientific disciplines. *Journal of Informetrics*, 12(3), 950–959. doi:https://doi.org/10.1016/j.joi.2018.07.010

Association for Computing Machinery. (2020). *About ACM digital library*. https://dl.acm.org/about/content#sec2

Clarivate. (2020). *Web of Science platform*. https://clarivate.com/products/web-of-science/databases/.

Dunn, K., Marshall, J. G., Wells, A. L., & Backus, J. E. B. (2017). Examining the role of MEDLINE as a patient care information resource: an analysis of data from the Value of Libraries study. *J Med Libr Assoc*, 105(4), 336–346. doi:10.5195/jmla.2017.87

Elsevier. (2020). *Scopus [fact sheet]*. https://www.elsevier.com/__data/assets/pdf_file/0017/114533/Scopus_GlobalResearch_Factsheet2019_FINAL_WEB.pdf.

EBSCO Health. (2020). *CINAHL Complete*. https://www.ebscohost.com/nursing/products/cinahl-databases/cinahl-complete.

Hersh, W. (2009). *Information retrieval: A health and biomedical perspective* (3rd ed.) NY: Springer. p. 121.

IEEE. (2019). *Learn about IEEE*. https://www.ieee.org/about/index.html

Institution of Engineering and Technology (2020). *Inspec: A scientific and technical database*. https://www.theiet.org/publishing/inspec/

JSTOR. (2020, Feb. 12). *How to use JSTOR (for students)*. https://guides.jstor.org/how-to-use-jstor/content

Levy, S. (2014, Oct. 7). *The gentleman who made Scholar*. Wired. https://www.wired.com/2014/10/the-gentleman-who-made-scholar/

Markey, K. (2019). *Online searching: A guide to finding quality information efficiently and effectively* (2nd ed.). Rowman & Littlefield.

Martín-Martín, A., Orduna-Malea, E., Thelwall, M., & Delgado López-Cózar, E. (2018). Google Scholar, Web of Science, and Scopus: A systematic comparison of citations in 252 subject categories. *Journal of Informetrics*, 12(4), 1160–1177. doi:https://doi.org/10.1016/j.joi.2018.09.002

Merkle. (2019). *Digital marketing report for Q4 2019*. https://www.merkleinc.com/thought-leadership/digital-marketing-report?utm_source=email&utm_medium=email&utm_campaign=2019_DMR_Q4.

Nahin, A. (2005, March 7). Links from commercial search engines to PubMed citations. *NLM Technical Bulletin*, 343. https://www.nlm.nih.gov/pubs/techbull/ma05/ma05_google.html

National Library of Medicine. (2018, August 22). *Key MEDLINE indicators*. https://www.nlm.nih.gov/bsd/bsd_key.html.

National Library of Medicine. (2019a, Dec. 2). *Fact Sheet: MEDLINE journal selection*. https://www.nlm.nih.gov/lstrc/jsel.html -->2019a.

National Library of Medicine. (2019b, Dec.2). *FAQ: Journal selection for MEDLINE indexing at NLM*. https://www.nlm.nih.gov/lstrc/j_sel_faq.html □ 2019b.

National Library of Medicine. (2019c, April 10) *MEDLINE®: Description of the database*. https://www.nlm.nih.gov/bsd/MEDLINE.html. --? 2019c.

National Library of Medicine. (2019d, September 9). *PubMed, and PMC (PubMed Central): How are they different?* https://www.nlm.nih.gov/bsd/difference.html □ 2019d.

National Library of Medicine, MEDLINEPlus. (2020, Feb. 13). Diabetes type 1. https://MEDLINEplus.gov/diabetestype1.html --? 2020a.

National Library of Medicine, MEDLINEPlus. (2020b, Feb. 13). *Diabetes type 2*. https://MEDLINEplus.gov/diabetestype2.html –2020b.

National Library of Medicine, MEDLINEPlus. (2020c, Feb. 26). *How to prevent diabetes*. https://MEDLINEplus.gov/howtopreventdiabetes.html --? 2020c.

Pariser, E. (2011). *Beware online "filter bubbles"*. [TED2011]. https://www.ted.com/talks/eli_pariser_beware_online_filter_bubbles/transcript?language=en.

PsycINFO. (2019). *Highlights*. https://www.nlm.nih.gov/bsd/MEDLINE.html.

Segev, E. (2010). *Google and the digital divide: The bias of online knowledge*. Chandos Publishing.

Sherman, C., & Price, G. (2001). *The invisible web: Uncovering information sources search engines can't see*. Information Today.

Yom-Tov, E. (2016, May 11). *Cancer and the internet: The strange, sad case of Wei Zexi*. https://mit-press.mit.edu/blog/cancer-and-internet-strange-sad-case-wei-zexi

CHAPTER 5

Trusted Information Sources

Catherine Arnott Smith

Lay individuals need support in evaluating the authority, objectivity, and trustworthiness of online health information. Consumer Health Informatics as a field can address this problem. Inaccurate health information proliferates on the Web, propagated through social media and emerging in online advertisements that are tailored to previous searches. This section reviews efforts for quality control of health information online; describes quality source markers such as the HONCode and DISCERN; and lists online information sources that incorporate these and other quality criteria.

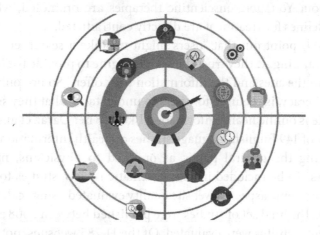

5.1 OVERVIEW: ACCURACY AND CHI

Users of CHI have many possible roles. They might be patients, friends, and family of patients, student researchers, patient advocates or health professionals, or developers of technologies connecting all these people with health information. One 2017 study from the Pew Research Center found that health or medical news was the second most popular topic of information US adults looked for online – right after the topic "schools and education" (Horrigan, 2017). Sixty-nine percent of those US adults in a different survey – HINTS, or Health Information National Trends – reported using "a computer, smartphone, or other electronic means" to find online health information (National Cancer Institute, 2018).

College students at Florida State University were surveyed by Stvilia & Choi (2015) about the sources they used when looking for mobile wellness apps. Ninety-six percent of them used websites and 90% used mobile apps; only 34% used social media. Search engines were the primary source of user information about the apps. These students clearly needed searching skills, as well as evaluation skills, to assess the credibility of the app and its developer.

When users like this are faced with health information on a device or a website, they may be assuming that this information has been vetted for accuracy, but the trust that users place in specific information sources has a lot to do with their health literacy and e-health literacy levels.

The concept of health literacy is addressed in much more detail in Part I, Chapter 3, of this book. It has been defined as the "degree to which individuals have the capacity to obtain, process, and understand basic health information and services needed to make appropriate health decisions" (IOM). Highly e-health literate people examine the information they find very carefully; people with low health literacy have "distorted" perceptions, seeing low-credibility sources as much better than they are. Thirty-one percent of adults polled in the 2018 HINTS (Health Information National Trends, conducted by the National Cancer Institute) had watched health-related YouTube videos. Paige et al. (2017) found significant differences according to health literacy levels in how much users trusted YouTube, which has no vetting for accuracy or quality, as a source of health information. Among the safety concerns about YouTube: unscientific therapies are promoted, while professional standards and guidelines for treatment are directly contradicted.

Allam et al. (2014) point out that "users might mistake a search engine's ranking of results as a quality ranking … they trust the search engine to provide the best websites and transfer this trust to the sites and the information they offer." So not only health literacy, but search engine literacy, is required for users to understand what they see online.

Just how accurate is online health information likely to be? Daraz et al. (2019) published a systematic review of 149 English-language studies of health information quality, focused on websites targeting the general public as opposed to physicians, nurses, or health professions students. To be included in this systematic review, studies to be published in English and report on some aspect of website quality evaluated using scales (both validated and non-validated). The final set of studies were published between 2008 and November of 2017; 11,785 different websites were evaluated. Of the 11,785 websites, not a single one had received an "excellent" rating according to the longstanding and widely used evaluation instrument called DISCERN (discussed below) (http://www.discern.org.uk/).

Sometimes, consumers themselves act as online information sources. How accurate are they? This is an open question. The health app called Iodine (www.iodine.com) provides consumer-facing medication information; Iodine features a mix of information from different sources, including the FDA label, as well as crowdsources user reviews obtained from Google Consumer Surveys – "real life experience from more than 100,000 people like you." Iodine was named "Best Health Website" in the 2018 Webby Awards. The Webbies are awarded in seven media-type categories: websites, videos, advertising, media/PR, social, apps, mobile/voice, games, and podcasts. Submissions are judged by more than 2000 of the "Internet's most brilliant movers and shakers"; for example, Anne Wojcicki of 23 and Me (see Chapter 8 of this book) was a judge in 2020 (Webby Awards, 2020).

Currently, FDA guidelines for consumer medication information, like that from Iodine, do not address the problem of accuracy and particularly the need for users to be able to distinguish between evidence-based information and user-provided content (Sage et al., 2017). Millenson et al. (2018) performed a scoping review of research into 30 diagnostic apps. They found that this research clustered into three categories: medical symptom checkers (20 studies); smartphone photo analysis (12 studies); and crowdsourcing (five studies). Millenson et al.'s conclusion: No studies reported on patient outcomes from app use and most simply reported the apps' attributes. The lack of an evidence base is a problem for the more than 250,000 health apps on the market. As McCartney (2013) puts it, "Straightforward information [is] not subject to [FDA] guidance." Lambert et al. (2017) evaluated 21 English-language mobile apps focusing on renal (kidney) diets, intended for use by patients living with chronic kidney disease (CKD). Just less than half (47.6%) of the apps contained information that was judged to be accurate and evidence-based. Fougerouse et al. (2017) cast a wider net and assessed the 100 most popular apps they found in the Apple Store and Google Play. Forty-four percent of the apps in their sample did not indicate the source of their medical information through a citation or reference, even though 71% of these apps provided medical information. Fifty-eight percent provided outdated medical content, and not one of the 100 apps were supported by a study demonstrating their effectiveness. For all these reasons, healthcare practitioners and researchers are calling for improvement in the evidence base around apps, which means paying attention not just to standards, but to the methods by which evaluation happens (for more on apps as a CHI technology, see Part II, Chapter 8 of this book).

5.2 EVALUATION GUIDELINES

Multiple stakeholders in the healthcare system have served as gatekeepers to health information and now see their position challenged by the widespread use of information technologies, particularly the internet and social media. What are their concerns about information quality online?

The very first evaluation study of medical information on the World Wide Web to appear in the professional literature of medicine was published in 1997. It was a study of recommendations for handling childhood fever, published in the BMJ, by Italian researchers Impicciatore et al. (1997). These researchers found that only four of the 41 webpages they examined conformed to pediatric practice guidelines. This was a much-cited article for some years and in fact is still being cited – 881 times, according to Google Scholar, in February of 2020. And ever since its publication, a diverse set of healthcare and information professionals have developed different standards and criteria for evaluating health information online.

5.2.1 General Criteria

Some general guidelines for evaluation of health information have been taught by librarians and educators for decades. They apply equally well to print and electronically based materials in all kinds of settings. Criteria from one commonly cited early article, well entrenched in higher education by now, were published in the *Journal of the American Medical Association* (Silberg et al., 1997).

5.2.1.1 Authority/Authors

Who is responsible for the information? Authors should be qualified to write about what they write about. By extension, website content providers should have staff, or affiliates, who have such qualifications. Some specific questions to ask to evaluate information authority are:

- Do you know who they are?

- Do they *tell you* who they are? (Are names of the individuals responsible for the information provided?)

- Do they tell you what their qualifications are?

- Are the qualifications themselves legitimate? (Board-certified, if a board exists? Degreed, if a degree exists?)

- Do they tell you institutions with which they are affiliated (research institutes, centers of excellence, government agencies?)

- Do they tell you if they themselves produced this information, or are they an information middle-person, passing on somebody else's work?

5.2.1.2 Purpose

Information is always produced with a purpose. If there were no purpose, people and organizations would not spend the time and resources to produce it. The trick in *evaluating* information's purpose is to make sure that one purpose is not hiding behind another. For example, while a magazine or a website may give the superficial appearance of an unbiased source of information, it may in fact be the product of a medical device maker who's interested in selling more devices. The careful evaluator will need to consider: How does the purpose of the site affect the information being provided? More questions to ask relating to purpose include:

- Is it to improve the quality of somebody's health?

- Is it to enable the author or the website maintainer or anybody else to make money?

- Is it to increase awareness of a specific diagnosis or health condition?

- Is it to raise money for research into the causes and/or prevention and/or cure of a specific diagnosis or health condition?

- Is it to educate people?

- Is it to promote a particular viewpoint or advocacy position?

- What people are the primary audience?

5.2.1.3 Recency

How current is the information? Note not only the date/year in which specific information was produced, but also how frequently webpages on a site have been updated. Remember that the journal article is the basic unit of scientific communication, including medicine, which includes consumer health (see Part I, Chapter 4, for details on journals). Old medical information is more than outdated; it may be actively harmful.

5.2.1.4 Citations

Are there sources provided for the information? The sources referenced in citations are all information resources themselves, and thus are additional material to assess! When a citation has gaps in it – an author, a journal or book title, or year of publication missing – it becomes more difficult for the reader to assess its quality. Good citations should not only support the author's claims, but also point the reader to additional information. Some questions to ask about citations include the following:

Can you see citations?
Are the citations complete, or are there gaps?
Are the citations used correctly, that is, to support the statements made by the author?

Over time, organizations and institutions have attempted to codify these quality guidelines to make it easier for consumers to evaluate specific kinds of health-related content. Two classic and long-running examples discussed in more detail below are DISCERN, from Oxford University, and the HONCode, from Switzerland's Health on the Net Foundation.

5.3 HEALTH-INFORMATION-SPECIFIC INSTRUMENTS

5.3.1 DISCERN

The DISCERN instrument was developed out of an extended collaboration of different kinds of information users: not only the usual physicians, but librarians, health communicators, representatives of patient support groups, members of the medical publishing industry, medical journalists, and researchers. The Project Team was funded in 1996–1997 by a combination of the British Library and the UK National Health Service (Charnock et al., 1999).The original motivation was to help both patients and professionals by providing them with a way to measure the quality of written health information about health treatments. DISCERN migrated to the Web just as treatment information did.

The instrument this team developed contains 15 individual items on which users can rank websites, from 1 – "Serious or extensive shortcomings" – through to 5 – "Minimal shortcomings." For content developers, it can serve as a benchmark and a checklist; for healthcare professionals, it can help determine what content to use for patient education; and for consumers and patients, it can work as a decision support tool. The current version of DISCERN can be found for free online at http://www.discern.org.uk/discern_instrument.php. The 15 questions that make up its evaluation criteria are:

1. Are the aims clear?

2. Does the publication achieve its aims?

3. Is it relevant?

4. Is it clear what sources of information were used to compile the publication (other than the author or producer)?

5. Is it clear when the information used or reported in the publication was produced?

6. Is it balanced and unbiased?

7. Does it provide details of additional sources of support and information?

8. Does it refer to areas of uncertainty?

9. Does it describe how each treatment works?

10. Does it describe the benefits of each treatment?

11. Does it describe the risks of each treatment?

12. Does is describe what would happen if no treatment is used?

13. Does it describe how the treatment choices affect overall quality of life?

14. Is it clear that there may be more than one possible treatment choice?

15. Does it provide support for shared decisionmaking?[i]

A 16th question asks the user to "rate the overall quality of the publication" based on answers to the 15 previous questions.

5.3.2 HONCode

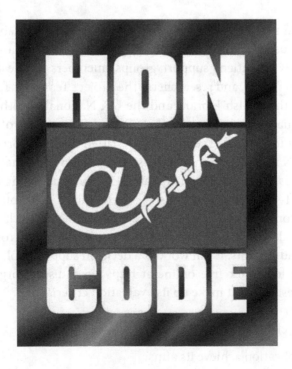

The Health On the Net, or HON, Foundation originated in Geneva, Switzerland, at a tele-medicine conference attended by a diverse set of physicians and researchers from organizations like the International Telecommunications Union, the World Health Organization, and the National Library of Medicine (Health on the Net, 2018). The standard instrument they developed, called the HONCode, is "a set of ethical, honesty, transparency and quality standards … the oldest and the most used ethical and trustworthy code for medical and health related information available on Internet [sic]" (Boyer et al., 2017). Website developers apply for HON membership, which is free for the first year and fee-based thereafter – with tiered pricing, the tier and costs depending on the commercial nature of the website and how visible it is. Credentialing is done by a HONCode review committee using the HONCode principles (see below) as a guide. Sites adhering to all eight of the principles receive a seal linked to a certificate stating compliance with the principles, and certified sites are monitored for continued compliance beginning one year later.

The Eight Principles of the HONCode are:

Authoritative: Any medical or health advice provided and hosted on this site will only be given by medically trained and qualified professionals unless a clear statement is made that a piece of advice offered is from a non-medically qualified individual or organization.

Complementarity: The information provided on this site is designed to support, not replace, the relationship that exists between a patient/site visitor and his/her existing physician.

Privacy: Confidentiality of data relating to individual patients and visitors to a medical/health website, including their identity, is respected by this website. The website owners undertake to honor or exceed the legal requirements of medical/health information privacy that apply in the country and state where the website and mirror sites are located.

Attribution: Where appropriate, information contained on this site will be supported by clear references to source data and, where possible, have specific HTML links to that data. The date when a clinical page was last modified will be clearly displayed (e.g., at the bottom of the page).

Justifiability: Any claims relating to the benefits/performance of a specific treatment, commercial product, or service will be supported by appropriate, balanced evidence in the manner outlined above in Principle 4.

Transparency: The designers of this website will seek to provide information in the clearest possible manner and provide contact addresses for visitors that seek further information or support. The Webmaster will display his/her E-mail address clearly throughout the website.

Financial disclosure: Support for this website will be clearly identified, including the identities of commercial and non-commercial organizations that have contributed funding, services, or material for the site.

Advertising policy: If advertising is a source of funding, it will be clearly stated. A brief description of the advertising policy adopted by the website owners will be displayed on the site. Advertising and other promotional material will be presented to viewers in a manner and context that facilitates differentiation between it and the original material created by the institution operating the site (Health on the Net Foundation, 2019a).

Health-related websites certified by the Foundation are accessible through a specialized search engine available on the HON site. Users can also arm their Web browsers with a HONcode toolbar that checks websites in real time (Boyer et al., 2017). As of September 2019, "over 7300" websites had been certified from 102 countries (Health on the Net Foundation, 2019a).

It is important to understand that neither DISCERN nor the HONCode can attest to the *accuracy* of website content in the scientific sense. Rather, these instruments focus on the provision of evidence with which the reader can *determine* trustworthiness for themselves. For example, the developers of DISCERN have always been careful to point out that "DISCERN cannot be used to assess the scientific quality or accuracy of the evidence on which a publication is based, as this would require checking against other sources" (DISCERN, 2019).

Similarly, the HONCode principles focus on the provision of evidence supporting the claims made on the webpage; they make no judgment about the quality of the evidence itself. The website "must back up claims relating to benefits and performance" (Health on the Net Foundation, 2019b).

5.4 OTHER WIDELY USED STANDARDS

In addition to the two popular instruments discussed above, other kinds of metrics for assessment of different attributes of health information have been developed over the years. Some have been imported from other domains outside healthcare. For example, the Flesch–Kincaid literacy test (see Table 5.1, below, and discussed in more detail in Part I, Chapter 3 of this book) originated in the US military but, like its differently weighted sibling the Flesch–Kincaid Reading Ease Test, is heavily used in education. The Gunning FOG (Frequency of Gobbledygook) tests were the invention of a publishing executive but are now used in the field of linguistics. These instruments are used in health and non-health website research and development to assess the reading level, and thus the difficulty level, of websites (for more on health literacy in health informatics, see Part I, Chapter 3; for a

TABLE 5.1   Instruments Used in Evaluation of Consumer Health Information

Evaluation instrument	Studies
DISCERN	45
HONCode	24
JAMA Benchmarks (Silberg et al., 1997)	18
Flesch–Kincaid	17
Flesch Reading Ease	13
Homegrown by authors or modification of published instruments by authors	11

comprehensive review of readability tools used in this domain of research, see Abdel-Wahab et al., 2019).

Abdel-Wahab et al. (2019) performed a scoping review of articles from the health sciences as well as the citation databases Scopus, Google Scholar, and Web of Science, identifying literature that described website quality evaluation instruments. From this, these authors developed a new instrument incorporating *usability* and *accessibility* as constructs, calling them an important part of evaluation because "the information on the internet can be beneficial only if it is easily conveyed to the audience."

Some reputable organizations do their own evaluations and make their criteria inspectable by users who can then decide if their personal preferences and values align with those of the website. For example, the National Library of Medicine consumer health website, MEDLINEPlus, publishes its own criteria here: http://www.nlm.nih.gov/MEDLINEplus/criteria.html

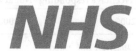

And the British National Health Service provides website and app developer guidelines that are useful for consumer users as well as builders here: https://digital.nhs.uk/services/nhs-apps-library/guidance-for-health-app-developers-commissioners-and-assessors/how-we-assess-health-apps-and-digital-tools#how-the-assessment-works

5.5 TRUSTED SOURCES OF HEALTH INFORMATION

Daraz et al. (2019), who looked at published reports of health information quality, were interested in what types of organizations produced higher-quality information. They found, to their surprise, that government sites were rated higher, in general ("very good" according to DISCERN) but academic sites lower – for example, the websites of medical schools and universities, academic medical centers, and professional medical organizations such as the AMA. "Poor" websites were, in general, those maintained by media organizations.

What is the public perception of these sources? The National Cancer Institute's HINTS (Health Information National Trends Survey, mentioned above) has been asking respondents about their trust in various health information sources since 2005, ending in 2017. HINTS asks: "How much would you trust information about health or medical topics in" or "from"… "Doctor or other healthcare professional" is quite consistently the most trusted source, followed by "government health agencies." During just one year, in 2011, HINTS respondents were asked why they *had not* visited the FDA website. Six and 7/10 percent indicated that they did not visit the site because they did not trust the FDA; 5.3 percent, that they did not trust government websites in general (National Cancer Institute, 2017). This suggests that there may be more distrust of that specific federal agency than other surveys have been able to determine. The *least* trusted source overall, according to HINTS, has consistently been "religious organizations and leaders," followed by "charitable organizations."

The most and least trusted sources appear below in Tables 5.2 and 5.3.

TABLE 5.2   HINTS Respondents' Most Trusted Sources for Health Information, 2005–2017

	Percentage responding "A lot"				
	2005	2008	2011	2013	2017
Newspapers and magazines?	*Question not asked*	7	2.9	*Question not asked*	2.1
Government health agencies?	*Question not asked*	30.5	25.1	25.6	28.3
Charitable organizations?	*Question not asked*	10.1	7	6.6	7.1
Religious organizations and leaders?	*Question not asked*	8.6	4.6	5	4.6
A doctor or other healthcare professional?	66.9	68.2	70.3	67.8	69.5

* Data drawn from various HINTS surveys at hints.cancer.gov.

TABLE 5.3   HINTS' Respondents' Least Trusted Sources of Health Information, 2005–2017

	Percentage responding "Not at all"				
	2005	2008	2011	2013	2017
Newspapers and magazines?	*Question not asked*	6	3.5	*Question not asked*	5.3
Government health agencies?	*Question not asked*	6.9	3.5	3.8	4.9
Charitable organizations?	*Question not asked*	15.8	16.2	14	15.7
Religious organizations and leaders?	*Question not asked*	28.6	30.9	30.2	36
A doctor or other healthcare professional?	1.6.	8	1.4	.8	1.4

* Data drawn from various HINTS surveys at hints.cancer.gov.

Health Topics   Drugs & Supplements   Videos & Tools

Home → Health Topics → Heart Diseases

Heart Diseases
Also called: Cardiac diseases

On this page

Basics
- Summary
- Start Here
- Diagnosis and Tests
- Prevention and Risk Factors
- Treatments and Therapies

Learn More
- Living With
- Related Issues
- Specifics
- Genetics

See, Play and Learn
- Health Check Tools
- Videos and Tutorials

Research
- Statistics and Research
- Clinical Trials
- Journal Articles

Resources
- Reference Desk
- Find an Expert

For You
- Children
- Men
- Women
- Older Adults
- Patient Handouts

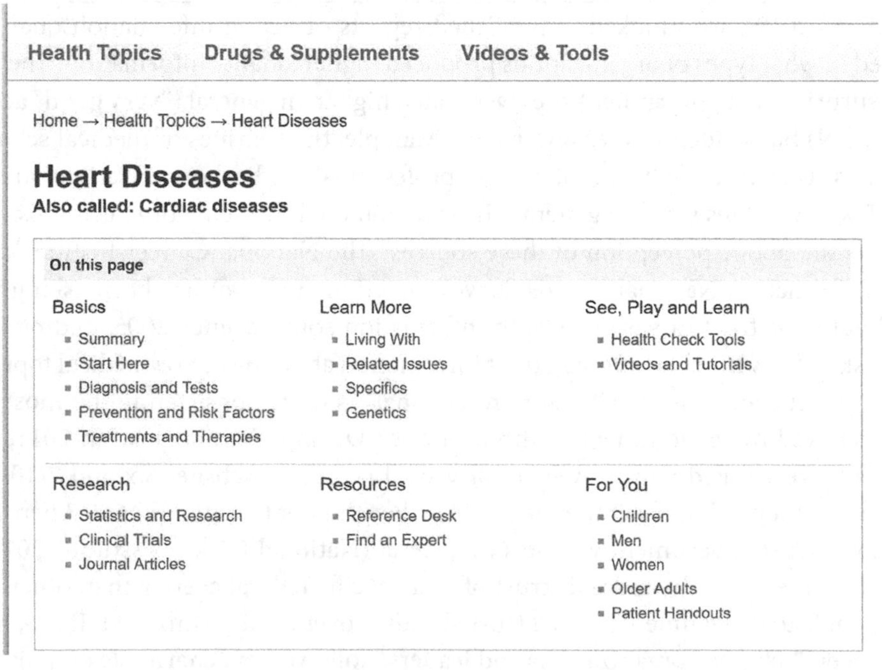

FIGURE 5.1 MEDLINEPlus information sources: health topic: Heart Diseases.

MEDLINEPlus, maintained by the National Library of Medicine, serves as the gateway to high-quality health-related US government agency websites – every institute at NIH, and others – as well as sites representing healthcare specialties. Over one million people visit it every day for features like the Health Topic pages specific to over 1000 different diseases and conditions. MEDLINEPlus' quality guidelines for site selection (see below) stress the importance of science-based information, original content, and low or no advertising. See Figure 5.1 for a graphical illustration of the sources available for one health topic: Heart Disease, the leading cause of death in the US for 2017 (most recent data available at this writing).

Source	Source Type
ABIM Foundation	Charitable corporation
American Association for Clinical Chemistry	Professional organization
American Heart Association	Voluntary health organization
Centers for Disease Control and Prevention	Federal agency
Mayo Foundation for Medical Education and Research	Charitable corporation
Medical Encyclopedia	[Feature of MEDLINEPlus]
Merck & Co., Inc.	Healthcare company
National Center for Complementary and Integrative Health	Federal agency
National Center for Health Statistics	Federal agency
National Heart, Lung, and Blood Institute	National Institutes of Health (NIH) Institute
National Institute of Biomedical Imaging and Bioengineering	NIH Institute
National Institute of Diabetes and Digestive and Kidney Diseases	NIH Institute
National Institute on Aging	NIH Institute
National Institutes of Health	NIH Institute
National Jewish Health	Healthcare facility
National Library of Medicine	NIH Institute
Nemours Foundation	Healthcare system
Texas Heart Institute	Healthcare facility

5.6 COMMON CRITERIA

Eysenbach et al. (2009) articulated the different kinds of criteria considered a "minimum requirement" when evaluating health information online. These criteria (illustrated in Figure 5.2) were:

Table 5.4 shows the points at which DISCERN, the HONCode, and the US National Library of Medicine's evaluation criteria intersect.

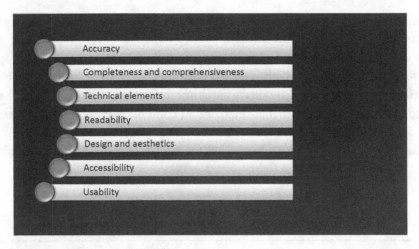

FIGURE 5.2 Domains to evaluate health information online. Modified from Eysenbach *et al.* (2002).

TABLE 5.4   Questions and Evaluation Criteria: DISCERN, HONCode, and NLM

DISCERN *[for evaluating treatment information in print and online]*	**HONCode** *[for evaluating health information websites]*	**National Library of Medicine** *[for evaluating health information websites]*
[questions to ask] Are the aims clear?	[questions to ask]	[questions to ask] Why are they providing the website?
Does it achieve its aims?		
Is it relevant?		
Is it clear what sources of information were used to compile the publication (other than the author or producer)?	[Does the site] cite the sources … of medical information?	Where does the information on the website come from?
Is it clear when the information used or reported in the publication was produced?	[Does the site] cite the… dates of medical information?	
Is it balanced and unbiased?	[Does the site] provide justification of claims/balanced and objective claims?	
Does it provide details of additional sources of support and information?	[Does the site] provide details of funding?	Where does the money to support the website come from?
Does it refer to areas of uncertainty?		
Does it describe how each treatment works?		
Does it describe the benefits of each treatment?		
Does it describe the risks of each treatment?		
Does it describe what would happen if no treatment is used?		

(Continued)

TABLE 5.4 (*Continued*)   Questions and Evaluation Criteria: DISCERN, HONCode, and NLM

DISCERN [for evaluating treatment information in print and online]	HONCode [for evaluating health information websites]	National Library of Medicine [for evaluating health information websites]
Does it describe how the treatment choices affect overall quality of life? Is it clear that there may be more than one possible treatment choice? Does it provide support for shared decisionmaking?		
	[Does the site] give qualifications of authors?	Do experts review the information that goes on the site?
	[Does the site intend] information to support, not replace [a physician]	
	[Does the site] respect the privacy of site users?	Does the site ask for your personal information?
	[Does the site] provide valid contact details?	Can you contact [the provider of the website]?
	[Does the site] clearly distinguish advertising from editorial content?	Does the site have advertisements? Are they labeled?
		Who is in charge of the website?
		How is the content selected?
		Does the site avoid unbelievable or emotional claims?
		Is it up-to-date?
		Are you comfortable with how [personal information] will be used?

5.7 RESOURCES DEVELOPED BY HEALTHCARE PROFESSIONALS AND OTHER TRUSTED SOURCES

Consumers taking care of themselves are generally information seekers, and they may be working either without a physician or in direct opposition to the advice of the physician. For this reason, physicians for a long time have worried a great deal about the health information their patients were getting, and from where they got it. Today, healthcare professional associations are beginning to publish guidelines for their members to use in educating patients and consumers about information evaluation online (see Table 5.5 for examples). So do non-profit research and advocacy organizations in diagnosis-specific areas, such as cancer, and institutions that produce professionals, such as Harvard's School of Public Health. Increased public interest in genetics and genetic testing prompted the National Human Genome Research Institute, one of the National Institutes of Health, to produce its own guidelines. Cancer Research UK launched its Science Blog to publicize

TABLE 5.5 Health Information Evaluation Guidelines: From Healthcare Association and Research/Advocacy Organizations

Sponsor	Website	Title
American Academy of Otolaryngology – Head and Neck Surgery	https://www.entnet.org/content/how-find-reliable-ent-info	How to Find Reliable ENT Info
American Academy of Family Physicians	https://familydoctor.org/health-information-on-the-web-finding-reliable-information/?adfree=true	Health Information on the Web: Finding Reliable Information
The American Cancer Society	https://www.cancer.org/cancer/cancer-basics/cancer-information-on-the-internet.html	Cancer Information on the Internet
T.H. Chan School of Public Health, Harvard University	https://www.hsph.harvard.edu/nutritionsource/media/	Diet in the News: Who to Believe?
National Human Genome Research Institute, National Institutes of Health	https://www.genome.gov/Genetic-and-Rare-Diseases-Information-Center/Finding-reliable-health-information	How to Find Reliable Health Information
National Center for Complementary and Integrative Health, National Institutes of Health	https://nccih.nih.gov/health/know-science/facts-health-news-stories?page=1	Know the Science: The Facts About Health News Stories
Federal Trade Commission	https://www.consumer.ftc.gov/articles/0167-miracle-health-claims	Miracle Health Claims
Genetic Alliance	http://www.trustortrash.org/	Trust It or Trash It?
National Cancer Institute	https://www.cancer.gov/about-cancer/managing-care/using-trusted-resources	Using Trusted Resources
National Institutes of Health	https://newsinhealth.nih.gov/2015/09/checking-symptom-checkers	Checking the Symptom Checkers

cancer research, but also to "debunk myths and media scares" (Abdel-Wahab et al., 2019). AHRQ, the Agency for Healthcare Research and Quality, is a federal agency tasked with producing evidence of healthcare effectiveness. AHRQ considers website evaluation part of patient education and bundles it into its *Health Literacy Universal Precautions Toolkit* (Agency for Healthcare Research and Quality, 2015).

Some of the resources listed in Table 5.5 focus on problems with health *news*, which is a common source of health information for the general consumer. However, the Federal Trade Commission is just as concerned about consumer fraud and health-related products.

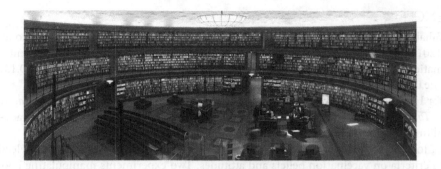

5.8 LIBRARIANS AS INTERMEDIARIES FOR QUALITY

Librarians work in settings from corporate offices to grade schools and universities, but the public librarian is the most accessible type for most consumers, including consumers doing general information seeking without interacting with a doctor or nurse. Public libraries get most of their funding from the communities they serve and are open to all. The public library was named by consumers in one 2018 poll as the most trustworthy source of general information – more than healthcare providers or local and national news organizations; social media was the least trusted source of all (Rainie, 2018). Thirty-eight percent of respondents 16 and older who had used a public library computer – or a public library's WiFi connection – were doing so because they needed health information (Pew Research Center for the People and the Press, 2016).

Medical librarians are equally trustworthy, but work in different places: hospitals and medical schools, which are not always open to the public and have as their primary mission the information needs of healthcare professionals (and student professionals). Medical librarians are experts in medical content and collaborate with public librarians on initiatives to better inform the public; for example, the ongoing Public Library Association campaign, "Healthy Community Tools for Public Libraries" (Public Library Association, 2019). Website evaluation has been a cornerstone of such educational initiatives for years. Guidelines developed by information professionals in different library settings appear in Table 5.6.

TABLE 5.6   Information Guidelines Online: Information Professionals

Sponsor	Website	Title
National Library of Medicine	https://MEDLINEplus.gov/webeval/webeval.html	Evaluating Health Information: A Tutorial from the National Library of Medicine
	https://MEDLINEplus.gov/webeval/ EvaluatingInternetHealthInformationChecklist.pdf	Checklist [of evaluation questions to ask]
Medical Library Association	https://www.mlanet.org/p/cm/ld/fid=398	Find Good Health Information

REFERENCES

Abdel-Wahab, N., Rai, D., Siddhanamatha, H., Dodeja, A., Suarez-Almazor, M.E., & Lopez-Olivo, M.A. (2019) A comprehensive scoping review to identify standards for the development of health information resources on the internet. *PLoS ONE*, 14(6): e0218342. https://doi.org/10.1371/journal.pone.0218342

Agency for Healthcare Research and Quality. (2015, February). *Use health education material effectively: Tool #12.* https://www.ahrq.gov/health-literacy/quality-resources/tools/literacy-toolkit/healthlittoolkit2-tool12.html

Allam, A., Johannes Schulz, P., & Nakamoto, K. (2014). The impact of search engine selection and sorting criteria on vaccination beliefs and attitudes: Two experiments manipulating google output. *Journal of Medical Internet Research*, 16(4), e100–e120. doi:10.2196/jmir.2642

Boyer, C., Gaudinat, A., Hanbury, A., Appel, R. D., Ball, M. J., Carpentier, M.,... Geissbuhler, A. (2017). Accessing reliable health information on the web: A review of the HON approach. *Studies in Health Technology & Informatics*, 245, 1004–1008.

Charnock, D. (1998). *The DISCERN Handbook: Quality criteria for consumer health information on treatment choices.* Radcliffe Medical Press. http://www.discern.org.uk/discern.pdf

Charnock, D., Shepperd, S., Needham, G., & Gann, R. (1999). DISCERN: An instrument for judging the quality of written consumer health information on treatment choices. *Journal of Epidemiology and Community Health*, 53(2), 105–111. doi:10.1136/jech.53.2.105

Daraz, L., Morrow, A. S., Ponce, O. J., Beuschel, B., Farah, M. H., Katabi, A., Alsawas, M., Majzoub, A.M., Benkhadra, R., Selsa, M.O., Ding, J.F., Prokop, L., & Murad, M. H. (2019). Can patients trust online health information? A meta-narrative systematic review addressing the quality of health information on the Internet. *Journal of General Internal Medicine*, 34(9):1884–1891. doi:10.1007/s11606-019-05109-0

DISCERN Online. (1997). *The DISCERN instrument.* http://www.discern.org.uk/discern_instrument.php

DISCERN Online. (2019) *Background.* http://www.discern.org.uk/background_to_discern.php

Eysenbach, G., Powell, J., Kuss, O., Sa, E.R. (2002). Empirical studies assessing the quality of health information for consumers on the world wide web: A systematic review. *JAMA*, 287(20):2691–2700.

Fougerouse, P. A., Yasini, M., Marchand, G., & Aalami, O. O. (2017). *A cross-sectional study of prominent US mobile health applications: Evaluating the current landscape. AMIA Annual Symposium Proceedings*, 715–723.

Health on the Net Foundation. (2018, Oct. 2). *About HON.* https://www.hon.ch/Global/index.html.

Health on the Net Foundation. (2019a). *The commitment to reliable health and medical information on the Internet.* https://www.hon.ch/HONcode/Visitor/visitor.html.

Health on the Net Foundation. (2019b). *Discover the 8 principles of the HONcode in 35 languages.* https://www.hon.ch/cgi-bin/HONcode/principles.pl

HONCode. (2017, May 2). *The HON Code of Conduct for medical and health Web sites (HONCode).* https://www.healthonnet.org/HONcode/Conduct.html

Horrigan, J. B. (2017). *How people approach facts and information.* https://www.pewinternet.org/2017/09/11/how-people-approach-facts-and-information-methodology/

Impicciatore, P., Pandolfini, C., Casella, N., & Bonati, M. (1997). Reliability of health information for the public on the World Wide Web: systematic survey of advice on managing fever in children at home. *BMJ 28*;314(7098):1875–1879.

Lambert, K., Mullan, J., Mansfield, K., & Owen, P. (2017). Should we recommend renal diet-related apps to our patients? An evaluation of the quality and health literacy demand of renal diet-related mobile applications. *Journal of Renal Nutrition*, 27(6), 430–438. doi:10.1053/j.jrn.2017.06.007

Madathil, K. C., Rivera-Rodriguez, A. J., Greenstein, J. S., & Gramopadhye, A. K. (2015). Healthcare information on YouTube: A systematic review. *Health Informatics Journal*, 21(3), 173–194. doi:10.1177/1460458213512220

McCartney, M. (2013). How do we know whether medical apps work? *BMJ*, 346, f1811. doi:10.1136/bmj.f1811

Millenson, M.L., Baldwin, J.L., Zipperer, L., & Singh, H. (2018). Beyond Dr. Google: The evidence on consumer-facing digital tools for diagnosis. *Diagnosis*, 5(3): 95–105.

National Cancer Institute. (2017). *Health Information National Trends Survey [Data file]*. https://hints.cancer.gov/view-questions-topics/question-details.aspx?qid=1188 .

National Cancer Institute. (2018). *Health Information National Trends Survey [Data file]*. https://hints.cancer.gov/view-questions-topics/question-details.aspx?PK_Cycle=11&qid=1352.

National Center for Health Statistics. (n.d.) *Leading causes of death*. https://www.cdc.gov/nchs/fastats/leading-causes-of-death.htm

National Library of Medicine (2020). *MedlinePlus: Health topics: Heart diseases. U.S. Department of Health and Human Services*, National Institutes of Health. https://MEDLINEplus.gov/heartdiseases.html

Paige, S.R., Krieger, J.L., & Stellefson, M.L. (2017). The influence of eHealth literacy on perceived trust in online health communication channels and sources. *Journal of Health Communication*, 22(1):53–65. doi: 10.1080/10810730.2016.1250846.

Pew Research Center for the People and the Press. (2016, Sept. 9) [survey]. *Polling the Nations [database]*.

Public Library Association. (2019). *Healthy community tools for public libraries*. https://publiclibrary.health/.

Rainie, L. (2018, April 9). *The information needs of citizens: Where libraries fit in*. https://www.pewinternet.org/2018/04/09/the-information-needs-of-citizens-where-libraries-fit-in/.

Sage, A., Blalock, S. J., & Carpenter, D. (2017). Extending FDA guidance to include consumer medication information (CMI) delivery on mobile devices. *Research in Social & Administrative Pharmacy*, 13(1), 209–213. doi:10.1016/j.sapharm.2016.01.001.

Science blog. (2019, June 13). https://scienceblog.cancerresearchuk.org/.

Silberg, W.M., Lundberg, G.D., & Musacchio, R.A. (1997). Assessing, controlling, and assuring the quality of medical information on the Internet: Caveant lector et viewor—Let the reader and viewer beware. *JAMA*, 277(15):1244–1245. doi:10.1001/jama.1997.03540390074039

Smith, C.A. (2018, November). [Panel]. The future ain't what it used to be: Negotiating the changing digital health ecosystem. *American Medical Informatics Association*, San Francisco, CA, Nov. 3–7.

Stvilia, B., & Choi, W. (2015). Mobile wellness application-seeking behavior by college students—an exploratory study. *Library & Information Science Research (07408188)*, 37(3), 201–208. doi:10.1016/j.lisr.2015.04.007

Webby Awards. (2019). *Winners*. https://www.webbyawards.com/winners/2018/websites/general/health/

Webby Awards. (2020). *Meet our new judges for the 24th annual Webby Awards*. https://www.webbyawards.com/news/meet-our-new-judges-for-the-24th-annual-webby-awards/

CHAPTER 6

People Engaging with Health Information Technology

Catherine Arnott Smith and Alla Keselman

CONSUMER HEALTH INFORMATICS IS a field that considers both consumer and patients *simultaneously* as users and beneficiaries of information systems that empower them to manage their own health – they are active agents, not passive recipients; they are not only users, but also people who are affected by information technology. The scope of CHI research and practice includes any information processes and technologies that have the potential to empower people to manage their own health. And "people" is literally the largest user group on the planet Earth. In this chapter, we will use the lens of age (children, teenagers, seniors) and role (intermediary, parent, caregiver) to consider how different people interact with CHI technologies. We will also present specific examples of such technologies. We begin by articulating some important differences between consumers and patients.

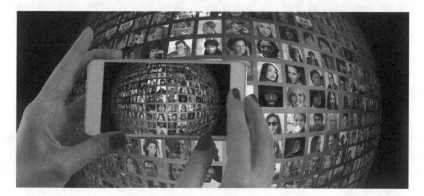

6.1 CONSUMERS

Consumer and *patient* are not synonymous terms. The origins of the term *consumer* are fundamentally economic: The Sears Roebuck Catalog for the year 1897 first used the word "consumer" to mean the opposite of a "producer," that is, a person who pays for goods or services as opposed to producing them. And it was in this economic sense that the word "consumer" first became attached to healthcare, when the first health maintenance organization, the ancestor of Kaiser Permanente, was formed in the 1930s and members purchased access to healthcare in advance of need (Cutting & Collen, 1992). A word like *consumer* is necessary because the word *patient* encodes the idea that the person is receiving medical treatment. One physician argues that "citizens will spend most of their life as 'owners' of their health, some time as 'participants' in and 'consumers' of healthcare, and, hopefully, a very small period during their lives as 'patients.'" (Gorman, 2018, p. 899). While the word *consumer* is intended to signal that the individual is an active participant in their care, this term is not without its own problems; for example, Deber et al. note that it can be "potentially more objectionable" than patient – "consumer," "customer," and "client" all encode the idea that "medical services are commodities to be managed in a market" (2005).

As problematic as the word *consumer* may be, what else can we call a person who is potentially in need of medical treatment, but has not sought out that treatment yet? Or a person who is not living with a diagnosis, but engages with health informatics tools or applications *relevant* to a diagnosis anyway? "Consumer" is thus a category that includes not only patients (see below) but also family and friends of patients and members of the general public. It is a category of users that *potentially* includes the entire world.

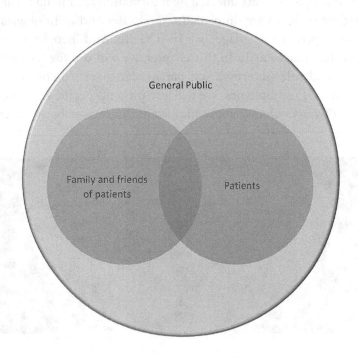

In the twenty-first century, many different civic, political, commercial, and nonprofit agents compete for the attention of consumers in different spheres: in digital and social media markets, and nonprofits like public libraries. Smith et al. (2020) conducted a scoping review of consumer health informatics research published between 2007 and

2015 to find that certain subgroups of consumers had been studied more than others. In that set of 271 empirical research studies, college and university students were the most frequently studied population – six times – and secondary school students twice. Members of the armed services appeared three times, as did people at risk of something (former smokers, for example). Consumers were also studied because they were users of Twitter or Yahoo! Answers; people who preregistered with market research panels; health information seekers; "key informants" for specific communities or affinity groups; had low socioeconomic status; were living in residential care; or had responded to the National Cancer Institute's HINTS (Health Information National Trends Survey).

Consumers are everywhere; they play multiple roles in multiple dimensions of society. They are simultaneously members of peer and affinity groups (by age, family status, sexual orientation, religious belief, culture, ethnicity, language, socioeconomic and educational status, for example) and clients of social service agencies and health-related agencies.

Consumers with access to consumer health information and CHI technologies, as well as skills to use these things, benefit because armed with evidence-based information to interpret their situation, they can be more active participants in self-care (e.g., following necessary dietary and exercise regimes, improving health behaviors); they can also be more effective caregivers.

6.2 PATIENTS

A patient is a person receiving services from a healthcare provider or system. It appears with this meaning as early as the fourteenth century, in Chaucer's *Canterbury Tales* (OED Online, 2019). A patient may be a resident of a healthcare facility (an inpatient in a hospital) or a resident in the community (an outpatient seen in a clinic).

Although this word is much older than *consumer, patient* has equally problematic overtones for some because of its other principal meaning: a person who has patience – and thus "carries connotations of passivity and deference to physicians, although that is not inherent in the definition" (Deber et al., 2005).

Because there are problems with *patient*, the question of just what else to call recipients of healthcare services has been the subject of some research over the years. Deber et al. (2005) surveyed 1,037 patients in four clinics – breast cancer, prostate cancer, fractures, and HIV – and asked these people which term they preferred to describe themselves: *customer, survivor, consumer, client, partner,* or *patient.* Respondents were largely negative about most of these terms, with the small exception of the group living with HIV, of which about one third liked the word *client.* But *customer* and *consumer* were strongly disliked by everybody. Dickens and Picchioni (2012) identified 11 published studies in which recipients of mental healthcare were asked their preferences; in eight studies, *patient* was preferred; in three, *client.* And in 2019, a large scoping review investigating preferences across healthcare contexts established that people continued to prefer *patient* consistently in 26 of 33 studies (Costa et al., 2019).

The patient is a potential user of CHI tools as well as a frequent subject of CHI research. Patients living with chronic illness have been of particular interest in the CHI space. However, the patient is only one type of user, because as discussed above, the patient exists in a social network. Patients no less than consumers can benefit from CHI technologies – and the consumer health information they access through these technologies – because they can be empowered to understand their diagnosis and course of treatment, as well as the medical testing they may undergo and resources to support and assist them. This, in turn, should help patients become active partners in managing their care as well as benefit from their partnerships with their healthcare providers (Coulter et al., 1999).

Smith et al.'s scoping review (2020) found that in 271 CHI studies, 109 (52%) involved patient participants. Sometimes, patients and consumers were compared to each other; for example, Koh et al. (2014) studied people who blogged about the experience of stroke, both as survivors and as caregivers. However, 17 other CHI studies illustrate the potential danger of failing to distinguish between consumers and patients. This is the problem for the evidence base in the CHI field. If the health status of the participant is not well understood, conclusions about the effectiveness of the technology will not be well-founded. In 12 of these studies reviewed by Smith et al., the method by which participants were recruited – from the clinic or the general population – was never specified. Some researchers categorized study participants extremely generically as "well, unwell, and disabled" (Lafky & Horan, 2011). Martinez-Pérez et al. (2015) studied mobile app users in the cardiology domain. The focus of their research was cardiology apps, but the users who participated in the study were never described nor any diagnoses mentioned, cardiac or not. In another interesting experiment, actors were hired to *simulate* patients having seizures because the university's Institutional Review Board would not give permission to use real patients (Spina et al., 2013).

6.2.1 Exemplar Technology: Consumers and Patients

An exemplar technology for both consumer and patient is the patient portal. As noted in Part II, Chapter 7, of this book, patient portal technologies document one person's encounters with the healthcare system; but because they are repositories of information, they also serve as two-way communication platforms enabling information provision, education, and dialog between a person and their healthcare team. Consumers access portals whether they are living with a diagnosis or not; 29% reported doing so to "monitor" their health when asked by the National Cancer Institute's HINTS survey in 2017. For example, they can use portals to make appointments for preventive screening (34% in 2017; National Cancer Institute, 2017b). Consumers download their personal health information to their personal computers and devices (25% in 2018; National Cancer Institute, 2018b). Patients can designate other people to have proxy access to their portals – friends, family, children, parents, and caregivers (see below) who are not necessarily patients themselves. While only 4% of consumers have sent their personal health information to family members (National Cancer Institute, 2018a), 50% of consumers had *accessed* that information through proxy access (National Cancer Institute, 2017a).

6.3 CAREGIVERS

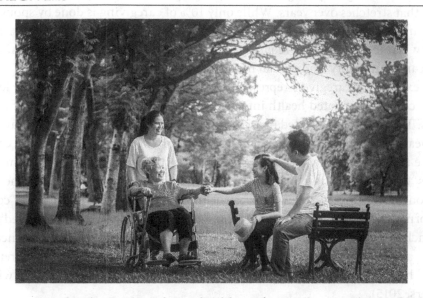

Caregivers are people who, without being health professionals, provide regular help with health maintenance and daily living activities to someone needing that help. Caregiving tasks encompass a range of activities and may include personal care (e.g., feeding, toileting), transportation, and household chores. Caregivers also often help with many tasks in the domain of health care and health information management: communicating with healthcare professionals, interpreting information, finding additional health resources, and managing medications. Caregivers help more fragile individuals perform more health-related tasks. For example, they often monitor the health status of the person they assist and advocate for that person with health providers and service agencies. In addition, they increasingly perform tasks that have traditionally done by nurses: for example, giving injections, helping with tube feeding, and colostomy care (Caregivers, 2015). Depending on the cognitive status of those needing assistance, caregivers sometimes have to assume decision making power.

Demographically, caregivers are a diverse group spanning age, gender, cultural background, and income categories. While parents of young children can be considered a subcategory of caregivers, their health information and technology needs are unique, and so are discussed in a separate subsection below.

Sometimes, an individual needing assistance has a primary caregiver who does most of the caregiving tasks. At other times, care can be provided by a network of unpaid family and friends and paid caregivers who coordinate their activities. According to the National Alliance for Caregiving and AARP "Caregiving in the US 2015" report (2015), approximately 16.6% of Americans are involved in unpaid caregiving of adults. Approximately 60% of caregivers were female, and 40% were male. The average age of a caregiver was 49 years. Most caregivers provide care for family members, often elderly parents or in-laws. Adult children caregivers often represent the "sandwich generation": people in their 40s, simultaneously caring for young children and aging parents. Caregiving is usually a long-term task that stretches over years. While only 10% of caregiving is done by spouses, these kinds of caregivers spend a greater number of hours weekly on caregiving tasks. The most commonly named conditions requiring caregiving are "old age," dementia, surgery/wounds, cancer, mobility, and mental health issues.

To the extent that caregivers represent the interests and well-being of those for whom they care, caregiving-related health information needs align with the needs of their care recipients. They may be interested in accessing informational websites or apps tailored to a specific health condition or an age demographic, for example, seniors. Some caregivers need more technical step-by-step guidance on caregiving procedures. For example, most caregivers who perform nursing tasks report being thrown into the routine without preparation or training. Caregivers overwhelmingly (84%) report that they "could use more information or help on caregiving topics" (p. 25). The most commonly cited topics of interest include home safety, challenging behaviors and toileting and incontinence in care recipients, as well as managing caregiver stress. But the majority of caregivers report that recipients' healthcare providers have not had conversations about these topics with them (Caregivers, 2015).

Caregivers may also need access to their care recipients' personal health information. Privacy and levels of access thus become important considerations in this population. For example, it might be helpful for caregivers to have access to some content within their family members' patient portals. Caregivers may wish to view test results, review prescriptions, and communicate with providers. At the same time, unless the recipient of care is not mentally competent to make decisions, that person should be the one defining the level of their caregivers' access to their personal information. This creates legal, ethical, and technical challenges for portal developers, as granting tiered access necessitates verification procedures and separate logins and access levels. Adult patients can grant proxy access to spouses, partners, and adult children; for patients who are under 13, access by parents is the default setting; but patients between 13 and 18 may, in some states of the US, not be allowed to have portals at all, while in other states, they can designate particular content to be viewable by parents. This confusing ethical and legal landscape means that in this age group, this CHI technology is currently unable to achieve its full potential (Ford et al., 2004).

Another type of personalized technology is both potentially very helpful to caregivers and ethically thorny for caregivers. This is smart medical home technology (see Part II, Chapter 9). Smart medical homes can monitor the health status of a fragile resident. For example, they can detect a resident's failure to take medication, their absence from their bed for more than a specified time interval, or a resident who has left the home without a key or identification. It can also alert a distant caregiver, for example, a remote family member, if any of these events occurs. While this technology can be invaluable for keeping a fragile family member with memory problems safe, it also takes away agency and control from the resident.

As people needing caregiving help are often rather sick, caregivers' health information needs are correspondingly complex and require managing medication regimens and other reminders (via apps, for example), ordering medication from online pharmacies, communicating with healthcare providers, and coordinating care among providers. In addition, caregivers often need to coordinate care with other caregivers. For example, several adult children may share responsibility for caring of an elderly parent. Each of these adult children needs access to relevant health information. Moreover, both caregivers and the people cared for need a convenient, secure way of sharing their information and using it to coordinate their efforts (e.g., helping with transportation to appointments and other chores). When it comes to these kinds of tasks, online scheduling assistants can be very helpful.

Finally and importantly, caregivers have unique health information needs related to their own well-being. Being a caregiver increases the likelihood of health information seeking. Seventy-two percent of caregivers do online health research, compared to 64% of non-caregivers (Fox et al., 2013). Taking care of a loved one is a difficult task that can leave even healthy adults physically and emotionally exhausted. This is particularly true for higher-hours caregivers – who are often elderly spouses with their own health issues – as well as for those combining caregiving with care of young children. Caregivers may feel fatigued, burned out, and isolated. They may also feel guilty for experiencing feelings and emotions that they may view as inappropriate and be unwilling to call attention to themselves and their own needs. The stress of intensive caregiving may exert a toll on the caregiver's own health. The multifaceted role of the caregiver, and the importance of considering the patient in the context of family, is one reason that a recent editorial called for a "family systems approach" to increase engagement of patients with CHI tools and interventions (Houston et al., 2019). As attention to this issue has been growing, numerous e-health support tools have begun to emerge for caregivers themselves. These tools support socialization and communication with other caregivers (e.g., online support groups and caregiver networks). Blogs of caregivers of PwD (people living with dementia) have been analyzed by nurse researchers and found to provide not just support, but a platform for information sharing about everything from clinical trials to service organizations (Anderson et al., 2016). Web-based education for caregivers has also been attempted in particular domains; for example, Arcia et al. (2019) involved Hispanic caregivers in design of an interactive web application for caregiver education about dementia (Arcia et al., 2019).

The remainder of this section provides examples of caregiver-used health information technology that aims to support caregiving experience: personal health record (PHR) portals that enables caregiver access, care-coordination apps, and technology-enabled psychosocial support tools for caregivers.

6.3.1 Exemplar Technology: PHRs and Portals for Caregivers

Health information management is another caregiver task receiving increasing attention in consumer health informatics. Holden et al. (2018) write that this activity involves acquisition and integration, maintenance and update, and finally sharing and communication of the patient's health information – all processes with implications for design of technology tools supporting the caregiver.

While informaticists are beginning to focus on caregivers' information needs when it comes to patients' information access, systems that actually allow such access are rare. For the most part, these are pediatric systems that allow access by patients and their parents or guardians. When it comes to PHRs and patient portals, it is unsurprising that pediatric tools constitute the cutting edge for caregiver engagement. For example, in 2014, Children's Healthcare of Atlanta (CHOA) released a patient portal product (MyChart; Epic Systems, Verona, Wisconsin; for more on patient portals, see Part II, Chapter 1) that supports separate accounts for teen patients and parents. While both parties access using the same interface, a parent's account can be connected to more than one child's. For patients between ages 13 and 18, mutual permissions are necessary for access. Once the patient turns 18, she needs to authorize parental access (Alshoumr et al., 2019).

A patient-centered toolkit (PCKT) developed at the Brigham and Women's Hospital is a tailored decision-support and education patient portal that targets caregivers of adult patients, as much as the patients themselves (Dalal et al., 2016). The tool explicitly includes caregivers as one of its target audiences because it is designed for the inpatient acute care setting, for example, for people at the bedside of ICU patients. As ICU patients may be very ill or incapacitated, caregivers' participation is crucial. PCKT enabled patients and caregivers view their care plan information, set recovery goals and priorities, access educational materials, review their health care team members, and communicate with providers via messages. The tool involved secure login access and did not differentiate between patient and caregiver interfaces. A study of the tool suggests that participants saw the tool as useful and easy to use. Yet, this tool is still rather far from the ideal that supports inpatient to outpatient care transition and coordination of caregiving.

6.3.2 Exemplar Technology: Apps for Coordinating Caregiving

In 2019, AARP published guidance for navigating "the clutter of an overwhelming amount of electronic aids" for caregivers (Saltzman, 2019). The AARP's list centers on general-purpose consumer health apps that can be used by caregivers, such as medication reminders. However, three of the apps listed are caregiver tools that allow coordinating and managing care of a loved one. These include CareZone, Caring Village, and Lotsa Helping Hands. Reliance on such tools may be particularly valuable in remote/geographically dispersed caregiving network. For example, SeniorNavigator, a Virginia Navigator website that provides support to seniors and their caregivers, promotes care coordinating sites as tools that "can help caregivers during COVID-19 and social distancing" (Virginia Navigator, 2020).

Caring Village, which includes an online dashboard and a mobile app, allows the user to create a networked group of "administrators," "inner circle" members, and "friends" of a care recipient. Different types of membership come with different levels of access. Administrators can create to-do tasks (e.g., driving to an appointment, preparing a meal) and ask other members to take responsibility for them. The tool supports other tasks, such as maintaining an up-to-date medications list, and includes a collection of uploaded reference documents that can be easily accessed from anywhere. The app also permits users to upload their own necessary documents and organize them into categories – for example, legal, financial, and medical forms such as home safety preparedness checklists.

6.3.3 Exemplar Technology: Psychosocial Support Networks for Caregivers

Online caregiver support groups help caregivers reduce stress and fight depression (Ploeg et al., 2017). They enable caregivers to connect to others and receive psychosocial support despite multiple demands on their time and difficulty leaving home. Social support networks differ in platforms (Facebook vs other forums), size, and focus (e.g., general vs. condition; demographic-specific). For example, the Dementia Caregivers Support Group, created in 2013, is a private Facebook Group that includes over 16,000 members. The group unites caregivers of individuals with dementia and Alzheimer's disease. The group description stresses that "people coming here are hurt and damaged; they need to vent" (Dementia Caregivers Support Group, 2020). The rules of the group require that members include photos in their profiles and treat one another with kindness. They also explicitly prohibit posting messages for survey recruitment or research purposes, as well as "pseudoscience from a questionable source."

6.4 PARENTS

As noted above, parents are a particular type of caregiver with their own needs and requirements for CHI. With children and teenagers, just as with seniors, the needs of the one who is cared for drive those of the caregiver. Parents, as a group, got online early. As early as 1999, the marketing research firm Cyber Dialogue found that parents were more likely than non-parents to use the internet for fun (73 vs. 64%) and also more likely to do their shopping online, as opposed to offline (Smith, 2008). In 2006, the Pew Internet and American Life Project found that 54% of health information seekers with children under 18 at home were searching for information on behalf of another person – and doing so more than the 44% who didn't have children at home (Fox, 2006).

Some parental information needs relate to keeping a healthy child healthy or prevention of illness, for example, topics like vaccination, exercise, and nutrition. ParentsPlace.com was one of the hundreds of communities on the site called iVillage, among the "most popular female-oriented" sites during the early years of the internet (Tierney, 1998). In 2005, iVillage contained 278 separate sub-bulletin boards devoted to parent-driven topics ranging from premature infants to night terrors, but a separate Adult Health section within ParentsPlace covered such completely adult issues as natural family planning and diabetes self-care (for parents, not children) (Smith, 2008).

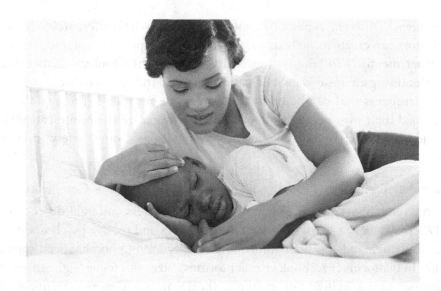

In 2019, Lee (2019) surveyed 851 mothers ages 18–45 (in three demographic groups: US-born, Korean-born residing in Korea, and Korean-born immigrants to the US). These were all parents of healthy children, a population that has been studied only very little in any country. Ninety-eight percent of these mothers had sought health information from *any* source in the last 6 months. Korean natives in both Korea and the US searched quite frequently for health information, 15% of the immigrants and 18% of mothers in Korea doing so more than once a day. In contrast, most US-born mothers looked online for this information just a few times a month.

Personal characteristics affect parental source preferences for health information. For example, the length of time that one has been a parent is significant. First-time mothers have been found to prefer electronic media (websites, mobile apps) over written materials or pamphlets as sources of health information – but personal contact with a healthcare provider is the most important source of all (Gazmararian et al., 2014). Lee (2019) asked her Korean residents, immigrants to the US and US-born survey respondents to rate 19 different sources in different media – including interpersonal sources like doctors and nurses, as well as digital sources, such as social media and social networks. In seeking health information, all three groups of mothers used the World Wide Web the most often. Both Korean subgroups, but not the US subgroup, used Twitter often. Lee (2018) also found a distinct preference for online communities as information sources among both Korean subgroups – probably due to the availability of Korean-language information online.

Parents of ill children have different needs: when a child is sick, their mothers or fathers need to communicate with pediatricians; that initial contact with the pediatrics practice (from a phone call to a Virtual Visit) often establishes whether further contact with the healthcare system is required. Parents are important mediators between their children and the healthcare system, even as children grow into adolescents. Eighty-three percent of logins to portals of adolescent patients were found, in one study, to be done by their parents (Steitz et al., 2017). For this reason, parents have been the subject of much research. The systematic review conducted by Morrison et al. (2013) revealed that about one third of parents presenting in US emergency departments with their children have low health literacy. A later review by Keim-Malpass et al. (2015) found that the majority of health literacy studies assessing parents of children with special healthcare needs had been done in the domain of asthma, but also for glaucoma, type 1 diabetes, and ADHD. The health literacy levels of parents are important to understand, not only because parents are caregivers, but because child health promotion campaigns need to be understood, and parents are gatekeepers of information for their families (Brega et al., 2016). Parents of children living with chronic illnesses are caregivers and consumers who engage with patients on a daily basis and mediate between the worlds. This requires a particular kind of informational support for caregivers, as well as support in discussing diseases and treatment options with their children.

Examples of consumer health informatics research done with parents of young patients include a personal health record (PHR) study focusing on chronic conditions (diabetes, juvenile idiopathic arthritis, and cystic fibrosis) (Byczkowski et al., 2014); social media as an information source for families of autistic children (Khudair & AlOshan, 2015); and search behaviors driving traffic to a website for parents of injured children called AfterTheInjury (Yang et al., 2011). The needs and demands of users of many different age groups and household compositions must be considered in design, rollout, and outreach about these technologies. Ronis et al. studied 184 parents in pediatric practice and found positive attitudes toward portals in this group – whether they used them or not – but 36% of these parents indicated that they had never used portals because they had not known they were available. The authors commented on "persistently low levels of awareness" on the part of patients and caregivers, simultaneous with "low levels of preparedness" on the part of healthcare providers. Healthcare systems have to promote these products in order for patients – and their family members – to become engaged (Ronis et al., 2015).

6.4.1 Exemplar Technology: MyChart Bedside

An example of a parent-centered CHI tool is MyChart Bedside. Bedside is a patient portal designed to be used in an inpatient hospital setting. Like MyChart, another Epic Systems™ product, Bedside allows users to view portions of the official medical record, including current medications (in real time). The difference with Bedside is that the users are parents of inpatients – or the patients themselves, if they are adolescents. Parent users of Bedside comment that Bedside helps them engage with their children's care team and gives them "a sense of control" (Kritz, 2019). The University of Wisconsin MyChart Bedside project and associated publications can be seen online at https://cqpi.wisc.edu/research/health-care-and-patient-safety-seips/mychart-bedside/#project-home. A toolkit for potential implementers can be found at https://www.hipxchange.org/InpatientPortal.

6.5 CHILDREN, ADOLESCENTS, AND YOUNG ADULTS

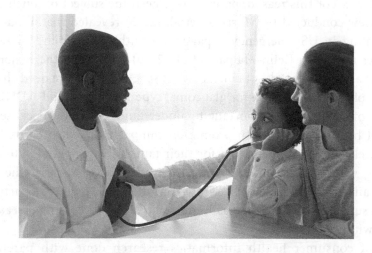

While children do not have legal authority to make crucial healthcare decisions, childhood is the time when many health and well-being practices are formed, particularly those related to nutrition and exercise. Childhood is also the time when individuals develop the foundation of health and science literacy essential for health functioning throughout the life span. A number of information tools can support such learning, from educational games to tools allowing children to create content that can be shared with others (e.g., health information outreach and classroom presentations). Children and adolescents living with chronic illnesses may need support in understanding their condition and handling their self-care. Young adulthood presents novel and unique health information challenges because it is the time of transition from pediatric to adult care. It is also the time of switching to health insurance policies that are not connected to the parents'. In addition, young adulthood is the time when sexual health and mental health constitute important health concerns. While young adults do have these prominent health information needs, they typically live busy lifestyles that make them underutilize information outreach programs, unless they are delivered in ways that are easy to integrate into the rest of their lives.

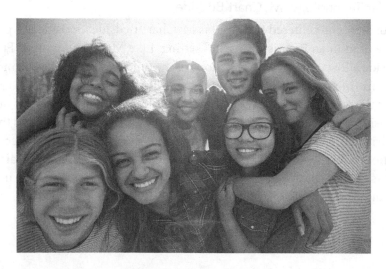

Living with chronic illness has been associated with an increase in PHR and portal adoption in the general population, and the same appears to be true of children and adolescents. People who grow up with a life experience of illness are not only the portal users of tomorrow, but the portal users of today. Yet less is known about the adolescent population and their portal usage than about other populations. A review of medical literature in PubMed published between 1991 and March 2019 done by the first author of this book yielded 26 studies of personal health records or patient portals in which children and young adults were involved. Since 2009, only five studies involved the young adult demographic. A large study of PHR adoption (75,056 patients) revealed, in the age group 18–35 specifically, that nonadopters (17%) were slightly more common than adopters (14%). (The highest proportion of adopters was in the age group 36–50) (Yamin et al., 2011). Yen et al. (2018) and Ali et al. (2018) included the same age bracket in usability studies. Only two studies focused on college students specifically (Walker et al., 2009; Whetstone & Goldsmith, 2009).

The health status of college students investigated thus far has been mixed. Walker et al. (2009) recruited healthy students. Whetstone and Goldsmith (2009) recruited from the general population, and not from hospitals or clinics; checking for health status, they found 15% were living with chronic illnesses. The American College Health Association conducts an annual survey of undergraduate students. Data from the Fall 2018 survey revealed that 8.5% of undergraduate respondents (N = 27,864) reported living with a chronic health problem or serious illness (e.g., diabetes, asthma, and cancer). Mental health diagnoses reported included anxiety (21.4%) and depression (16%) (American College Health Association, 2018). This is a demographic composed of people likely to be early and avid adopters of CHI technologies. For more on college students and chronic health issues, see below in the section on Intermediaries.

6.5.1 Exemplar Technology: College Students

An example of an app for college students is MyFitnessPal, an UnderArmour product. This app is one of many self-monitoring technologies that give users feedback and track their food intake and weight. In May 2018, it was ranked the second most popular "health and fitness" app by 20,000 US respondents aged 18 and up, with over 19 million active users (Clement, 2019). MyFitnessPal's website includes such health-supporting features as a food diary, a searchable food database providing caloric estimates, and a personalized diet profile (MyFitnessPal, n.d.). Use of trackers to count calories is highest among members of the Millennial generation, according to a 2018 survey (Mintel, 2019). One recent study (Patel et al., 2020) defined Consistent Trackers as users who fulfilled all the self-monitoring tasks established by the researchers (weight and diet tracking) at least 6 days a week for at least 75% of the weeks of the trial. MyFitnessPal was the app used in this study. The researchers' conclusion: Consistent Trackers lost twice as much weight as the Inconsistent Trackers, and even more so at the 6-month point.

6.6 INTERMEDIARIES

Intermediaries are middle-people between consumers, caregivers, patients, and various societal systems. In their professional roles, they are not patients; nor are they friends or family members of patients. Nor are they health professionals, although they may be parahealth professionals (i.e., people in occupations that assist in healthcare systems without being professionally licensed). Rather, they are individuals who work with personal health information in the course of their jobs.

Intermediaries work in the intersecting spaces of the world: social services offices (Social Security Disability, for example), camps and extracurricular sports programs, student disability centers in higher education, school systems, libraries, and community centers for clients of all abilities, ages and stages.

Sometimes, intermediaries are gatekeepers: they assess clients for eligibility for certain services. Service coordinators in Social Security offices are an example. Others are Disability Benefit Specialists (such as found in Aging and Disability Resource Centers, which serve clients in the elderly and disabled subpopulations); case managers, care coordinators, and social workers. One author calls them SLBs, or "street-level bureaucrats ... [who] strive to advocate for their clients yet often experience conflict between their own beliefs, commitments, work demands, and limited resources" (Keesler, 2015). Both the advocacy and the demands of the work necessitate access to other people's health information in the form of medical documentation. Sometimes, intermediaries do health information seeking to help consumers and patients. In order to effectively meet the needs of these other people, a certain amount of private or personal health information must be shared by the client. Public librarians are an example: While "Do I have cancer?" is not answerable by a librarian, "Where is the closest specialist in my cancer?" is answerable but requires the client to share.

Documentation of disabilities for the purpose of academic accommodation has many similarities to that required for US SSDI (Social Security Disability Insurance) benefits. Both of these systems rely on health information as "a primary input to facilitate movement." Students and SSDI claimants alike may have to "recall a vast amount of information." Service coordinators have to wrestle with documentation just as their student clients do. Lytle-Kosola and colleagues concluded their study of SSDI documentation with a recommendation that consumer health IT be used to reduce the "information-gathering" burden on SSDI claimants (2012). Disabled college students could benefit from the same recommendation. Advocates for PHRs argue: since other consumer-facing health IT applications have been found to have positive effects, for example, on patient engagement, PHRs may hold the same promise for this particular subtype of consumer.

6.7 SENIORS

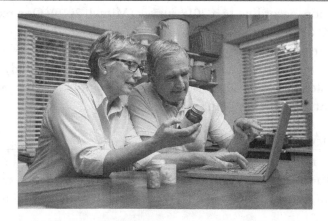

The health of older adults, usually defined as those 65 and older, is a significant focus of US healthcare and biomedical research. The definition sets its boundary age at 65 because this is the age when Americans first qualify for Social Security benefits. Within that definition, there is a broad range of lifestyles and health statuses.

Sixty-five was set as the minimum age for retirement benefits in 1935, when average life expectancy in the US was 61. Today, it is 79 years. Americans are living longer, and many today's 65-year-olds are enjoying healthy, socially engaged lives. At the same time, today's greater life expectancy generally means longer involvement with healthcare in the later years. Older adults are among the population groups with the greatest utilization of healthcare, and, thus, the greatest health information needs. As consumer health information technology holds promise of improving health functioning, targeting this group in consumer health information tools research and development is a promising enterprise. At the same time, on average, older adults are less likely than their younger counterparts to be among early adopters of new technology. Successful tools development for this population group requires close attention to information needs and preferences of target users, and a particularly strong emphasis on usability.

Older adults represent a large and growing segment of the market. According to HealthyPeople2020, in 2014, 14.5% of US residents were 65. This proportion is projected to grow to 23.50% by 2060. The majority of older adults live with two or more chronic illnesses, the five most common being heart disease, cancer, chronic bronchitis or emphysema, stroke, diabetes mellitus, and Alzheimer's disease (Ward et al., 2014). Managing multiple conditions typically means multiple medications, often taken on different schedules, multiple healthcare visits to different professional and specialists, a lot of care coordination, and, in some cases, periods of hospitalization. As people age, they may need more assistance with activities of daily living, such as self-care and household chores. This assistance is often provided by caregivers: spouses, adult children, and paid helpers. In matters of health information and health communication, caregivers often represent interests of their loved ones (see Caregivers section in this chapter).

For many older adults, continuing to live independently in their home is a desired goal. If the burden of independent living becomes too high, other housing options include, in order of increasing support, retirement communities, assisted living communities, and nursing homes. Residents of retirement communities own or rent their units and may have amenities such as meals, transportation, and group activities (e.g., exercise classes). Assisted living communities are similar, but also include help with activities of daily living, such as bathing or organizing medicines. Nursing homes usually provide professional nursing services that are available 24 hours a day, as well as assistance with all aspects of daily functioning. Consumer health technology, particularly smart medical home features (see Part II, Chapter 9), may be instrumental in enabling independent living as the age advances.

Health information content of particular interest to older adults includes (but is not limited to) healthy aging, wellness, information on the diseases and conditions common in the aging population, cognitive health, home care, managing multiple health problems, dental and eye health, urinary health, and falls prevention. Falls prevention and continuous health monitoring are important healthy aging topics in which emergent technology solutions are expected to play a significant role (see Part II, Chapter 9). But while health concerns faced by older adults can be effectively supported by technology, researchers and developers targeting this demographic group should be aware of a number of special considerations. For example, older adults are less likely to use computers and smartphones than other age groups. On the positive side, the technology adoption rate is growing rapidly. According to Pew Research Center, in 2016, use of internet by those 65 and older was 67%, up from 14% in early 2000. Use of smartphones by the same age group was 40%, having more than doubled compared to 2013. Adoption is not even across subgroups of this population, however. Older adults who use technology the most are relatively younger, wealthier, and more educated. Income-related and age-related disparities are sizable. For example, 81% of older adults with annual household income over $75,000, and only 27% of those with household income below $30,000, owned a smartphone. While 82% of those 65–69 used the internet, only 44% of those 80 and over did (Anderson & Perrin, 2017).

Older adults who do use information technology and the internet often do it via more traditional, "web 1.0" tools, and resources. For example, while 67% of older adults used the internet in 2016, only about a third of them had ever used social media (Anderson & Perrin, 2017). LeRouge et al. (2014) asked individuals of different ages about their willingness to use various health information technologies. While 60% of older adults were ready to use websites, the percentage of potentially willing users was much lower for videoconferencing (26%), texting (20%), podcasts (21%), blogs (19%), wikis (14%), and smartphones (11%). Reasons for reluctance included unfamiliarity with a particular technology, or not knowing how to use it. Other barriers to use of information technology by older adults include a lack of confidence in their ability and feeling the need for training or support (Gordon and Crouch, 2019). Older adults may not see the advantage of using technological over the non-technological solutions to which they are used (e.g., use of a portal vs. paper record-keeping system) (Young et al., 2014). This underlines the importance of training initiatives and social support in addition to usability. In the absence of such supports, health professionals should never assume that an online "information prescription" will be filled by their older adult patients.

But once older adults start using the internet, it often becomes a regular part of their routine. When older adults are directed to quality online health information resources, their knowledge of relevant health topics improves (Freund et al., 2017). They also view the internet as a positive influence on society and on their lives (Anderson & Perrin, 2017. Generally, studies suggest that older adults are willing to accept new technologies that they consider useful (Joe et al., 2018). To be seen as useful, however, technologies need to be developed with user input from their targeted users. This is especially important when developing for older adults, because technology designers and developers rarely belong to that demographic group.

Designing for older adults requires taking into consideration biological changes that happen with aging, such as a decline in vision and manual dexterity. Aging also affects memory and ease of learning new information. Thus, designs for older adults should simple and clear, with good color contrasts. Font and button size should be large enough for easy reading and comfortable clicking. As older adults may be less familiar with symbolic conventions, icons should be accompanied by text. In focus groups with older adults, Joe et al.

(2018) also found that participants valued such design features as portability (e.g., wearable devices, tablets, or smartphones), simplicity, and easy access to the information they needed. Participants also appreciated the social connectivity and communication features allowed by health information technology, valuing features that connected them to friends and family, as well as to healthcare providers. It is essential to assess user needs prior to starting the design process and then test intermediate and near-final products with users. There is also an important ethical consideration of data privacy and security in this population. While older adults may be less concerned about privacy of their online data than other users, it may be because of lack of awareness of issues around online data security and privacy (Le). It is extremely important that those who recommend information technology to older adults employ a proper informed consent mechanism, explaining security considerations in plain language.

We now review two examples of health information resources targeting older adults: the health information section of the National Institute on Aging website (https://www.nia.nih.gov/health), and the Medisafe app.

6.7.1 Exemplar Technology: National Institute on Aging Website

The health information section of the National Institute on Aging website (https://www.nia.nih.gov/health) provides up-to-date authoritative evidence-based information about health and wellness topics for older adults. The site has a simple layout, with the homepage featuring several topics relevant to the health of this population. Among them are dementias and cognitive health, caregiving, healthy eating, exercise and physical activity, doctor-patient communication, end of life, and participation in research. Beyond the home page, the site covers over 90 topics, accessible via an easy Browse A-Z Health Topics feature. Health topics pages are not identical in their format, which retracts somewhat from their usability. Furthermore, the site is written for multiple audiences, rather than specifically for older adults. For example, next to each other are "Talking with your doctor" and "Talking with your older patient." Pages use plain language guidelines, chunking content into sections with headers and short paragraphs, and using bullet lists and examples. They also include boxed sections with case studies or special highlights. For example, *Talking with Medical Specialists: Tips for Patients* has a highlighted section titled "Seeking a Second Opinion." The page's Flesch–Kincaid readability level is 7.9, which means that reading skills required by the text are possessed by an average reader with 8th grades of schooling (for readability levels, see Part I, Chapter 3 of this book). While reading formula designations should be interpreted with caution, this level falls into the range recommended by most guidelines for consumer health materials (e.g., Johns Hopkins, 2016). Most importantly, this site's coverage is comprehensive for all aspects of aging and health, including normal age-related changes (such as bladder health, eyes and vision, falls and falls prevention), specific diseases and conditions (e.g., diabetes), wellness (e.g., healthy eating, exercise), support of activities of daily life (e.g., driving and transportation, medication management), caregiving, and administrative support (e.g., legal planning). As such, it constitutes an excellent resource for older adults and their families and caregivers.

6.7.2 Exemplar Health Technology: Medisafe

Medisafe is a medication management app, identified by a leading trends-in-digital-health report as the top free and publicly available app in its category (Aitken et al., 2017). While there is a paid premium version of the app, the free version includes all the features mentioned below. Although Medisafe does not target a specific demographic group, it appears on many lists of "top health apps for older adults" (Langone, 2018).

The app was developed in 2012, by two brothers, Omri and Rotem Shor, after their father, living with diabetes, accidentally took an extra dose of his insulin and ended up in critical condition. At the time of the writing of this chapter, in January 2020, Medisafe was rated 4.6 out of 5.0 in Google Play store for Android apps and 4.7 out of 5.0 in Apple App Store. These ratings were by 196,000 and 32,000 users, respectively.

In addition to providing timed medication reminders for pre-set dose schedules, Medisafe includes a drug interaction checker function and a refill reminder. It also allows recording health measurements, recording health providers' contact information, and tracking medical appointments. The app has an educational component that provides information about medications and has "medfriend" feature that sends an email to a user-approved friend when a medication dose is skipped (not marked as "taken").

Medisafe is rather intuitive for habitual app users, as evidenced by its high ratings. But a cognitive walkthrough and heuristic evaluation usability analysis, conducted by Stuck et al. (2017) from the perspective of an older adult user persona, identified several usability issues with Medisafe. These included the absence of a "home" screen, small buttons that are potentially difficult to see, invisibility of some settings and function, difficulty figuring out the "Medfriend" function, and poor color contrast. Older adults who are not as comfortable with apps may need help installing it, entering their medications, and getting oriented to the app's functions. In some cases, such assistance may be provided by tech-savvy family members and friends, in others, by online volunteers. For example Jim Schrempp publishes a step-by-step Medisafe guide in his Tech-enhanced Life blog (2020). Perhaps, as app technology matures, apps like Medisafe will take into account design considerations for demographic groups that are generally not currently broadly represented among app users.

WEB RESOURCES

MEDLINEPlus
The National Library of Medicine's online health topics can help you familiarize yourself with these populations.

Children and Teenagers
https://MEDLINEplus.gov/childrenandteenagers.html
Older adults
https://MEDLINEplus.gov/olderadults.html

College students
Contraceptive information targeting college-age people
https://www.bedsider.org/

Crohn's and Colitis Foundation
Parents:

An example of a website for children and teenagers living with serious chronic illness: inflammatory bowel disease, which is often diagnosed between ages 15 and 25.
https://www.crohnscolitisfoundation.org/youth-parent-resources
This companion website is for college students with the same illness:
https://site.crohnscolitisfoundation.org/campus-connection/

National Alliance on Caregiving
"An objective national resource on family caregiving." Funds research studies on caregivers and disseminates findings; studies are "one of the most authoritative resources available to describe the American caregiver."
https://www.caregiving.org/research/

REFERENCES

"patient, adj. and n." (2019, December). *OED Online*. Oxford University Press.

Aitken, M., Clancy, B., & Nass, D. (2017). The growing value of digital health: Evidence and impact on human health and the healthcare system. IQVIA Institute for Data Science https://www.iqvia.com/insights/the-iqvia-institute/reports/the-growing-value-of-digital-health

Ali, S. B., Romero, J., Morrison, K., Hafeez, B., Ancker, J. S. (2018). Applying a task-technology fit model to adapt an electronic patient portal for patient work. *Applied Clinical Informatics*, 9(1), 174–184. https://doi.org/10.1055/s-0038-1632396

Alshoumr, B., Yu, P., Cui, T., & Song, T. (2019). Using inpatient portals to engage family caregivers in acute care setting: A literature review. *Studies in Health Technology and Informatics*, 264, 1627–1628. https://doi.org/10.3233/shti190567

American College Health Association. (2018). *National College Health Assessment II: Undergraduate Student Reference Group Data Report*. Silver Spring, MD: American College Health Association.

Anderson, J. G., Hundt, E., & Dean, M. (2016). "The Church of Online Support": Examining the use of blogs among family caregivers of persons with dementia. *Journal of Family Nursing*, 23(1), 34–54.

Anderson, M., & Perrin, A. (2017). Tech adoption climbs among older adults. https://www.pewresearch.org/internet/2017/05/17/technology-use-among-seniors/

Arcia, A., Suero-Tejeda, N., & Bakken, S. (2019). Development of pictograms for an interactive Web application to help Hispanic caregivers learn about the functional stages of dementia. *Studies in Health Technology & Informatics*, 264, 1116–1120.

Brega, A. G., Thomas, J. F., Henderson, W. G., Batliner, T. S., Quissell, D. O., Braun, P. A., Wilson, A., Bryant, L. L., Nadeau, K. J., & Albino, J. (2016). Association of parental health literacy with oral health of Navajo Nation preschoolers. *Health Education Research*, 31(1), 70–81. https://doi.org/10.1093/her/cyv055

Byczkowski, T. L., Munafo, J. K., & Britto, M. T. (2014). Family perceptions of the usability and value of chronic disease web-based patient portals. *Health Informatics Journal*, 20(2), 151–162.

Clement, J. (2019, November 20). Leading health and fitness apps in the U.S. 2018, by users. Statista. https://www.statista.com/statistics/650748/health-fitness-app-usage-usa/

Costa, D. S. J., Mercieca-Bebber, R., Tesson, S., Seidler, Z., & Lopez, A. L. (2019). Patient, client, consumer, survivor or other alternatives? A scoping review of preferred terms for labelling individuals who access healthcare across settings. *BMJ Open*, 9(3), e025166. https://doi.org/10.1136/bmjopen-2018-025166

Coulter, A., Entwistle, V., & Gilbert, D. (1999). Sharing decisions with patients: is the information good enough? *BMJ (Clinical research ed.)*, 318(7179), 318–322. https://doi.org/10.1136/bmj.318.7179.318

Cutting, C. C., & Collen, M. F. (1992). A historical review of the Kaiser Permanente medical care program. *Journal of Social Health Systems*, 3(4), 25–30.

Dalal, A. K., Dykes, P. C., Collins, S., Lehmann, L. S., Ohashi, K., Rozenblum, R., Stade, D., McNally, K., Morrison, C. R., Ravindran, S., Mlaver, E., Hanna, J., Chang, F., Kandala, R., Getty, G., & Bates, D. W. (2016). A web-based, patient-centered toolkit to engage patients and caregivers in the acute care setting: A preliminary evaluation. *Journal of the American Medical Informatics Association: JAMIA*, 23(1), 80–87. https://doi.org/10.1093/jamia/ocv093

Deber, R. B., Kraetschmer, N., Urowitz, S., & Sharpe, N. (2005). Patient, consumer, client, or customer: What do people want to be called? *Health Expectations*, 8(4), 345–351. https://doi.org/10.1111/j.1369-7625.2005.00352.x

Dementia Caregivers Support Group. (2020, March 4). About this group. https://www.facebook.com/groups/672984902717938

Dickens, G., & Picchioni, M. (2012). A systematic review of the terms used to refer to people who use mental health services: User perspectives. *International Journal of Social Psychiatry*, 58(2), 115–122. https://doi.org/10.1177/0020764010392066

Ford, C., English, A., & Sigman, G. (2004). Confidential health care for adolescents: Position paper for the Society for Adolescent Medicine. *Journal of Adolescent Health*, 35(2), 160–167.

Fox, S. (2006, October 29). Online health search 2006. Pew Internet & American Life Project. https://www.pewinternet.org/wp-content/uploads/sites/9/media/Files/Reports/2006/PIP_Online_Health_2006.pdf.pdf

Fox, S., Duggan, M., & Purcell, K. (2013, June 20). Family caregivers are wired for health. Pew Research Center. https://www.pewinternet.org/wp-content/uploads/sites/9/media/Files/Reports/2013/PewResearch_FamilyCaregivers.pdf

Freund, O., Reychav, I., McHaney, R., Goland, E., & Azuri, J. (2017). The ability of older adults to use customized online medical databases to improve their health-related knowledge. *International Journal of Medical Informatics*, 102, 1–11. https://doi.org/10.1016/j.ijmedinf.2017.02.012

Gazmararian, J., Dalmida, S., Merino, Y., Blake, S., Thompson, W., & Gaydos, L. (2014). What new mothers need to know: Perspectives from women and providers in Georgia. *Maternal & Child Health Journal*, 18(4), 839–851.

Gordon, N. P., & Crouch, E. (2019). Digital information technology use and patient preferences for internet-based health education modalities: Cross-sectional survey study of middle-aged and older adults with chronic health conditions. *JMIR Aging*, 2(1), e12243. https://doi.org/10.2196/12243

Gorman, D. (2018). Citizens, consumers or patients: What's in a name? *Internal Medicine Journal*, 48(8), 899–901. https://doi.org/10.1111/imj.13983

Holden, R. J., Karanam, Y. L. P., Cavalcanti, L. H., Parmar, T., Kodthala, P., Fowler, N. R., & Bateman, D. R. (2018). Health information management practices in informal caregiving: An artifacts analysis and implications for IT design. *International Journal of Medical Informatics*, 120, 31–41.

Houston, T. K., Richardson, L. M., & Cotton, S. R. (2019). Patient-directed digital health technologies: Is implementation outpacing evidence? *Medical Care*, 57(2), 95–97. https://doi.org/10.1097/MLR.0000000000001068

Joe, J., Hall, A., Chi, N. C., Thompson, H., & Demiris, G. (2018). IT-based wellness tools for older adults: Design concepts and feedback. *Informatics for Health & Social Care*, 43(2), 142–158. https://doi.org/10.1080/17538157.2017.1290637

Johns Hopkins Medicine, Office of Human Subjects Research – Institutional Review Board. (2016, April). II. Informed consent guidance – How to prepare a readable consent form.

https://www.hopkinsmedicine.org/institutional_review_board/guidelines_policies/guidelines/informed_consent_ii.html

Keesler, J. M. (2015). Applying for Supplemental Security Income (SSI) for individuals with intellectual and developmental disabilities: Family and service coordinator experiences. *Intellectual & Developmental Disabilities*, 53(1), 42–57.

Keim-Malpass, J., Letzkus, L. C., & Kennedy, C. (2015). Parent/caregiver health literacy among children with special health care needs: A systematic review of the literature. *BMC Pediatrics*, 15, 92. https://doi.org/10.1186/s12887-015-0412-x

Khudair, A. A., & AlOshan, M. S. (2015). Caregivers of autistic children: Seeking information in social media. *Proceedings of the International Conference on Information Society* 68–72.

Koh, S., Gordon, A. S., Weinberg, C., Sood, S. O., Morley, S., & Burke, D. M. (2014). Stroke experiences in weblogs: A feasibility study of sex differences. *Journal of Medical Internet Research*, 16(3), e84. https://doi.org/10.2196/jmir.2838

Kritz, F. (2019, April 7). For hospital patients, bedside tablets and apps are providing some control over care. *Washington Post*. https://www.washingtonpost.com/national/health-science/for-hospital-patients-bedside-tablets-and-apps-are-providing-some-control-over-care/2019/04/05/9d545de0-3c67-11e9-aaae-69364b2ed137_story.html

Lafky, D. B., & Horan, T. A. (2011). Personal health records: Consumer attitudes toward privacy and security of their personal health information. *Health Informatics Journal*, 17(1), 63–71. https://doi.org/10.1177/1460458211399403

Langone, A. (2018). The best apps for older adults you should download right now. https://money.com/the-best-apps-for-older-adults-you-should-download-right-now/

Lee, H. S. (2018). A comparative study on the health information needs, seeking and source preferences among mothers of young healthy children: American mothers compared to recent immigrant Korean mothers. *Information Research*, 23(4). http://www.informationr.net/ir/23-4/paper803.html

Lee, H. S. (2019). Health information-seeking behavior among mothers of healthy infants and toddlers: A comparative study of U.S.-born, Korean-born, and immigrant Korean mothers (Order No. 27669038). Available from ProQuest Dissertations & Theses Global. (2337136494). http://search.proquest.com.ezproxy.library.wisc.edu/docview/2337136494?accountid=465

LeRouge, C., Van Slyke, C., Seale, D., & Wright, K. (2014). Baby boomers' adoption of consumer health technologies: Survey on readiness and barriers. *Journal of Medical Internet Research*, 16(9), e200. https://doi.org/10.2196/jmir.3049

Lytle-Kosola, N., Feldman, S. S., Horan, T. A., Elias, E., & Gaeta, R. (2012). Investigation of a consumer focused health IT system: The role of claimant information in the Social Security determination process. *HICSS*, 2012, 2706–2713.

Martinez-Pérez, B., de la Torre-Díez, I., & López-Coronado, M. (2015). Experiences and results of applying tools for assessing the quality of a mHealth app named Heartkeeper. *Journal of Medical Systems*, 39, 42.

Mintel. (2019, January). *Health management trends – US*. Mintel Research.

Morrison, A. K., Myrvik, M. P., Brousseau, D. C., Hoffmann, R. G., & Stanley, R. M. (2013). The relationship between parent health literacy and pediatric emergency department utilization: A systematic review. *Academic Pediatrics*, 13(5), 421–429. https://doi.org/10.1016/j.acap.2013.03.001

MyFitnessPal. (n.d.) About. https://www.myfitnesspal.com/welcome/learn_more

National Alliance for Caregiving & AARP Public Policy Institute. (2015). *Caregiving in the U.S., 2015*. https://www.aarp.org/content/dam/aarp/ppi/2015/caregiving-in-the-united-states-2015-report-revised.pdf

National Cancer Institute. (2017a). How did you access a family member or close friend's personal health information? Used a login and password assigned to me to access their record. https://hints.cancer.gov/view-questions-topics/question-details.aspx?PK_Cycle=10&qid=1671

National Cancer Institute. (2017b). In the past 12 months, have you used your online medical record to make appointments with a health care provider? https://hints.cancer.gov/view-questions-topics/question-details.aspx?PK_Cycle=10&qid=1654

National Cancer Institute. (2018a). Have you electronically sent your medical information to a family member or another person involved with your care? https://hints.cancer.gov/view-questions-topics/question-details.aspx?PK_Cycle=11&qid=1665

National Cancer Institute. (2018b). In the past 12 months, have you used your online medical record to download your health information to your computer or mobile device, such as a cell phone or tablet? https://hints.cancer.gov/view-questions-topics/question-details.aspx?PK_Cycle=11&qid=1661

Patel, M. L., Brooks, T. L., & Bennett, G. G. (2020). Consistent self-monitoring in a commercial app-based intervention for weight loss: Results from a randomized trial. *Journal of Behavioral Medicine*, 43, 391–401. https://doi.org/10.1007/s10865-019-00091-8

Ploeg, J., Markle-Reid, M., Valaitis, R., McAiney, C., Duggleby, W., Bartholomew, A., & Sherifali, D. (2017). Web-based interventions to improve mental health, general caregiving outcomes, and general health for informal caregivers of adults with chronic conditions living in the community: Rapid Evidence Review. *Journal of Medical Internet Research*, 19(7), e263. https://doi.org/10.2196/jmir.7564

Ronis, S. D., Baldwin, C. D., McIntosh, S., McConnochie, K., Szilagyi, P. G., & Dolan, J. (2015). Caregiver preferences regarding personal health records in the management of ADHD. *Clinical Pediatrics (Phila)*, 54(8), 765–774. https://doi.org/10.1177/0009922814565883

Saltzman, M. (2019). These apps for caregivers can help you get organized, find support. https://www.aarp.org/home-family/personal-technology/info-2019/top-caregiving-apps.html

Schrempp, J. (2020). How to use the Medisafe app. https://www.techenhancedlife.com/citizen-research/how-use-medisafe-app

Smith, C. A. (2008). The ten thousand questions project. *Journal of Consumer Health on the Internet*, 11(1), 33–47.

Smith, C. A., Yu, D., Maestre, J. F., Backonja, U., Boyd, A. D., Buis, L. R., Chaudry, B. M., Huh-Yoo, J., Hussain, S. A., Jones, L. M., Lai, A. M., Senteio, C. R., Siek, K. A., & Veinot, T. C. (2020). Consumer health informatics research: A scoping review of informatics, information science and engineering literature. [Unpublished manuscript submitted for publication.]

Spina, G., Roberts, F., Weppner, J., Lukowicz, P., & Amft, O. (2013). CRNTC+: A smartphone-based sensor processing framework for prototyping personal healthcare applications. *Pervasive Health '13: Proceedings of the 7th International Conference on Pervasive Computing Technologies for Healthcare* 252–255. https://doi.org/10.4108/icst.pervasivehealth.2013.252039

Steitz, B., Cronin, R. M., Davis, S. E., Yan, E., & Jackson, G. P. (2017). Long-term patterns of patient portal use for pediatric patients at an academic medical center. *Applied Clinical Informatics*, 8(3), 779–793.

Stuck, R. E., Chong, A. W., Mitzner, T. L., & Rogers, W. A. (2017). Medication management apps: Usable by older adults? *Proceedings of the Human Factors and Ergonomics Society … Annual Meeting. Human Factors and Ergonomics Society. Annual Meeting*, 61(1), 1141–1144. https://doi.org/10.1177/1541931213601769

Tierney, J. (1998, December 17). The big city: Women ease into mastery of cyberspace. *The New York Times*, B1.

Virginia Navigator. (2020). Senior Navigator, a Virginia navigator website: How tech tools can help caregivers during COVID-19 and social distancing. https://seniornavigator.org/article/74273/how-tech-tools-can-help-caregivers-during-COVID-19-and-social-distancing

Walker, J., Ahern, D. K., Le, L. X., & Delbanco, T. (2009). Insights for internists: "I want the computer to know who I am". *Journal of General Internal Medicine*, 24(6), 727–732.

Ward, B. W., Schiller, J. S., & Goodman, R. A. (2014). Multiple chronic conditions among US adults: A 2012 update. *Prevention of Chronic Diseases*, 11, 130389.

Whetstone, M., & Goldsmith, R. (2009). Factors influencing intention to use personal health records. *International Journal of Pharmaceutical and Healthcare Marketing*, 3(1), 8–25. https://doi.org/10.1108/17506120910948485

Yamin, C. K., Emani, S., Williams, D. H., Lipsitz, S. R., Karson, A. S., Wald, J. S., & Bates, D. W. (2011). The digital divide in adoption and use of a personal health record. *Archives of Internal Medicine*, 171(6), 568–574. https://doi.org/10.1001/archinternmed.2011.34

Yang, C. C., Winston, F., Zarro, M. A., & Kassam-Adams, N. (2011). A study of user queries leading to a health information website – AfterTheInjury.org. *Proceedings of the iConference*. https://doi.org/10.1145/1940761.1940798

Yen, P. Y., Walker, D. M., Smith, J. M. G., Zhou, M. P., Menser, T. L., & McAlearney, A. S. (2018). Usability evaluation of a commercial inpatient portal. *International Journal of Medical Informatics*, 110, 10–18. https://doi.org/10.1016/j.ijmedinf.2017.11.007

Young, R., Willis, E., Cameron, G., & Geana, M. (2014). "Willing but unwilling": Attitudinal barriers to adoption of home-based health information technology among older adults. *Health Informatics Journal*, 20(2), 127–135. https://doi.org/10.1177/1460458213486906

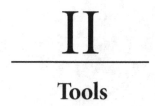

II

Tools

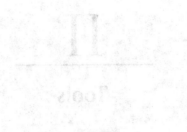

CHAPTER 7

PHRs and Patient Portals

Catherine Arnott Smith

THIS CHAPTER CENTERS ON patient portals and personal health records, which are variants and subsets of the Electronic Health Record. Topics discussed include PHR/portal history and standards; key organizations; typical content, features, and functions; and current challenges, including issues of patient access to medical record content.

7.1 DEFINITIONS

Somner, Sii, Bourne, Cross, and Shah (2013) describe a "spectrum" of personal health record products ranging from simple paper passports and wallet cards through full-blown patient portals such as MyChart™ (Epic Systems, Verona, Wisconsin). The principal types of *patient-facing* medical record products are the Personal Health Record (PHR) and the Patient Portal.

7.1.1 Personal Health Record (PHR)

Personal Health Records, or PHRs, have been defined as "collections of health or wellness data arising from multiple sources about an individual's health that are managed, controlled or shared by that individual or designate" (Archer et al., 2011, p. 515). Intended users are not healthcare practitioners, but patients and/or their designates, a category which can include patients' spouses, partners, adult children, and adult parents (see the "Caregivers" section of Part I: Chapter 6 for more). PHRs can be paper-based or digital and exist in various formats of both types. Paper-based PHRs can take the form of journals, logs, or diaries; some are developed by healthcare providers with particular populations in mind, to serve as "passports" carried by the patient from one provider to another. Digital PHRs might be apps, devices, or Web-based products. Major players in the internet and tech industries have developed PHRs of this type with varying degrees of success. Google Health, for example, released to the public in May 2008, after a pilot collaboration with the Cleveland Clinic, lasted only until January 2012 (Moore, 2011). Microsoft launched HealthVault, a free PHR permitting sharing across multiple providers, in 2007; after several name changes, the platform and associated apps were terminated in November of 2019 (Foley, 2019).

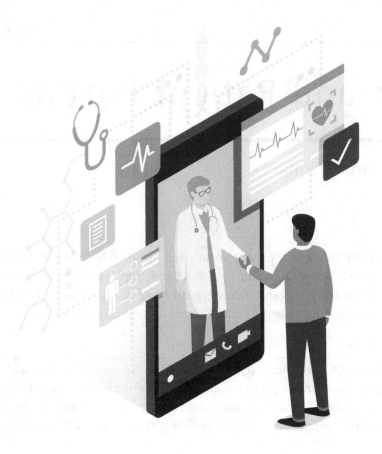

7.1.2 Patient Portals

Portals are more than straightforward documentation of one person's healthcare encounters, but place those encounters in a real-life context by serving as platforms for content and thus for information provision, education, and communication technologies. Portals typically allow the user to view test results and to communicate with their healthcare team through an electronic mail feature. Portals can also include multimedia patient education content customized by the system for the individual patient; for example, diabetes education for people living with diabetes. Portals can also be dedicated to use by particular *groups* of people; for example, a pediatric patient portal might be locked down for use only by family members of inpatients in a particular wing of a hospital and contain links to vetted information targeting the needs of those patients. Another patient portal might feature its own gated and hyperlocal online community for parents and other caregivers of pediatric patients.

7.1.3 "Tethered" versus "Untethered"

It is important to understand that neither PHRs nor patient portals provide patients with their complete medical record. Instead, the patient is an intended co-creator and targeted user of the medical record content. EHRs, on the other hand, are medicolegal repositories created by and used by healthcare providers.

"Tethered" PHRs and portals are products that connect to, and contain updated information from, the patient's official EHR maintained by the patient's healthcare providers.

"Untethered" PHRs are products that do not connect to any official medicolegal records. The content found in untethered PHRs is contributed entirely by the user.

Personal health records and their offspring patient portals are one of the main components of patient-centered e-health (discussed in detail in Part I: Chapter 1). This positions personal health information management – or PHIM – as an important factor not only on the World Wide Web, but on smartphones via both apps and text messaging (Brown, Patrick, & Pasupathy, 2013; Neyens & Childers, 2017). The guiding assumption behind the creation of both PHRs and portals is the same: that participating in creating, managing, and using their health information not only increases individuals' health knowledge, but leads consumers and patients to assume more responsibility for their individual health and well-being. Advocates for PHRs argue that because other consumer-facing health IT applications have been found to have positive effects, such as increasing patient engagement with their care, PHRs may hold the same promise.

PHR and portal technology development – and industry interest – was greatly accelerated by the HITECH Act of 2009. This federal legislation was part of the American Recovery and Reinvestment Act of 2009 (ARRA; Public Law 111–5, 2009). Under this Act, the US Centers for Medicare & Medicaid Services (CMS) Electronic Health Record Incentive Program was able to incentivize healthcare professionals and hospitals to adopt "Meaningful Use" of EHRs. Meaningful Use (MU) took place in three sliding stages. For Stage 1, beginning in 2014, healthcare providers were required to give patients access to health information; Stage 2, required that the provider's system support not just access, but *interaction* by patients with that system and with their providers. The Core Measures established for Stage 2 included two measures specific to patients:

#7. Provide patients the ability to view online, download, and transmit their health information.

#17. Use secure electronic messaging to communicate with patients on relevant health information (Office of the National Coordinator, 2019).

Note that the specific term "patient portal" never appeared in the MU requirements. However, portals appeared to be the most effective and efficient technology to fulfill both the criteria noted above.

In 2017, MU was replaced by a different CMS program, the Medicare Access and CHIP Reauthorization Act (MACRA), which continues to incentivize clinicians' use of certified health IT. Under MACRA, clinicians target two performance categories, Advancing Care Information and Quality Measures Reporting. Provision of patient access to health data and patient engagement are still goals of the program and criteria by which clinicians are assessed (Office of the National Coordinator, 2017a, 2017b).

These technologies will continue to evolve as consumer and patient empowerment movements, healthcare industry, and economic incentives continue to push more information out of the clinic and hospital and onto the end-user. In March 2020, new regulations were announced from the Center for Medicare and Medicaid Services, as well as companion updates to ONC's Health IT Certification Criteria. The combined effect of these regulations will make patient sharing of health information easier through third party software, such as apps (Office of the National Coordinator, n.d.; Rankin, 2020).

7.2 PORTALS: AN OVERVIEW

7.2.1 History

Patients have kept records of family illnesses as long as they have been able to read and write; one family health record was a page in the family Bible or other religious text (Genetic Alliance, 2006). But the idea that an individual should maintain something as formal as a medical record is more recent. In 1912, the American pediatric neurologist John Madison Taylor (1855–1931) (Hinsdale, 1932) wrote in *Science* about the "practical advantages" of keeping family history records. Taylor suggested that heads of households should document medical content that included not just data about the growth and development of children, but information about their illnesses, injuries and surgical operations, weight and height charts, clinical data and laboratory findings, and photographs and various memoranda relating to the person's anatomy and teeth (p. 482). Dr. Taylor argued that this would enable the collection of accurate data. However, Taylor's designated audience for that data seems to have been not the head of the household themselves, but rather specialists like Dr. Taylor: families that collected data would benefit "the scientific research worker, especially the physiologist, the psychologist, eugenist, human-economist and sundry others" (Taylor, 1912, p. 481).

The first published research into medical records designed for and *stored* by patients, as opposed to healthcare practitioners, was a pilot study in 1964, involving public health practitioners and migrant farmworkers (Zusman, 1964). This "patient-held record" in this study was still authored and controlled by healthcare providers, not patients, but because of the mobility of this population, the innovation was that this record was carried by and then handed over by patients *to* healthcare workers whenever they required care at a different clinic. Twenty years later, a number of studies investigated the effect of providing patients with copies of their medical records (Giglio & Papazian, 1987), a practice considered quite controversial at the time and, even in 2020, it remains a point of debate (see *Challenges*, below).

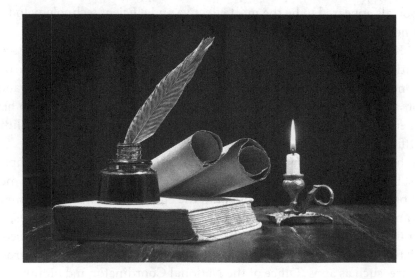

7.2.2 Current Status

Since the advent of Meaningful Use (MU) and its successor MACRA, PHR and portal products are referred to by the health IT industry under the umbrella term *patient engagement*. The HIMSS (Health Information Management Systems Society) Leadership Survey polls health IT leaders in healthcare and technology organizations in the US. The 2019 Survey asked respondents to rate health IT priorities for the coming year on a 1–7 scale, with 7 the highest priority. "Consumer/Patient Engagement & Digital/Connected Health" [the two priorities appear in one item] was ranked 4.95 by vendors and consultants, 4.80 by hospitals, and 4.44 by providers (HIMSS, 2019). Enthusiasm for the portal in the industry continues to grow. In 2016, a separate HIMSS survey revealed that 58% of industry leaders had mobile-optimized patient portals in their hospital or health system (HIMSS, 2016). In 2020, 70 healthcare professionals – Chief Information Officers, executives, and directors in 65 US healthcare systems – were asked about their key patient engagement strategies; 82% named the patient portal as their top technology, followed by telemedicine (33%) and secure communication (18%) (Center for Connected Medicine, 2020). These figures attest to the importance of patient engagement to the industry, and thus to the importance of patient portals. Most telling, perhaps, is *Medical Economics* magazine's 2018 EHR Report Card (the most current available at this writing). Ninety-four percent of physician respondents had been using an EHR for more than a year, and 49% had used three or more systems (Economics, 2018). Only 28% felt that their EHR had improved the quality of care in the practice. Despite this, 33% of respondents indicated that their EHR had improved communication with their patients via portals – 26% agreed that it had improved patient access to their records.

How many patients use portals? Statistics are difficult to find, in part because "usage" means different things to different researchers. Potential interest in a technology and *adoption* of a technology are also two different things – registration for portals is not the same thing as using them (Archer et al., 2011). Small wonder that with only 17% of organizations reporting high engagement through health IT, patients were named by Connected Medicine's health IT leaders (2020) as "the biggest roadblock" to patient engagement (p. 7).

Woods et al. (2017) argue that what is needed to understand takeup of portals is evidence of "sustained usage over time" (para 1). Fraccaro et al. (2017) was the first study to summarize portal adoption rates. These authors reviewed 40 published studies of portals, the majority published after 2010 and representing research primarily done in the United States. Their definition of adoption was "the % of eligible patients who logged in at least once or – if this information was not available – had an active account during the study period" (p. 80). Fraccaro et al. found a range of adoption rates from 42% to 62%. They distinguished between two kinds of portal studies. In "controlled" experiments, patients were recruited to participate, and the patient portal was marketed to these prospective users. Conversely, in "real-world" experiments, no recruitment or even marketing occurred, and the portal system was simply observed without any intervention by the researchers. There proved to be a large difference between the two types of studies. In the 24 controlled experiments, the mean adoption rate was 71%, but in the other 16 real-world experiments, the mean adoption rate was 23%.

The largest real-world study to date focused on the very large Kaiser Permanente system, with over 2.4 million adult members in California (Gordon & Hornbrook, 2016). Users aged 65–79 were surveyed; of these, 72% had registered to use their portal.

The Veterans Administration (VA) portal, My HealtheVet, is one of the longest-running and most investigated portal systems. It is free to everybody in the United States, regardless of their veteran status; however, only veterans receiving care through the VA healthcare system are able to view portions of their medical record using this portal, making it a *tethered* system for veterans and an *untethered* system for everybody else. In the first quarter of 2019 (Oct-Dec), the VA reported 113,713 new registrations; 2,482,661 active users; and 1,457,123 downloads of medical records. Thirty-seven percent of these users are accessing their portal using a mobile device; the VA has a suite of apps for veteran health (Veterans Administration, 2019).

The HINTS (Health Information National Trends Survey) data from 2019 revealed that 60% of the patients surveyed who *could* access their medical records online, presumably through a portal, did look at those records; 20% viewed them more than three times (Health Information National Trends Survey, 2019).

Despite all this activity, there is little empirical evidence for positive *clinical* outcomes of PHR usage. Tenforde, Jain, and Hickner (2011) conducted an extensive literature review of research on PHRs and chronic disease management, published between 2000 and 2010, and found mixed and inconsistent results. Only three of 1417 articles focused on clinical outcomes, and all of these were studies of type 2 diabetes. However, none of those three studies investigated the effect of PHR access *alone*, but rather looked at PHRs in the context of other forms of care tools. Two studies published after Tenforde et al.'s review have demonstrated clinical effects. Shimada, Allison, Rosen, Feng, and Houston (2016) examined the role of secure messaging on users living with type 2 diabetes and found that *sustained* use of the messaging within the patient portal was significantly associated with control of blood sugar levels. Mortimer, et al. (2015) deployed a personal health record as part of a platform called Healthy.me. This system targeted young people aged 18–29. Its features included not only PHIM supports such as a schedule, but a "pillbox" medication minder, appointment scheduler, social features, and an educational intervention to prevent sexually transmitted infections (STI). The researchers found a significant increase in STI testing among participants who used Healthy.me.

Despite the limited and mixed evidence for clinical outcomes, patients still tend to be positive about increased access to information through their portals, and the greater amount of medical record content that they acquire once they log on (Archer et al., 2011). Seventy-eight percent of the low-income, ethnically diverse consumers surveyed by Patel et al. (2011) believed the information they viewed in their PHRs would help their own understanding of their healthcare. PHRs seem to have a motivational effect on patients to serve as monitors of their own health data. And information and communication are necessarily intertwined. The cancer patients investigated by Komura et al. found writing in a paper PHR easier than talking to their physicians – they could know that staff "understood what they felt" by reading their PHR (Komura et al., 2013).

Less is known about portal users than the statistics quoted above would suggest. Adults living with diabetes have received most of the attention in what research literature exists (Byczkowski, Munafo, & Britto, 2014). Comparatively little research has been done on patients not living with diabetes. However, inpatient portals – that is, patient portals for use in the hospital – are an emerging area of interest. A study of all patients admitted for surgery at Vanderbilt University between 2012 and 2014 focused on inpatient portals. The most frequent usage was by patients who were White and male, which contradicted outpatient portal studies that found only slight gender differences. Four percent of all surgical patients, but 16% of all registered patients, used their portals during this time period (Robinson, 2016). Inpatient portals are now being investigated in pediatric practice; see the section on children and young adults in Part I: Chapter 6.

Patient portals began as Web-based services, intended for access outside of clinical settings. However, they have begun their migration into the hospital, where inpatients can read the results of their own lab tests just minutes to hours after the test was conducted. MyChart Bedside is an inpatient application of the MyChart patient portal. Seventy-four percent of patients in one 2017 study (Winstanley et al., 2017) reported that MyChart Bedside improved communication with their nurse – not so much with their physician (52%) – as well as their understanding of medications (90%). This technology has potential for improving – in real time – not only the patient's understanding of the healthcare process and the course of their illness, but that of their family members and other home support as well.

7.2.3 Exemplar Users of Patient Portals

From the beginning, patient portal users have been described as members of three principal groups: "people with disabilities and chronic conditions, frequent users of healthcare services, and people caring for elderly parents" (Archer et al., 2011, p. 518). Clearly these three groups overlap a good deal. People living with chronic illness were found in one study to be 25% more likely to adopt these technologies (Madrigal & Escoffery, 2019).

The author's perusal of medical literature published between 1991 and 2017 about personal health records – paper-based or electronic – as well as the related technologies, patient-held records, and patient portals, yielded 26 studies in which children and young adults were either involved, or represented by their parents. The vast majority of logins to portals were found, in one study, to be done by parents and other surrogates – even in the case of adolescents (Steitz et al., 2017). The role of "caregiver" has grown to encompass not only family members caring for seniors, but parents of children and adolescents, for example, children living with special healthcare needs. These are children with developmental, physical, or mental disabilities (Rocha et al., 2007), for example, those on the autism spectrum (Bush et al., 2016) or living with inflammatory bowel disease (Schneider et al., 2016). Parents and family members of children on multiple medications face not only a burden of caregiving, but the burden of "recalling and explaining the history and medication lists" (Jubrai & Blair, 2015); My Medication Passport, began as a patient-held record for elderly patients, then evolved into an app, and was eventually deployed among families with children to meet their health information management needs (My Medication Passport, n.d.). Inpatient use of portals is now attracting interest in pediatrics. A team at the University of Wisconsin-Madison, with investigators drawn from pediatrics, informatics, and engineering, is evaluating the use of MyChart Bedside for families of inpatients at a local children's hospital (Kelly, 2017; Smith et al., 2020). For a general discussion of the interaction between caregivers and CHIT, see Part I: Chapter 6.

Ronis et al. comment that few PHRs have been developed for pediatric patients and families, in part because of "persistently low levels of awareness" on the part of patients and caregivers, while on the other hand, healthcare providers showed "low levels of preparedness" for engagement with these technologies (2015, p. 766). Unsurprisingly, although attitudes toward patient portals were generally positive among the parents surveyed in this study, whether they used portals or not, 36% indicated that they had not used portals because they had not known they were available. Healthcare systems have to promote these products in order for patients – and their family members – to become engaged. Children who grow into adulthood with the experience of illness, and whose parents use portals to help manage their care, may be more likely to become portal adopters themselves. The needs and demands of users in many different age groups and household compositions must be considered in design, rollout, and outreach about these technologies.

7.3 STANDARDS AFFECTING PHRS/PORTALS

Patient portal content relies on content of electronic health records (EHR) and, for this reason, the standards that inform EHRs also inform portals. Portal user interfaces, however, have been shown to be a significant obstacle to portal use. Third-party development in portals is typically not permitted by vendors (Baldwin, Singh, Sittig, & Giardina, 2017), but as noted above, recent updates to ONC's Health IT Certification Program are expected to smooth the way (Office of the National Coordinator, n.d.). For one example of an open platform supporting app development drawing on EHR content, see SMART Health IT at https://smarthealthit.org. For an example of a standards framework for health IT, investigate FHIR at Fast Healthcare Interoperability Resources: hl7.org/fhir.

While PHR vendors can use various proprietary formats that are not inspectable from the outside, there are also open standards used to organize the data in these products. Roehrs, da Costa, Righi, and de Oliveira (2017) point to standards in nomenclature and terminology (e.g., the Unified Medical Language System; see Part I, Chapter 3); privacy (e.g., HIPAA); structure and semantics (e.g., the Health Level 7 or HL7 family of standards); and templates and technology platforms (e.g., OpenMRS at openMRS.org).

7.3.1 Key Standards Organizations and Resources for Standards Development in Healthcare

HL7 (www.hl7.org): This ANSI-accredited, not-for-profit organization develops frameworks and standards for "exchange, integration, sharing, and retrieval of electronic health information." Members are drawn from more than 50 countries and include stakeholders not only from healthcare but the government, the pharmaceutical industry, vendors, and consultants.

Office of the National Coordinator of Health IT (ONC) (www.healthit.gov): Mandated through the Health Information Technology for Economic and Clinical Health Act (HITECH Act) of 2009, ONC is "the principal federal entity charged with coordination of nationwide efforts to implement and use the most advanced health information technology and the electronic exchange of health information."

7.4 PORTAL CHARACTERISTICS AND CONTENTS

Bouayad, Ialynytchev, and Padmanabhan (2019) analyzed PHR and portal research literature published from 1950 to 2015. These authors defined as the PHR as "an electronic record designed for patients to self-manage care" – a definition that includes both apps and portals – and developed an exhaustive list of data elements they found reported there.

The data elements occurring most frequently in the systems researched were health history, treatments, patient general information, and diagnostics. Details appear in Table 7.1.

Data formats used ranged from text and metadata (email) through images (radiology results, lab tests) to audio and video (recorded visits with healthcare providers, for example) (Bouayad, Ialynytchev, & Padmanabhan, 2017).

Typical functions of PHRs and portals include appointment scheduling, prescription refills, and messaging to specific clinics and healthcare providers. Users can view test results, medication lists, notes generated at prior visits, and, increasingly, small portions of text from clinical documents in their official record (see *Challenges* below). Links to external web resources, such as Laboratory Tests Online and other patient education sites, enhance the content of the record. While core functions are similar across PHR and portal products, external resources vary, based largely on decisions made by healthcare systems and health insurance companies. Some of these features are more popular than others. Consider this snapshot from the VA's My HealtheVet service, data collected from July 2017 to June 2018. Fifty-one percent of users refilled prescriptions, 38% looked at appointment information, 25% tracked delivery of prescriptions, 23% reviewed their history of medications, and 19% viewed lab test results (Veterans Administration, 2019).

7.5 CHALLENGES

As PHRs and patient portals continue to evolve with technology, the principal challenges for both the health IT and healthcare industries arise because of human factors: privacy and disparities in access.

7.5.1 Privacy

Concerns over *data privacy* and *confidentiality* affect the chances of a potential user adopting, then using, these technologies. For example, Pevnick et al. (2016) investigated the attitudes of people using personal fitness trackers (PFTs) in a large non-profit hospital setting. Of 66,105 registered patients, with very little promotion on the part of the healthcare

TABLE 7.1   Typical PHR and Portal Data Elements, 1950–2015*

Category	Elements
Patient general information	Personal information
	Psychographics
	Genetic data
	Preferences
	PHR settings
Scheduling	Appointments
	Facility information
	Personalized search results
	Provider information
Visits	Outpatient visit information
	Visit preparation information
Diagnostics	Vital signs and anthropometric data
	Physiological information
	Results
History of present illness	Allergies
	Diagnostic
	Health state

* From Bouayad et al., 2019.

system, only .8% uploaded data in the first 37 days and displayed little interest in sharing their PFT data with their healthcare team. People who *were* interested in sharing were likely to be younger, male, White, lower-income, and have a higher body mass index. The worse a user's health status, the less likely that user was to share their health data (see Part II: Chapter 11 for an extended discussion of privacy concerns as they relate to consumer health informatics technologies).

7.5.2 Digital Divide

Well-documented disparities between technology skills and usage across racial/ethnic and socioeconomic groups play a role in uptake of PHRs and portals as well. Patel et al. (2011) conducted an outpatient study and found decreased use of portals by minorities, especially African Americans. Patients from populations with greater medical need are "significantly less likely" to use portals (Sarkar et al., 2014). Wallace et al. (2016) investigated adoption and use of Epic MyChart during the first year of deployment in a large underserved patient population in 13 US states. Only 29% of patients accessed their portals, with 6% of those identified as "superusers" logging in at least twice a month. Men, non-Whites, and Latinx patients were much less likely to log in than women, Whites, or non-Latinx.

Peacock et al. found that healthcare providers had a large role to play in adoption of portals by patients. Ninety-two percent of respondents to a national survey (N = 3677) considered access to portals important, only 34% reported that they had been offered such access by their healthcare providers, and only 28% had accessed that information. While Black and Latinx respondents were just as likely to consider access important, they were less likely to have heard about it from their providers (Peacock et al., 2017).

However, an overall interest in health information seeking and managing personal health information were characteristics associated with patient portal usage in an underserved population (Nambisan, 2017). To increase adoption, Lyles et al. (2016) recommend that healthcare systems require user-friendly design and content in multiple languages for portals, as well as engage not only in training for portal users, but outreach to the family members and caregivers who support patients at home.

In 2017, Woods et al. investigated portal usage by VA patients and considered the effects not only of race but of gender. Women were represented at a rate larger than the proportion of women in the VA population generally. "Usage" was operationalized not as registration for the VA portal, but as actual logins to the system. These researchers found no statistically significant differences in log in behavior by age, gender, education level, marital status, race/ethnicity, or distance from a VA facility. Self-reported health status, having a specific chronic condition, smoking status, or having previously obtained copies of health records were not significantly associated with variation in usage. Instead, the three statistically significant factors correlated with portal usage were all related to the internet itself. Patients in this study were more likely to use portals if they:

(1) had broadband access to the internet;

(2) indicated a high self-rating of their ability to use the internet; and.

(3) indicated "high" internet use behavior, measured by activities such as using email, shopping, banking, using social networks, and searching for health information.

This study has many implications not only for the future of patient portals and PHRs, but of consumer health informatics tools in general (Woods et al., 2017).

7.6 EXPANDING TECHNOLOGICAL HEALTH ACCESS

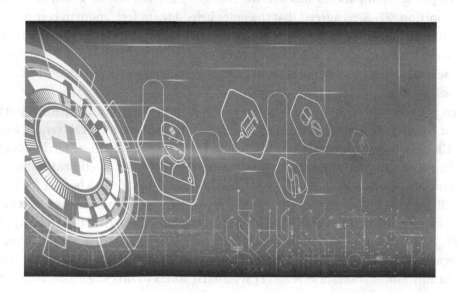

7.6.1 Future Directions

7.6.1.1 Expanding Markets

Market researchers at Rock Health report that venture funding for digital health in 2019 received nearly one of every ten venture dollars in the US – that year startups in this category raised $7.4 billion (Day & Gambon, 2020). Patient engagement and patient empowerment is big business (for more on older adults as a market opportunity, see Part I: Chapter 6). After some initial stumbles in the 2000s (see above), not only Google but Samsung, Apple, and Microsoft have developed health self-monitoring platforms to become "hubs" for individuals' sensor data; that data can then be shared with healthcare providers (see also Part II: Chapter 9). Their platforms are, respectively, Google Fit, Apple HealthKit, Microsoft Band, and the Samsung Digital Health Initiative. The Apple Watch Series 4, for example, was the first product to receive clearance from the US Food and Drug Administration (FDA). It enables the wearer's electrocardiogram (ECG) readings to be sent to their physicians via the PHR feature, Apple Health Records. Healthcare partners with Apple include Epic Systems and the Mayo Clinic (for a growing list of healthcare institutions that can work with Apple's Health app, see https://support.apple.com/en-us/HT208647; for more on apps as a CHI technology, see Part II: Chapter 8).

7.6.1.2 Expanding Access

The question of how much of their medical records patients should be able to see has been a longstanding debate in healthcare. Consumer health informatics technologies have the potential to greatly affect the balance of power between physician and patient simply by providing the patient with more information about themselves. In 2010, a movement called Open Notes began as a collaborative experiment between hospitals in Boston, Pennsylvania, and Seattle. Twenty thousand patients were given the opportunity to read their clinical notes – textual summaries of their doctor visits – using their patient portals. In two of the study sites – Pennsylvania and Boston – 82% of patients opened the notes, while in Seattle, only 47% did.

The response from patients was overwhelmingly positive (Walker et al., 2011). A very high proportion (77–87%) agreed that the notes helped them feel "more in control of their care." Clinical outcomes were also positive: by self-report, 60–78% reported increased adherence to their medications. As a result of this early success, many health systems in the US and several Canadian systems are now engaging in Open Notes (for an up-to-date map, see https://www.opennotes.org/join/map/).

When patients and their families access health information through patient portals, a small but consistent minority of them experience confusion over medical terminology (see Part I: Chapter 3 for a discussion of the relationship between medical terminology and health literacy). That terminology has been a barrier not just for clinical notes but for understanding laboratory test results (Byczkowski et al., 2014). It was a barrier for 1–10% of the 20,000 patients in the original Open Notes experiment who reported their notes caused them "confusion, worry or offense" and for 18% of respondents to the HINTS study of 2017 (Bazzoli, 2018; Walker et al., 2011). The challenge for the future, then, is how to meet the needs, reassure the fears, educate and reach out to that small minority. In August 2016, the Kaiser Family Foundation surveyed 1211 registered voters to investigate the demographic characteristics of patients accessing their medical records or personal information online. The higher the level of education and income, the greater the likelihood of access; conversely, 49% of respondents with a high school education or less had not accessed their records or information, nor had 47% of those with incomes below $40 K. The original Open Notes study enrolled mostly patients who were already experienced in using portals. Does their experience resemble that of the portal-naïve, non-internet savvy, and generally less healthy consumers referred to by Lyles et al.? (Lyles et al., 2016). Only time – and a considerable investment of research – will tell.

WEB RESOURCES

Open Notes
"Movement Hub" for patient access to medical record content in real time.
https://www.opennotes.org/

HealthIT.gov

Patient Access to Health Records
One-stop shop for all issues involving patient PHRs and portals. Explanation of patient rights of access, and information for the developer and vendor community.
https://www.healthit.gov/topic/patient-access-health-records/patient-access-health-records
The Guide to Getting and Using Your Health Records
Comprehensive guide to rights and access, with links to HIPAA information, guides to requesting copies and correcting errors in your record, and other useful tools.
https://www.healthit.gov/how-to-get-your-health-record/

REFERENCES

Archer, N., Fevrier-Thomas, U., Lokker, C., McKibbon, K. A., & Straus, S. E. (2011). Personal health records: A scoping review. *Journal of the American Medical Informatics Association*, 18(4), 515–522. doi:10.1136/amiajnl-2011-000105

ARRA; Public Law 111–5, 2009, *American Recovery and Reinvestment Act of 2009. Public Law 111–5.* https://www.gpo.gov/fdsys/pkg/PLAW-111publ5/html/PLAW-111publ5.htm.

Baldwin, J. L., Singh, H., Sittig, D. F., & Giardina, T. D. (2017). Patient portals and health apps: Pitfalls, promises, and what one might learn from the other. *Healthcare(Amst)*, 5(3), 81–85. doi:10.1016/j.hjdsi.2016.08.004

Bazzoli, F. (2018, October 8). *Individuals' use of online medical records is on the rise.* Available online: https://www.healthdatamanagement.com/list/individuals-use-of-online-medical-records-is-on-the-rise. Date accessed: 10/10/2018.

Bouayad, L., Ialynytchev, A., & Padmanabhan, B. (2017). Patient health record systems scope and functionalities: Literature review and future directions. *Journal of medical Internet research*, 19(11), e388. doi:10.2196/jmir.8073

Bouayad, L., Ialynytchev, A., & Padmanabhan, B. (2019). Multimedia appendix correction: Patient health record systems scope and functionalities: Literature review and future directions. *Journal of medical Internet research*, 21(9), e15796. doi:10.2196/15796

Brown, G.D., Patrick, T.B., & Pasupathy, K.S. (2013). *Health informatics: A systems perspective.* Chicago: Health Administration Press.

Bush, R. A., Stahmer, A. C., & Connelly, C. D. (2016). Exploring perceptions and use of the electronic health record by parents of children with autism spectrum disorder: A qualitative study. *Health Informatics J*, 22(3), 702–711. doi:10.1177/1460458215581911

Byczkowski, T. L., Munafo, J. K., & Britto, M. T. (2014). Family perceptions of the usability and value of chronic disease web-based patient portals. *Health Informatics J*, 20(2), 151–162. doi:10.1177/1460458213489054

Center for Connected Medicine (2020). Patient portal is the primary engagement tool employed by health systems, survey finds. https://connectedmed.com/blog/content/patient-portal-the-primary-engagement-tool-employed-by-health-systems

Day, S., & Gambon, E. (2020). *In 2019, digital health celebrated six IPOs as venture investment edged off record highs.* https://rockhealth.com/reports/in-2019-digital-health-celebrated-six-ipos-as-venture-investment-edged-off-record-highs/

Delbanco, T., Walker, J., Bell, S.K., et al. (2011). Inviting patients to read their doctors' notes: a quasi-experimental study and a look ahead. *Ann Intern Med*. 157(7):461-470. doi:10.7326/0003-4819-157-7-201210020-00002

Fraccaro, P., Vigo, M., Balatsoukas, P., Buchan, I. E., Peek, N., & van der Veer, S. N. (2017). Patient portal adoption rates: A systematic literature review and meta-analysis *Studies in Health Technology & Informatics*, 245, 79–83.

Genetic Alliance. (2006). Does it run in the family? A guide to family health history. http://www.geneticalliance.org/sites/default/files/publicationsarchive/book1ga_ll022309.pdf

Giglio, R.J., & Papazian, B. (1987). Acceptance and use of patient-carried health records. *Journal of the American Medical Record Association*, 58(5):32–36.

Gordon, N. P., & Hornbrook, M. C. (2016). Differences in access to and preferences for using patient portals and other ehealth technologies based on race, ethnicity, and age: A database and survey study of seniors in a large health plan. *J Med Internet Res*, 18(3), e50. doi:10.2196/jmir.5105

HIMSS (2016). *2016 Connected Health Survey Executive Summary.* https://www.himss.org/2016-connected-health-survey/executive-summary.

HIMSS (2018, January). *2018 HIMSS U.S. Leadership and Workforce Survey.* https://www.himss.org/sites/himssorg/files/u132196/2018_HIMSS_US_LEADERSHIP_WORKFORCE_SURVEY_Final_Report.pdf.

HIMSS (2019, February). *2019 HIMSS U.S. Leadership and Workforce Survey.* https://www.himss.org/resources/himss-leadership-and-workforce-survey-report.

Hinsdale, G. (1932). Dr. John Madison Taylor. *Transactions of the American Climatological and Clinical Association*, 48, xli.

HINTS (Health Information National Trends Survey). (2019). https://hints.cancer.gov.

Jubrai, B., & Blair, M. (2015). Use of a medication passport in a disabled child seen across many care settings. *BMJ Case Rep*, 2015. doi:10.1136/bcr-2014-208,033

Kelly, M. (2017, April 18). *Partnering with parents of hospitalized children using an inpatient portal.* https://www.hipxchange.org/InpatientPortal.

Komura, K., Yamagishi, A., Akizuki, N., Kawagoe, S., Kato, M., Morita, T., & Eguchi, K. (2013). Patient-perceived usefulness and practical obstacles of patient-held records for cancer patients in japan: OPTIM study. *Palliative Medicine*, 27(2), 179–184. doi:10.1177/0269216311431758

Lyles, C. R., Sarkar, U., Schillinger, D., Ralston, J. D., Allen, J. Y., Nguyen, R., & Karter, A. J. (2016). Refilling medications through an online patient portal: consistent improvements in adherence across racial/ethnic groups. *Journal of the American Medical Informatics Association : JAMIA*, 23(e1), e28–e33. https://doi.org/10.1093/jamia/ocv126

Madrigal, L., & Escoffery, C. (2019). Electronic health behaviors among US adults with chronic disease: Cross-sectional survey. *Journal of Medical Internet Research*, 21(3), e11240. https://doi.org/10.2196/11240

Medical Economics. (2018). EHR Report Card. https://www.medicaleconomics.com/ehr/2018-ehr-report-card.

Moore, J. (2011). *RIP Google Health*. Retrieved from https://www.chilmarkresearch.com/rip-google-health/

Mortimer, N. J., Rhee, J., Guy, R., Hayen, A., & Lau, A. Y. (2015). A web-based personally controlled health management system increases sexually transmitted infection screening rates in young people: A randomized controlled trial. *J Am Med Inform Assoc*, 22(4), 805–814. doi:10.1093/jamia/ocu052

My Medication Passport, n.d. http://myhealthapps.net/app/details/398/My-Medication-Passport

Nambisan P. (2017). Factors that impact Patient Web Portal Readiness (PWPR) among the underserved. *International Journal of Medical Informatics*, 102, 62–70. https://doi.org/10.1016/j.ijmedinf.2017.03.004

Neyens, D. M., & Childers, A. K. (2017). Determining barriers and facilitators associated with willingness to use a personal health information management system to support worksite wellness programs. *Am J Health Promot*, 31(4), 310–317. doi:10.4278/ajhp.140514-QUAN-204

Office of the National Coordinator. (2017a, September 21). *Advancing Care Information reporting*. https://www.healthit.gov/topic/federal-incentive-programs/MACRA/MIPS/advancing-care-information-reporting.

Office of the National Coordinator. (2017b, September 5). *Meaningful Use: Meaningful Use and the shift to the merit-based incentive payment system*. https://www.healthit.gov/topic/federal-incentive-programs/meaningful-use.

Office of the National Coordinator. (2019, January 7). *2015 Standards Hub*. https://www.healthit.gov/topic/certification/2015-standards-hub

Office of the National Coordinator. (n.d.) *Application Programming Interfaces (APIs): Certification criterion and associated conditions*. https://www.healthit.gov/sites/default/files/nprm/ONCCuresNPRMAPICertification.pdf.

Patel, V. N., Dhopeshwarkar, R. V., Edwards, A., Barron, Y., Likourezos, A., Burd, L.,. .. Kaushal, R. (2011). Low-income, ethnically diverse consumers' perspective on health information exchange and personal health records. *Inform Health Soc Care*, 36(4), 233–252. doi:10.3109/17538157.2011.554930

Peacock, S., Reddy, A., Leveille, S. G., Walker, J., Payne, T. H., Oster, N. V., & Elmore, J. G. (2017). Patient portals and personal health information online: perception, access, and use by US adults. *Journal of the American Medical Informatics Association : JAMIA*, 24(e1), e173–e177. https://doi.org/10.1093/jamia/ocw095

Pevnick, J.M., Fuller, G., Duncan, R., & Spiegel, B.M.R. (2016) A large-scale initiative inviting patients to share personal fitness tracker data with their providers: Initial results. *PLoS One*, 11(11): e0165908. https://journals.plos.org/plosone/article?id=10.1371/journal.pone.0165908

Rankin, J. (2020, April 15). It's time to expand our thinking about interoperability. *Health IT Outcomes*. https://www.healthitoutcomes.com/doc/it-s-time-to-expand-our-thinking-about-interoperability-0001.

Robinson, J. R., Huth, H., & Jackson, G. P. (2016). Review of information technology for surgical patient care. *The Journal of Surgical Research*, 203(1), 121–139. https://doi.org/10.1016/j.jss.2016.03.053

Rocha, R. A., Romeo, A.N., & Nortlin, C. (2007). Core features of a parent-controlled pediatric medical home record. In *Medinfo* (pp. 997–1001): IOS Press.

Roehrs, A., da Costa, C. A., Righi, R. D., & de Oliveira, K. S. (2017). Personal health records: A systematic literature review. *J Med Internet Res*, 19(1), e13. doi:10.2196/jmir.5876

Sarkar, U., Lyles, C. R., Parker, M. M., Allen, J., Nguyen, R., Moffet, H. H., Schillinger, D., & Karter, A. J. (2014). Use of the refill function through an online patient portal is associated with improved adherence to statins in an integrated health system. *Medical Care*, 52(3), 194–201. https://doi. org/10.1097/MLR.0000000000000069

Schneider, H., Hill, S., & Blandford, A. (2016). Patients know best: Qualitative study on how families use patient-controlled personal health records. *Journal of Medical Internet Research*, 18(2), e43. doi:10.2196/jmir.4652

Shimada, S. L., Allison, J. J., Rosen, A. K., Feng, H., & Houston, T. K. (2016). Sustained use of patient portal features and improvements in diabetes physiological measures. *J Med Internet Res*, 18(7), e179. doi:10.2196/jmir.5663

Smith, C. A., Coller, R. J., Dean, S. M., Sklansky, D., Hoonakker, P., Smith, W., Thurber, A. S., Ehlenfeldt, B. D., & Kelly, M. M. (2020). Parent perspectives on pediatric inpatient OpenNotes. AMIA. *Annual Symposium Proceedings*: 812–819.

Somner, J. E., Sii, F., Bourne, R., Cross, V., & Shah, P. (2013). What do patients with glaucoma think about personal health records? *Ophthalmic Physiol Opt*, 33(6), 627–633. doi:10.1111/opo.12084

Steitz, B., Cronin, R. M., Davis, S. E., Yan, E., & Jackson, G. P. (2017). Long-term patterns of patient portal use for pediatric patients at an academic medical center. *Appl Clin Inform*, 8(3), 779–793. doi:10.4338/aci-2017-01-ra-0005

Taylor, J.M. (1912). Personal registration of family memoranda: A plea for the making and preserving of homely annals. *Science*, 36(928): 480–482.

Tenforde, M., Jain, A., & Hickner, J. (2011). The value of personal health records for chronic disease management: What do we know? *Fam Med*, 43(5), 351–354.

Veterans Administration. (2019, Nov. 29). *VA mobile apps*. https://www.myhealth.va.gov/ mhv-portal-web/mobile-apps

Walker, J., Leveille, S. G., Ngo, L., Vodicka, E., Darer, J. D., Dhanireddy, S., Elmore, J. G., Feldman, H. J., Lichtenfeld, M. J., Oster, N., Ralston, J. D., Ross, S. E., & Delbanco, T. (2011). Inviting patients to read their doctors' notes: Patients and doctors look ahead: Patient and physician surveys. *Annals of Internal Medicine*, 155(12), 811–819. https://doi.org/10.7326/0003-4819-155-12-201112200-00003

Wallace, L. S., Angier, H., Huguet, N., Gaudino, J. A., Krist, A., Dearing, M., Killerby, M., Marino, M., & DeVoe, J. E. (2016). Patterns of electronic portal use among vulnerable patients in a nationwide practice-based research network: From the OCHIN Practice-based Research Network (PBRN). *Journal of the American Board of Family Medicine : JABFM*, 29(5), 592–603. https://doi. org/10.3122/jabfm.2016.05.160046

Winstanley, E. L., Burtchin, M., Zhang, Y., Campbell, P., Pahl, J., Beck, S., & Bohenek, W. (2017). Inpatient experiences with MyChart Bedside. *Telemed J E Health*, 23(8), 691–693. doi:10.1089/ tmj.2016.0132

Woods, S. S., Forsberg, C. W., Schwartz, E. C., Nazi, K. M., Hibbard, J. H., Houston, T. K., & Gerrity, M. (2017). The association of patient factors, digital access, and online behavior on sustained patient portal use: A prospective cohort of enrolled users. *J Med Internet Res*, 19(10), e345. doi:10.2196/jmir.7895

Zusman, J. (1964). A study of use of health records by 83 California families. *Am J Public Health*, 54, 908–917.

CHAPTER 8

There Is an App for That

The Universe and the Promise of Consumer Health Mobile Apps

Alla Keselman

MOBILE APPS ARE SOFTWARE applications designed to run on phones and tablets, taking advantage of these devices' unique features, such as touch screen interface. Growing presence of smartphones has resulted in the emergence of mobile apps in a variety of domains, including consumer health. This chapter overviews the existing universe of consumer health apps, including their content domains and functions, and presents several approaches to classifying apps in order to think about their development and evaluation systematically. These approaches include classifying apps on the basis of the tasks they perform (e.g., data collection and processing), on the basis of a phase of patient experience they support (e.g., aftermath of receiving a diagnosis), or on the basis of their integration with a healthcare system. The chapter discusses challenges of health apps' quality assessment and control, such as scarcity of reliable, accessible (non-proprietary) rating systems, and absence of certifying organizations. It then overviews important health apps quality criteria such as content accuracy, theoretical grounding, usability and responsiveness to user needs, and clinical effectiveness. At the present, very few app developers conduct research into clinical effectiveness of their products, but such practice of building evidence base is starting to emerge. The chapter also discusses issues of privacy and security of the data that individuals contribute into their health apps. These privacy and security issues are complicated by the fact that most app developers and owners are not covered by existing laws governing healthcare information exchanges. Lastly, the chapter discusses practical challenges of findings good health apps, related to difficulty of searching app stores and doctors' limited familiarity with apps and reluctance to recommend them.

8.1 INTRODUCTION: WHY APPS?

The term "mobile application," or simply "app," refers to software programs specifically designed to run on operating systems of tablets and smartphones. Unlike mobile websites, which largely mirror features and functionality of computer websites, apps take advantage of unique features of mobile devices, most notably, the touch screen. A mobile app is "usually smaller in scope than a mobile website, offers more interactivity, and presents more specific information in a format that's easy and intuitive to use on a mobile device" (Viswanathan, 2019).

The ubiquity of smartphones has resulted in the emergence of mobile apps in many areas of human activity including personal finance, education, and entertainment. Health is also becoming an area where the number and functional diversity of apps are growing rapidly. In addition to ubiquity and portability, smartphones have several unique technical characteristics that greatly increase their consumer health information service potential. These include the ability to serve as sensors/monitors/recorders, ability to take photo images, and GPS function. They can also interface with other specialized sensors and devices. As a result, patient- and consumer-oriented mobile health apps can provide a much broader range of services than computer applications.

8.2 THE EVOLVING UNIVERSE OF CONSUMER HEALTH APPS

8.2.1 What Topics Are Covered in Consumer Health Apps?

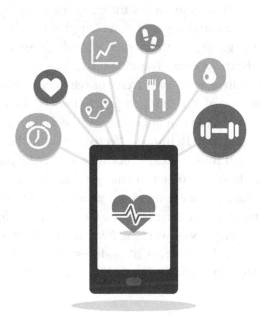

The universe of consumer health apps is an unruly one. Apps are designed and developed by a variety of very different groups with different interests, ranging from individuals driven by their own or loved ones' personal experience with a particular condition to pharmaceutical companies and academic research groups. Apps also span a broad range of domains. IQVIA (Aitken et al., 2017), a global company specializing in innovative technology solutions research, published a report of trends in digital health focusing on mobile consumer health apps. The report noted that 318,000 health apps existed on the market at the time of its publication, with 200 new apps being added every day. Most of these apps were general wellness apps, such as MyFitnessPal produced by Under Armour. The subcategories with the greatest numbers of apps included:

- exercise and fitness (30%)

- lifestyle and stress (19%)

- diet and nutrition (12%)

While wellness apps are the most prevalent, the number of apps dedicated to users' management of their diseases and conditions is growing. At the time of the IQVIA report, these constituted 40% of all health apps. The categories in order of frequencies, were:

- specific diseases (16%)

- medication reminders and information (11%)

- women's health and pregnancy (9%)

- healthcare providers and insurance (4%)

Of the disease-specific apps, 28% focused on mental health and behavioral disorders, 16% on diabetes, 11% on heart and the circulatory system, 7% each on the nervous system and musculoskeletal system, 5% each on cancer and the respiratory system (Aitken et al., 2017). These frequencies are likely to reflect a number of factors, such as prevalence of the diseases and conditions in the population, complexity of their management, and various spurious market and awareness drivers.

In this multitude, different apps fare very differently when it comes to their actual usage. The IQVIA report points out that "just 41 apps with over 10 million downloads each account for nearly half of all downloads while over 85% of all health apps have fewer than 5000 installs" (Aitken et al., 2017, p. 1). Navigating the universe of apps with little guidance, users frequently choose the apps with the highest number of downloads, thus contributing to the bimodal trend. For developers, especially small independent ones, this means that breaking into the market with good ideas is quite a challenge.

8.2.2 Features: What Do Apps Do?

Mobile technology affords the functionality that allows apps to have a range of features. For example, two research teams that independently analyzed features of consumer health apps in the context of diabetes management described a combination of the following (Arnhold et al., 2014; Årsand et al., 2012):

- **Data recording**

  - This feature enables the user to enter user-generated data or measurements. The data may include food and exercise selections or notes, blood glucose and heart rate measurements, number of steps, mood ratings, and more. Data entries may be done via a variety of forms, from manual entry to automated integration with sensors and other devices.

- **Data display and analysis**

  - This feature provides the capability to graphically display the entered data. The display may also present averages and temporal trends, making it easier for users to construct the big picture behind the individual records.

- **Data sharing/transfer**

  - Apps can have the capability of sharing the data with healthcare providers, either via automated transfer or via push by user (Årsand et al., 2012).

- **Bidirectional communication**

  - This feature involves a communication channel through which a provider can respond to a user's message or something noteworthy in the shared data. Apps can also support forum features through which users interact and support one another.

- **Reminders**

  - This very useful feature, often connected with the data recording function, reminds the user to take medication, enter data, and exercise, for example.

- **Education/information provision**

  - This feature involves providing relevant health-related information or teaching users to perform procedures.

- **Tailored advice**

  - Apps can provide specific tailored recommendations, such as nutritional guidance or a recommendation to see a doctor, based on users' recorded habits and vital signs.

While all of the above features are technically possible, it does not mean that they are common in an average app. Arnhold et al. (2014) note that when it comes to diabetes, a disease that involves complex medical and lifestyle management, most apps only include a single feature from the above list. The most common feature among the 656 diabetes apps analyzed by these authors is the ability to record data (53% of apps reviewed), followed by information provision (35%), and data transfer and communication (31% of apps). Data analysis (18%), reminders (11%), and tailored support (9%), while very potentially useful for supporting actual health behaviors, are rare.

As health management is complex, and different features support its different aspects, most effective apps combine multiple features. For example, Årsand et al. (2012) note that effective diabetes apps preferred by patients involve diverse data recording features, have sensor-enabled functions such as step counters, and include automatic data transfer capabilities. They also provide easy-to-read educational materials, enable online communication with providers and family members, and are context-sensitive. At the same time, designing multi-feature apps without sacrificing usability is a challenge. While most diabetes apps included in the review by Arnhold et al. (2014) received high ratings from experts, the more features an app included, the lower its usability score.

8.3 CLASSIFYING CONSUMER HEALTH APPS: AN ATTEMPT TO THINK SYSTEMATICALLY

When we design, support, or promote consumer health apps, understanding their relationship to the big picture of health/disease management and healthcare can help us decide what features to include. While no universally agreed-upon classification scheme exists for categorizing consumer health apps, several such schemes have been attempted and can be useful in different situations.

Many researchers studying apps and their functionality classify apps based on tasks they support (see, for example, Höhn et al., 2016). Examples of tasks may include data collection and analysis (e.g., diaries, trackers, decision support tools), appointment management, and information provision. Unfortunately, this way of categorizing apps does not provide ready insights for designers because it draws together apps from very different contexts. For example, blood glucose monitors, calorie intake calculators, and mood diaries are all data collection and processing tools. However, it is unlikely that they can meaningfully inform one another's design process. In addition, as discussed previously, the most effective apps are those that support multiple tasks, which makes classifying apps by task a challenge. For instance, a single app for diabetes patients can provide information about the disease, support food tracking, calculate needed insulin dose based on nutrition data entered by the user, send blood glucose reading to a provider, and enable communication with that professional.

The 2017 IQVIA report proposes a more useful way to categorize digital health tools, of which apps are a subcategory, in terms of their relevance to one of the locations on the spectrum of the "patient journey" (Aitken et al., 2017, p. 1). These locations, or points, include (1) Wellness and Prevention, (2) Symptoms Onset and Seeking Care, (3) Diagnosis, (4) Condition Monitoring, and (4) Treatment. Each of the points triggers unique information needs that can be met with specific mobile tools and features. While "patient journey" is an unfortunate name (living with diabetes or cancer is not exactly exotic travel), this classification system is very practical and can help structure design and development process by calling attention to identifying target users, their health status, the tasks related to that health status, and the corresponding information support that can be provided via apps. Table 8.1 provides examples of apps supporting users at different points of their "patient journey."

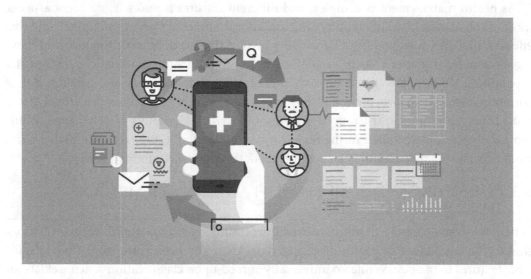

Another way to classify apps is from the perspective of their role in, and their integration into, the larger healthcare system. This perspective is most useful for developers working for the healthcare industry and/or those concerned not only with supporting patients in the larger context of their care, but with taking workload off healthcare providers. In an influential book on consumer health informatics, Wetter (2015) describes four levels of consumer health informatics services, which also apply to services provided via apps.

Wetter's Level 0 is only marginally a "service." Activity at this level is straightforward, unidirectional provision of non-tailored health-related information to a searching or browsing user. An example of a Level 0 app is a mobile app providing general narrative information about a disease or condition.

Level 1 health information service supports an existing relationship between a patient and a healthcare provider. Examples of such services include medication management tools and patient portals that collect information that may be shared with healthcare providers for review and feedback. Level 1 apps are usually produced by health insurance companies and healthcare organizations, which then offer them to their patients/clients. They may include capabilities to access medical records, send questions to providers, and manage appointments.

Level 2 are virtual services that aid care via providing screening/prevention services and supporting logistics, and, thus, do not involve interactions with healthcare providers. Examples include doctor finder and internet pharmacy apps.

Level 3 services similarly do not involve interactions with providers, but include interactions with other patients/lay individuals offering support and advice. Examples of such apps include tools that support patient forums and communities.

Wetter's taxonomy is helpful for understanding the healthcare system's sometimes uneasy relationship with mobile health technology. While providers' support and endorsement

TABLE 8.1   Apps Supporting Users at Different "Patient Journey" Points

Patient Journey Point	Types of Apps	Possible Features	Example*
Wellness and Prevention	Support tool for: - smoking cessation - diet and nutrition - exercise - sleep - meditation	- data recording - data display and analysis - reminders - education / information provision - tailored advise	MyFitnessPal - diet and exercise tracker Headspace - meditation app
Symptoms Onset and Seeking Care	Support tools for: - symptoms checking - doctor finding - appointment scheduling - general information seeking	- reminders - education / information provision	ZocDoc - medical appointment booking tool
Diagnosis**	NA	NA	NA
Condition Monitoring	Support tools for: - performing new tasks (e.g., taking measurements) - tracking vitals - recording notes - sharing data with providers	- data recording - data display and analysis - reminders - education / information provision	mySugr - diabetes data logbook and tracker Diabetes: M - diabetes data logbook and tracker Treatment / Possible features - data recording - data display and analysis - reminders - education / information provision
Treatment	Support for: - prescription filling - medication management adherence	- data recording - data display and analysis - reminders - education / information provision	Medisafe - medication reminder and tracker

* Apps are identified by their primary functions, but typically include other functions and features.
** Diagnosis happens during an interaction with a physician and is usually not supported by consumer health apps, so it is not included in this table.

could potentially help consumers with app selection and use, these professionals may be more comfortable supporting Level 1 and 2 services, as those more closely parallel doctor-patient relationships in traditional healthcare. At the same time, health insurance reimbursement systems are typically not set up to cover Level 1 services (more on this later).

8.4 CHALLENGES OF QUALITY CONTROL AND ASSESSMENT

8.4.1 Challenges of Apps Certification

In many areas of healthcare, certification agencies issue quality criteria and certify technological products that meet them. Thus, they provide a highly regarded and broadly recognized seal of approval. Examples are the Magnet and Joint Commission certifications for nursing and hospitals, respectively (American Nurses Credentialing Center, n.d.; Joint Commission, 2020). This certification can be done by government agencies in cases when it is deemed essential to safety, or by non-profit or for-profit organizations that charge fee for certification. For example, all medical devices in the US need to be reviewed and approved by the Food and Drug Administration, a federal organization. No device can make it to the market without this approval. In other areas of healthcare technology, approval is not mandatory, but serves as a well-recognized indicator of quality, which provides the developers with the incentive to seek certification. For example, The Office of the National Coordinator for Health Information Technology (Office of the National Coordinator for Health Information Technology [ONC], 2019) (https://www.healthit.gov/topic/about-onc) is a federal office that provides certification for Electronic Medical Records. While the certification is not legally mandated, virtually no healthcare facility will sign a contract with a vendor whose product is not certified. In contrast, Health on the Net Foundation (HON, 2020) is a non-governmental organization based in Switzerland that certifies health information websites. HONcode certification signals to a health-related website's users that the site had been reviewed and found to meet a number of specified quality criteria (for a more detailed review of qualified sources and HON, please refer to Part I: Chapter 5).

Despite nascent efforts, there are currently no established entities certifying health apps. The US FDA is concerned with those apps that can be classified as medical devices or accessories to medical devices, but determining which apps fit into that category is challenging on both conceptual and policy levels. Overall, apps that make specific diagnostic and treatment recommendations (e.g., calculate insulin dose based on blood glucose values) are considered devices and require regulatory oversight, while apps that provide general information and wellness recommendations are not (Powell et al., 2014). However, FDA regulation is limited to that subset of apps and is primarily concerned with safety. For example, BlueStar from Welldoc Inc (n.d.), a diabetes management app that is FDA-cleared as a medical device, provides tailored coaching and education in response to user-entered data. In contrast, an app that provides non-tailored diabetes information is not considered a device and is not regulated by the FDA.

The challenge to establishing consistent, reliable ways of certifying apps is the cost of certification. Since certification is not required by law, someone has to have an incentive to pay for it. In the case of traditional medical technology, such as devices with purely clinical functions (e.g., an infusion pump), the payers are hospitals, because they are highly interested in having quality ratings of expensive tools. In the case of apps, app users who download the apps for free or for a a small fee are not motivated to absorb the cost. If the cost is paid by developers, however, this creates a conflict of interests, as they are paying for certification of their own products. Perhaps both for that reason and because there is tradition of professional peer review in the professions that develop physician-facing technologies, more effort has gone into certifying apps oriented toward health professionals than apps oriented toward consumers.

A few entities attempted to overcome these challenges and develop app certification systems. The first was in 2013, by a company called Happtique (Kao & Liebovitz, 2017). Unfortunately, as developers were not eager to pay for certification, the Happtique library had opened with only 19 apps, several of which were hacked during the library's brief existence. Also in 2013, a leading medical informatics journal, the Journal of Medical Internet Research, or JMIR, developed and launched a process for peer-reviewing apps. App developers or manufacturers completed a questionnaire about their app and submitted the app for review by "medical and mHealth experts" who received a small fee for providing the review (a copy of the JMIR review form is listed in the Web Resources section at the end of this chapter). Certified apps could be featured in JMIR or one of its spin-off publications (e.g., JMIR mHealth). Eventually, JMIR stopped peer-reviewing apps because the model in which apps designers paid for reviews of their products proved problematic. However, JMIR mHealth and uHealth (n.d.) currently maintains a collection of JMIR-published peer-reviewed papers that includes app reviews by independent investigators (to see the collection, visit https://mhealth.jmir.org/themes/217). Other apps libraries with inclusion criteria akin to certification are described at the end of the chapter.

8.4.2 Developing Authoritative and Reliable Rating Criteria

Reliable, authoritative rating criteria that can be used to assess apps are essential to any attempt at quality control for apps, whether it be credentialing, certification, or simple assessment. Even in the absence of agreed-upon certifying organizations, the existence of agreed-upon quality rating criteria for consumer health apps could guide designers and developers, as well as users and health professionals wishing to select and recommend apps. Of course, the problem of evaluating quality of e-health resources is much older than the apps themselves. Consumer health informatics as a field has long been concerned with developing quality information criteria. Traditional information quality markers such as designer qualifications, support of claims by evidence, and transparency of designers' financial interests, codified by schemes such as HON code and DISCERN, all pertain to apps (Charnock and Shepperd, n.d.; Health On the Net Foundation [HON], 2020); see Part I: Chapter 5 for more on these standards. However, as apps are more diverse in goals and functionality than traditional websites, quality rating criteria developed for other types of health sources are unlikely to be sufficient for them.

Ultimately, good apps are the ones that contribute to their users' health and well-being. However, few apps have this kind of effectiveness data, and few developers have the resources to collect them. The most readily available and commonly used quality assessment is, thus, the user rating, available in app stores such as Android Google Play Store or iOS App Store. These ratings are subjective holistic assessments lacking clear criteria. It is not apparent what apps' characteristics are being rated, which may differ from user to user. Wetter (2015) points out that customer preferences are not necessarily a sign of either information accuracy or effectiveness. For example, although research suggests that hypnosis is not effective for smoking cessation, many self-hypnosis smoking cessation apps feature numerous endorsements by satisfied customers.

Several apps rating services have attempted to design more transparent, systematic, and comprehensive health apps rating systems based on specific criteria. Although these services are volatile and their criteria are often proprietary, the emphasis on identifying specific benchmarks for evaluating apps is very valuable. For example, Stoyanov et al. (2015) conducted a comprehensive review of papers with apps and websites quality criteria and synthesized their findings into the Mobile App Rating Scale, or MARS. This assessment instrument includes subscales such as engagement (entertainment and interactivity), functionality (performance and ease of use), esthetics (visual appeal), and information (quality and quantity). Each subscale is rated by expert reviewers on a five-point scale, which lends itself to easy comparison with app stores' user ratings systems. MARS has good reliability, which means different raters tend to agree with each other in their ratings, and has been used in reviewing apps in a variety of health domains (Kim et al., 2018).

In another approach, IQVIA developed AppScriptScore quality rating ranging from 1 to 100 that combines six sub-scores: patient rating, professional rating, functional rating, developer rating, endorsement rating, and clinical rating (Aitken et al., 2017). Each sub-score is complex, combining several quantitative measures. For example, *patient rating* sub-score is computed based on the app's user ratings in app stores, download counts, and proprietary data on the length of the app's retention on a mobile device. *Professional rating* is derived from frequency with which the app is recommended to patients by healthcare providers via an IQVIA platform. *Functional rating* assesses specific available app functionalities. *Developer ratings* take into account frequency of app updates and the app's interoperability with sensors. *Endorsement rating* weighs the apps' endorsement by credible health organizations. Finally, *clinical rating* takes into account the app's effectiveness as evidenced in peer-reviewed publications, as well as the quality of research designs featured in those publications.

While IQVIA scores are much more comprehensive, informative, and uniquely tailored to the health domain than simple user ratings, they are also extremely labor-intensive to obtain, and reliant on proprietary data. Consequently, while these scores provide useful information for IQVIA-rated apps, developers and consumers can not apply the methodology to new apps. Moreover, IQVIA does not provide validity data on its rating system, and we cannot know whether the importance it assigns to different quality indicators is optimal. Still, IQVIA's approach suggests that a good app is the one that gets frequently updated, has a range of functions (e.g., connects to sensors), is highly rated by users, recommended by doctors, respected by developers, endorsed by healthcare organizations, and has quality research evidence of effectiveness.

8.4.3 So, Are These Apps Any Good?

From the preceding section, we see that the answer to this question is not a simple one, since "good" is neither easy to define nor simple to measure. Good apps are the ones that set good goals, which they then meet successfully, while making the experience easy and enjoyable for the user. In addition, they do not misinform, and do no harm. The rest of this chapter will focus on unpacking different aspects of app quality and functionality, and the challenges of evaluating these qualities. However, while we cannot say whether the existing apps are, on the whole or on average, "good", we CAN say that they seem to be getting better. For example, IQVIA 2017 report notes that while before August 2015 only 31% of apps received app store user ratings above 4 out of 5 stars, in the next two years (2015–2017), this number rose to 55%. Yet, while by 2017 each existing app category had at least one high-quality app according to more reliable expert reviews (rather than user ratings), the average scores within each category of apps remained low. To put it plainly, the majority of health apps in the vast universe of what is available are not great. Patient experience (e.g., doctor finders, records management) and wellness and prevention categories generally have higher quality scores than do specific condition management apps.

8.5 AN IN-DEPTH LOOK AT IMPORTANT APP CHARACTERISTICS

8.5.1 Content Accuracy

Whatever criteria we choose for evaluating quality of consumer health information apps, accuracy of information is a prerequisite of good quality. Like any health information, health information contained in the apps can be accurate or inaccurate. Because apps present information in a complex, non-linear flow that is very different from traditional text, assessing accuracy of health apps in a systematic review is not easy. We know that accuracy of health information is tied to the authors' qualifications. However, many apps are currently being developed without involvement of health professionals or testing with patients (Arnhold et al., 2014).

Accuracy of health information in apps requires more than just avoiding conveying inaccurate facts and statistics. It is also avoiding provision of inappropriate information that would lead users to incorrect inferences. For example, many general wellness programs include calorie counters that prompt users to record caloric value of their food. The counters typically have stored databases of caloric values of many pre-packaged foods (e.g., a specified brand of a granola bar). In addition, they provide caloric estimates for home-made foods. Although such estimates are helpful, they may lead to significant over- and underestimates, because the number of calories in a "medium size pancake" can differ a lot depending on the pancake. This may ultimately sabotage a weight loss program.

The effect of inaccuracies is potentially more serious in disease management apps. For example, in a review of diabetes tools, Arnhold et al. (2014) describe an app with a documentation feature that prompts users to record their blood glucose values after meals. Unfortunately, insulin amounts are typically adjusted based on blood glucose values before, rather than after meals. While this feature does not technically involve erroneous numbers, it may lead to bad decisions nonetheless.

The above examples demonstrate that seriousness of consequences of apps' inaccuracies may differ. As we will discuss further, some apps are closer to medical devices than to information resources, and so involve correspondingly greater potential risks. Yet, most apps are not currently considered medical devices and do not require certification.

8.5.2 Usability

Usability has to do with how easy or difficult apps' interfaces are to learn and navigate, as well as how enjoyable the experience of doing so is for the user. The concept grew out of web interface design theory and practice, a field that has developed a number of methods for assessing and ensuring usability. As apps potentially involve a greater range of functionalities than traditional websites, addressing their usability assessment entails some unique challenges. Nevertheless, established interface design usability principles are generally applicable to apps, and if you are a designer/developer, you are well advised to become familiar with them (Nielsen, 2013).

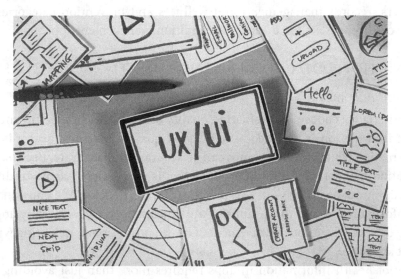

How usable are the health apps that are currently on the market? The majority of these apps do not have formal usability evaluation data. For those that do, the answer depends on the type of app and the complexity of its features and functions. For example, studies suggest good app usability in domains such as hypertension management, pregnancy support, and physical activity promotion (Alessa et al., 2018; Bondaronek et al., 2018). At the same time, achieving good usability may be trickier for apps that attempt to provide support for managing complex conditions. A number of studies analyzing apps for diabetes self-management, which is notoriously complex, found their usability low (Fu et al., 2020; Veazie et al., 2018). Finally, in an extensive systematic review, Arnhold et al. (2014) found that usability of diabetes consumer health apps is related to the number of functions they support. While the majority of single-function (usually, data recording) apps had adequate usability, multi-function apps were both less common and less usable. As diabetes management is a complex multi-function process, what we are seeing here is a trade-off between usability (ease of use) and usefulness.

Rather than being merely attributes of apps, ease of use and enjoyability are the matter of a fit between the app and the user. In many domains (e.g., games, online stores), app designers draw on market research findings to find out how factors such as gender, age, geography, prior technology experience, and others affect user preferences. But in consumer health app design, the only characteristic that is heeded by the designer is often the prospective user's health status and goals. Thus, a designer imagines his target audience as "people who want to lose weight," or "individuals living with diabetes."

It is highly likely that "wellness apps" and "disease management apps" address rather different segments of the users' market, and, therefore, should involve different usability considerations. Data on who uses health apps are scarce. A study from the Pew Research Center, a highly authoritative public opinion polling fact tank, suggested that, at the time the study was released, users of smartphone health apps were much more likely to be teens and young adults (Fox & Duggan, 2012). Most of the health apps users had on their phones had to do with fitness, diet, and weight control. Other studies confirm that when it comes to fitness and lifestyles apps, their users tend to be younger, as well as more educated and female. These individuals also tend to be in excellent health (Carroll et al., 2017; West et al., 2012).

In contrast, many people living with chronic diseases, who are targeted by designers of "condition management apps," do not fit the demographic profile of healthy, educated young adults. Using apps may be less habitual and intuitive to them, and they may need more support dealing with interface and literacy requirements. As with internet use in the previous decades, the gap in usage between demographic groups is likely to be closing; nevertheless, audience considerations remain important.

8.5.3 Responsiveness to User Needs

Users may have no trouble getting the app to do what it is designed to do, but the app may still fail to support what users actually want and need to accomplish. The best way of assessing and meeting user needs is by engaging users in all phases of app design. This approach to design and development is called user-centered design. User-centered design involves focusing on the user, the task, and the environment in which the user will be performing the task.

As most apps are developed as proprietary commercial entities, we do not know to what extent designers of most apps involve their potential users. However, analyzing the ways in which different apps with comparable functionalities fit into users' lifestyles can present an interesting case study of different responsiveness to users' needs. A common type of consumer health apps involves medication tracking and reminders. TecTrack app, developed by Biogen (2019), a pharmaceutical company, is a medication tracker a reminder for Tecfidera, a Biogen-manufactured drug for treating multiple sclerosis (MS). While the app is easy to use, because its interface only accommodates one drug – Tecfidera – it is a poor fit for anyone taking and wishing to track more than one medication, which is the case for the majority of individuals living with MS. For example, in a study of medication practices of people living with MS, conducted by Frahm et al. (2019), all participants took medications daily, and only 11% of them took just one daily medication. The average number of medications taken by a participant was 3.6 a day. It appears that TecTrack app's objectives were driven by the developer's identification with a specific medication much more than by its focus on the three-dimensional user.

In contrast, Medisafe medication tracker and reminder by Medisafe Inc. (Figure 8.1) allows users to schedule multiple medications on different schedules, import them from health records, and check drug interactions (Medisafe, 2020). For most users living with MS, Medisafe is likely to be a much better fit to their needs than TecTrack. Indeed, IQVIA 2017 lists Medisafe as a top free and publicly available medication management app (Aitken et al., 2017).

When potential users are asked about what features they want to see in health apps, they ask for multiple functions supporting a broad range of actions (e.g., data recording and data transfer to providers for disease management apps), motivational support, ability to tailor the interface and behavioral objectives, social networking functionality, and intuitive interfaces (Alnasser et al., 2015; Årsand et al., 2012; Giunti et al., 2018). Another feature

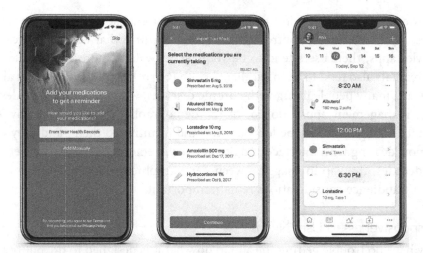

FIGURE 8.1 Medisafe Medication Management App. [*Note.* From "Media resources: Download our media kit: Medisafe-health-records-three-main-screens-.jpg," by Medisafe, 2020 (https://www.medisafe.com/media-resources/). Copyright 2020 by Medisafe. Reprinted with permission.]

that users wish to see in consumer health apps is cultural sensitivity. For example, while apps are available internationally, most highly rated wellness and prevention apps are tied to Western lifestyle, making them difficult to use in other cultures. For example, Alnasser and colleagues interviewed Saudi women about their perception of the most popular weight loss apps. Women had trouble with American tools' nutritional guidelines that were centered around American diet, as well as exercise suggestions that were a poor fit for their climate and traditional clothing.

Engaging users is essential throughout all stages of app design. Users are the ones who know what they need the apps to do and under what circumstances. They are also the ones who can provide the designers with feedback about the apps' ease of navigation and comprehensibility. However, it is important to remember that potential users come from a variety of demographic and cultural backgrounds, and that different user personas may have different needs and interact with the app in different ways.

8.5.4 Health Professionals' Involvement in Design

Previous sections suggest that potential users have a lot of unique knowledge for strengthening the quality of consumer health apps. Another group with essential knowledge – of health topics, healthcare flow, and points at which health can be supported and enabled by mobile consumer health technology – is healthcare professionals.

At the time of writing this chapter, we are not aware of any surveys presenting statistics on the prevalence of health professionals' involvement in consumer health app development. Assessing such involvement from the information provided in consumer health app store descriptions is difficult. The challenge is much greater than with consumer health websites, which usually include the About section providing information about their authors and sponsors. The absence of such information on a website is an indicator of untrustworthiness (for a more detailed review, refer to Part I: Chapter 5). By contrast, the rapidly evolving field of mobile apps has no implicitly or explicitly agreed-upon standards for provision of, or content of, such background information. Users can glean some insights from their knowledge of app designers: apps produced by clinics and pharmaceutical companies are likely to lean on professionally endorsed and reviewed content.

Even when one ventures beyond the mobile store product descriptions, finding information about the details of health professionals' involvement in development is very challenging, even for popular, highly rated apps. Although such apps usually have dedicated websites with the About sections referred to earlier, the level of detail provided about the designer team's expertise is often cursory. These gaps are not unique to apps and are true of health information websites in general. However, as apps – unlike websites – often offer information that is both tailored and highly actionable, the transparency and accountability bar should be high.

Fortunately, many app development companies engage health professionals, even if it is not obvious from their products' app store listings. For example, the website promoting mySugr (n.d.), listed by the IQVIA's report (Aitken et al., 2017) as the top free and publicly available diabetes management app, states that the app is informed by "advice from highly trained Certified Diabetes Educators who live with diabetes." Another top free app (hypertension) listed by Aitken et al. is SmartBP by Evolve Medical Systems, LLC, which states on its site, "Our team comes from diverse backgrounds and are comprised of Biomedical Engineers, Physicians and Computer Scientists" (Evolve Medical Systems, 2012, About Us section). Headspace, an extremely popular meditation app with millions of users around the world, has a chief medical officer, a UK-trained MD, David Cox, who maintains a blog on the Headspace site (Cox, 2017).

8.5.5 Fit to Behavioral Change Theory

Some consumer health apps are tools that make a specific straightforward function easier (e.g., making doctors' appointments, calculating medication dosages). Others, however, aim to support complex health behavioral change, such as smoking cessation or weight loss. The field of behavioral change has developed many effective strategies for producing positive change. In order to effectively change behavior, apps with this aim should ground themselves in behavioral change theories, supporting execution of their actionable components, making them easier and less expensive to carry out (e.g., by performing caloric calculation and sending reminders for weight loss programs). This tying of behavioral change apps to theories of behavioral change does not always happen, and technology-enabled app features often outpace theoretical knowledge of what is likely to produce a behavioral difference (Pagoto & Bennett, 2013).

Sometimes, apps take a component of a proven approach and isolate it, even though the effect of such isolation has never been tested. For example, although research evidence suggests that weight loss programs that involve food tracking are effective, interventions targeting weight loss include many components, with food tracking being only one. It is not clear whether food tracking works alone, yet many apps that claim weight loss support are single-feature in design. Overall, Pagoto et al. (2013) show that weight loss mobile apps usually incorporate only a small percentage of behavioral strategies that have been shown to work for weight loss. West et al. (2013) offer similar findings. Strategies that are most utilized in apps are not the ones that are most effective, but instead are the easiest to implement. For example, supporting the user to set a target weight goal and track food intake and weight progress is a technically straightforward task, so these features are common. In contrast, helping users control stress and address triggers that lead them to "slip" from healthy eating habits is more difficult, and therefore, much rarer. The two latter strategies, however, are very important for relapse prevention in evidence-based weight loss interventions (Pagoto et al., 2013).

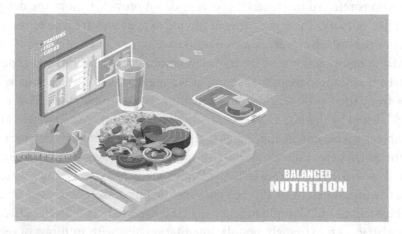

Of course, the imperfect fit to theory does not render an app useless. Rather, it raises the question of the place of mobile consumer health technology in the larger context of health and healthcare. As previously mentioned, Wetter (2015) categorized mobile technology on the basis of its interaction with/independence from healthcare. Perhaps, to the extent that behavioral change apps cannot fully adhere to evidence-based models of behavioral change, they are better viewed as supplements, rather than alternatives, to provider-driven programs. We should also be cognizant that as technology matures and becomes less of a barrier, more and more behavioral change program functions may become relegated to it.

So far, we have addressed the technological capabilities of apps, as well as their theoretical base. A third and related consideration becomes a factor: the background of the design team. Many designers/developers of commercial apps do not have the expertise for grounding their work in theory. In the meantime, research-driven apps that emerge from behavioral health research programs often have the foundation, but are tied to short-term grant funding cycles that curtail their beyond-prototype release and continuous maintenance (Barnett et al., 2015). In this situation, collaboration between research and commercial app developers could be mutually beneficial.

8.5.6 Clinical Effectiveness

For some apps, such as doctor finders and reminders, satisfied customers are the best evidence of quality. For lifestyle and disease management apps, however, the ultimate quality marker is their impact on users' health behaviors and health outcomes. Lifestyle apps are only truly good to the extent that they lead their users to exercise more, sleep better, feel less stressed, control their weight, and eat healthier. Similarly, disease management apps are only truly good to the extent that they help their users feel better and stay healthier. The only way to assess consumer health apps' impact on users' health and behavior is via rigorous research comparing app users and non-users, or individuals' functioning during periods of use and non-use.

Ideally, we would want to have user impact data on two levels: (1) for specific apps and (2) for categories of apps pertaining to specific content domains or stages in the healthcare "journey." The second level is gleaned via meta-analytic generalization of individual studies conducted on the first level. The challenge is to correctly attribute apps' effectiveness or ineffectiveness to their specific features and characteristics reviewed throughout this chapter. This challenge is both common and unique. On the one hand, the same is true for assessment of impact of any medication, device, or procedure. On the other hand, two different diabetes management apps differ from one another on more dimensions than do two different insulin pumps or medication regimens.

Accumulating this valuable knowledge is the matter of much time and effort, and mobile health is an emerging field. Moreover, as most apps are not classified as medical devices, their producers may have no motivation to conduct effectiveness studies, as long as the apps are successful on the market. Yet, the tide may be turning, as app developers increasingly are held accountable for the claims they make. In January of 2016, Lumos Labs, a company behind a brain training app Lumosity, paid $2 million to settle the Federal Trade Commission's charges of deceptive advertising. According to the statement by the Director of the Federal Trade Commission (FTC) Bureau of Consumer Protection, "Lumosity preyed on consumers' fears about age-related cognitive decline, suggesting their games could stave off memory loss, dementia, and even Alzheimer's disease. But Lumosity simply did not have the science to back up its ads" (Federal Trade Commission [FTC], 2016, para. 3).

As the field of mobile health matures, not only do app developers wish to avoid negative attention from regulatory organizations, but they also want to attract positive attention of healthcare professionals who may recommend their products to patients. As research evidence is of paramount importance to doctors, it may become a priority to companies seeking to integrate their apps into healthcare.

Commercial developers may have their apps evaluated via a variety of models. For example, the developers of a leading meditation app, Headspace, state that the company has a "seven-person, in-house science department led by Chief Science Officer Dr. Megan Jones Bell, who has +14 years of experience running National Institute of Health (NIH) and European Research Council (ERC)-funded clinical trials on digital health interventions" (Headspace, 2017, Our Approach section). The site also states that the organization is "currently in-process on 65+ research studies to scientifically validate the Headspace approach to meditation" (Headspace, 2017, Our Approach section). According to the site, the majority of these studies are done by third-party experts.

Few companies are able to engage in this degree of validation research. Depending on our outlook, research into clinical evidence of mobile health apps' effectiveness can be characterized as sparse or rapidly emerging. When it comes to categories of apps, several, though far from all, categories have accumulated sufficient evidence to suggest their clinical effectiveness. When it comes to individual apps, however, the vast majority remain untested.

In healthcare, the gold standard of clinical evidence comes from the experimental design called the randomized controlled trial, or RCT. This method reduces bias by randomly assigning participants to groups receiving and not receiving treatment (e.g., using an app), and then comparing their outcomes along variables of interest (e.g., specific health behaviors). Randomized controlled trials of consumer health apps are rare, but their number is growing rapidly. The IQVIA report (Aitken et al., 2017) states that 234 qualitative randomized controlled studies have been published between 2007 and 2017. Throughout this period, the rate of such publications increased in a non-linear fashion, with a lot more appearing in the later years. Later years also saw an increase in the number of published observational studies and systematic reviews. As of March 6, 2020, PubMed lists 627 clinical trials involving mobile apps – as well as 190 systematic reviews, a testament to just how much clinical literature is appearing on the topic (for more information on PubMed, refer to Part I: Chapter 4).

According to IQVIA, the mobile health areas with the most mature supportive research evidence of effectiveness are in the domains of diabetes, depression, and anxiety. These three areas have scientific backing for IQVIA to recommend that digital health apps are included as standard of care recommendations by professional medical societies that issue clinical guidelines. Beyond that, the report notes 24 areas that have at least one RCT with positive findings, and many areas were only observational data or no data are available. Lastly, IQVIA notes six areas that have studies with disappointing results, in which more conclusive evidence is needed (exercise, pain management, dermatological conditions, schizophrenia/bipolar, multiple sclerosis, and autism) (Aitken et al., 2017).

While IQVIA interprets the existence of many clinically oriented apps with at least one RCT in a very positive light, one RCT per area is best viewed as a good start in a vastness of future research opportunities. IQVIA also does not comment on the quality of the RCTs. In contrast, other reviews focused on quality of RCTs in areas such as self-management in chronic obstructive pulmonary disease and asthma (Marcano Belisario et al., 2013; McCabe et al., 2017). These studies identified two RCTs of apps in each area. While two pulmonary studies and one asthma study provided evidence of the apps' effectiveness, these reviews concluded that the studies were at a high risk of being biased and thus did not provide conclusive evidence. This does not mean that the apps are ineffective, only that the studies attempting to assess their effectiveness were methodologically flawed.

While some existing RCTs of consumer health apps may be biased, the majority of consumer health apps have never been formally validated. In the absence of such data, assessing their usefulness relies on observational data, consumers' and health professionals' intuition, and many of the features discussed throughout this chapter – user reviews, professional reviews, usability, etc. Yet, the fact that many areas now have at least one RCT-supported app, and that the evidence body is growing rapidly, is encouraging.

8.5.7 Data Privacy and Security

Unlike most traditional consumer health websites on which information flow is unidirectional, from the page to the user, many apps collect personal information. This makes data privacy and security important considerations. While the concepts of privacy and security are related, they are not the same thing. *Privacy* is a legal term referring to how the data are collected, stored, and used and who is authorized to access data. For example, an app's privacy policy should state whether the data may be sold or transferred to third parties. *Security* is a technical term that describes how the data are protected from breach by unauthorized users (e.g., encryption).

The main US law that regulates how personally identifiable information should be protected in healthcare is the federal Health Insurance Portability and Accountability Act (HIPAA, 1996). As the law is decades old, interpreting its application to mobile health can be challenging. Moreover, HIPAA laws only apply when personally identifiable information is stored or managed by "HIPAA-covered entities," such as healthcare organizations and insurance companies, and developers need to take care to determine whether their tool's information operations are addressed by HIPAA or any other relevant laws.

Privacy and security of mobile health apps remain a concern. While the Federal Trade Commission recommends that mobile health apps have privacy policies that are easy for users to read and understand, the large majority of apps do not have such policies at all (Kao & LIebovitz, 2017). Moreover, not much attention is given to readability and comprehensibility of the policies, or whether users even read them, instead of scrolling through them and checking off the agreement box.

When it comes to personal health information, security considerations are of paramount importance. Data breaches may result in privacy loss and identity theft for consumers and significant reputation and financial losses for healthcare organizations behind the apps (Adu et al., 2018). While overall data breaches in healthcare records are going down significantly, apps represent new technology that may be more prone to hacking (Bitglass, 2018). Data hacking incidents are common in healthcare: while a review of technology for ensuring apps data security is beyond the scope of this chapter, security considerations should be part of the design process from the start. For a discussion of privacy as an ethical consideration in CHI work, review Part II: Chapter 11.

8.6 CHALLENGES OF FINDING GOOD APPS

Throughout this chapter, we saw that while mobile health tools can have much to offer, developing effective apps involves overcoming many challenges, and not all apps are created equal. How, then, is one to find good apps?

8.6.1 Searching App Stores

One way to look for apps is by searching app stores. Unfortunately, app stores are notoriously difficult to search. Unlike the web, which search engines search on the basis of all of their content, apps stores are searched on the basis of descriptor keywords provided by apps developers. Consequently, many relevant apps do not emerge among the top results unless very precise search terms are used.

Moreover, as mentioned above, outcomes of app store searches are difficult to evaluate, as they often provide little information about the developer's health-related expertise, and the only apparent quality criteria are user ratings.

8.6.2 Asking a Doctor

Asking healthcare professionals for recommendations is a good idea, and if you are a healthcare professional, you probably want to be able to recommend apps to your patients. Unfortunately, providers are often reluctant to do that. According to a study by a consulting firm Manhattan Research (2014), only a third of doctors recommended that their patients use apps. Of those, a half did not recommend specific apps, but suggests searching app stores. This is not surprising: doctors' do not have time to explore and vet apps. Holtz et al. (2019) comment that there is only limited research on primary care practitioners' opinions of health tracking digital technologies; in contrast, the opinions of consumers have been much better investigated. Moreover, in today's healthcare system, "prescribing" apps is not a reimbursable service, which limits doctors' motivation and ability to recommend apps.

8.6.3 Advocacy Organizations

Advocacy organizations focused on particular diagnoses are good ways to find apps tailored to the needs of particular patient communities, as well as caregivers of those patients. These organizations publicize apps. Such apps are usually of high quality. For example, Read and Muza-Moons (2017) reviewed five apps dedicated to management of symptoms and community networking for people living with inflammatory bowel disease (Crohn's and ulcerative colitis). Their review assigned the highest rating to GI Buddy, a free app from Crohns & Colitis Foundation of America.

8.6.4 Finding App Libraries

If app store searches are suboptimal in terms of completeness and quality of what they produce, and if doctors cannot be expected to be consumer health app experts, then experts-vetted app libraries could be a solution. Creating an app library encompasses developing something akin to a certification system, addressed above in the section on quality control, but it also involves developing a taxonomy into which the apps are organized, creating an interface through which users can learn about the apps, and maintaining the system and the interface up-to-date (e.g., by removing references to retired apps).

Several initiatives around the world have attempted to create such libraries. For example, MyHealthApps.net, formerly the European Directory of Health Apps, is maintained by Patient View, a UK-based consulting firm (Patient View, nd). Apps in this directory are nominated and reviewed by patient and consumer groups. In addition, app developers provide public information about pricing, funding, and medical consultants involved in development. The UK National Health Service (NHS) maintains an app library (see Figure 8.2). App providers submitting their apps for consideration by the NHS library have to provide information about their app's effectiveness, clinical safety, data protection and security, usability and accessibility, and more. Apps included in the NHS library display one of three badges. The highest-level badge is reserved for apps that provide

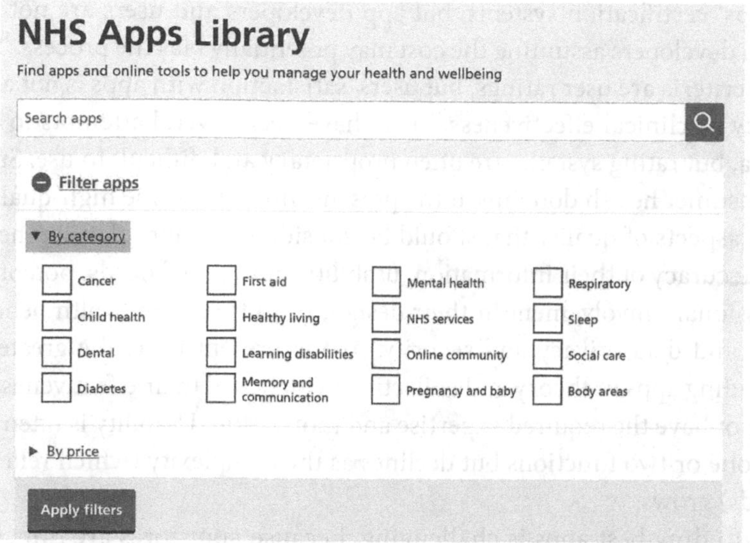

FIGURE 8.2 The UK National Health Service (NHS) Apps Library. [*NOTE*. From NHS Digital, *NHS Apps Library*, by NHS Digital, 2020 (https://www.nhs.uk/apps-library/). Copyright Crown 2020. Open Government License (OGLv3.0). Reprinted with permission.]

supporting evidence for their clinical effectiveness (NHS Digital, 2019). The online Journal of Medical Internet Research (JMIR) maintains an e-collection of mobile health apps reviews, as discussed above (https://mhealth.jmir.org/themes/217).

The process of building and curating a collection of mobile health apps is not without challenges. Curation requires a kind of certification, many challenges of which were described above. For example, the NHS Apps Library launched for the first time in 2013, but was closed two years later after an independent published study revealed privacy and security concerns in the majority of the libraries' apps (Huckvale et al., 2015). The library then relaunched in 2017, with data protection and security as specific inclusion criteria.

8.7 CONCLUSIONS

The world of mobile consumer health is both exciting and unruly. At this point, apps cover all general areas of health and wellness and handle a range of tasks, including (but not limited to) data recording, display and analysis, data sharing, communication, reminders, education, and advice. The number of health apps keeps growing, while the number of downloads and the quality differ tremendously.

Placing apps within broader taxonomies or classification schemes may help developers, reviewers, and users think about the desired features and functionalities. Depending on the context, most useful classification schemes may be organizing apps by tasks, points in the patient "journey," or engagement with healthcare.

Apps' quality is difficult to assess, because no agreed-upon quality guidelines exist. Some apps are considered medical devices and are, therefore, reviewed and approved by the FDA. However, FDA approval only signifies safety, and, in any case, most apps are not considered devices. Other, non-governmental, entities have attempted to implement voluntary apps' certification systems, but app developers and users are not motivated to pay for it, and developers assuming the cost may potentially bias the process. The most easily accessible criteria are user ratings, but users' satisfaction with apps is not a guarantee of their accuracy or clinical effectiveness. There have been several attempts to develop apps rating criteria, but rating systems are often proprietary and difficult to use. Still, it appears that most consumer health domains at the present time have some high-quality apps.

Important aspects of quality that should be considered in apps development and selection involve accuracy of their information, usability, fit to users' needs, potential users' and health professionals' involvement in their design, fit to theory of health behavior, clinical effectiveness, and data privacy and security. At the present time, the greatest challenges involve grounding apps in theory and collecting evidence of their effectiveness, as developers often do not have the required expertise and motivation. Usability is often good in apps that include one or two functions but declines as the complexity (which reflects greater fit to users' needs) grows.

Presently, finding best apps is challenging, because app stores are difficult to search, health professionals are often reluctant to recommend specific apps, and apps libraries are rare. However, as the field is relatively new and very rapidly developing, over the next decade we are likely to see important advances in every aspect of mobile health technology.

WEB RESOURCES

Journal of Medical Internet Research (JMIR)
E-collection 'Quality Evaluation and Descriptive Analysis/Reviews of Multiple Existing Mobile Apps'.
https://mhealth.jmir.org/themes/217
This is a collection of JMIR-published peer-reviewed papers that include health app reviews and analysis, including many systematic reviews.

JMIR Submission Form for Health Apps
https://docs.google.com/forms/d/e/1FAIpQLSdQfn9_fa3jfxOUeuzAH-wHQvy9VD-TU4m6Aj0FTkSNrcxZUUg/viewform?formkey=+dEY0YThtT2lXTXVUQ2VuUHRzSkh5a2c6MQ
This is a submission form for medical apps used by the *Journal of Medical Internet Research* for app quality assessment purposes.

iPrescribeApps
https://iprescribeapps.com/
This is a platform through which physicians can select vetted apps to recommend to their patients; run by physicians-staffed iMedicalApps online publication.

UK National Health Service (NHS) App Library
https://www.nhs.uk/apps-library/
This is a collection of NHS-reviewed apps "to help you manage your health and well-being," organized by category (e.g., cancer, diabetes, mental health) and price.

REFERENCES

Adu, M. D., Malabu, U. H., Callander, E. J., Malau-Aduli, A. E. O., & Malau-Aduli, B. S. (2018). Considerations for the development of mobile phone apps to support diabetes self-management: Systematic Review. *JMIR mHealth and uHealth*, 6(6), e10115. https://doi.org/10.2196/10115

Aitken, M., Clancy, B., & Nass, D. (2017). The growing value of digital health: Evidence and impact on human health and the healthcare system. *IQVIA Institute for Data Science* https://www.iqvia.com/insights/the-iqvia-institute/reports/the-growing-value-of-digital-health

Alessa, T., Abdi, S., Hawley, M. S., & de Witte, L. (2018). Mobile apps to support the self-management of hypertension: Systematic review of effectiveness, usability, and user satisfaction. *JMIR Mhealth Uhealth*, 6(7), e10723. doi:10.2196/10723

Alnasser, A. A., Alkhalifa, A. S., Sathiaseelan, A., & Marais, D. (2015). What overweight women want from a weight loss app: A qualitative study on Arabic women. *JMIR mHealth and uHealth*, 3(2), e41. doi:10.2196/mhealth.4409

American Nurses Credentialing Center. (n.d.) *ANCC magnet recognition program*. https://www.nursingworld.org/organizational-programs/magnet/

Arnhold, M., Quade, M., & Kirch, W. (2014). Mobile applications for diabetics: A systemic review and expert-based usability evaluation considering the special requirements of diabetes patients age 50 years or older. *Journal of Medical Internet Research*, 16(4), e104. https://doi.org/10.2196/jmir.2968

Årsand, E., Frøisland, D. H., Skrøvseth, S. O., Chomutare, T., Tatara, N., Hartvigsen, G., & Tufano, J. T. (2012). Mobile health applications to assist patients with diabetes: Lessons learned and design implications. *Journal of diabetes science and technology*, 6(5), 1197–1206. https://doi.org/10.1177/193229681200600525

Barnett, J., Harricharan, M., Fletcher, D., Gilchrist, B., & Coughlan, J. (2015). myPace: An integrative health platform for supportive weight loss and maintenance behaviors. *IEEE Journal of Biomedical and Health Informatics*, 19(1). 109–116. https://doi.org/10.1109/JBHI.2014.2366832

Biogen. (2019). *Stay on track with Tecfidera: get reminders, tools, and more with TecTrack, an appr for Tecfidera (dimethyl fumerate)*. Retrieve March 4, 2020 from https://www.tecfidera.com/en_us/home/getting-started/tectrack-app.html?cid=aff-tectrack-redirect-tta.

Bitglass (2018). *Bitglass report: Breached healthcare records hit four-year low*. https://www.bitglass.com/press-releases/healthcare-breach-report-2018

Bondaronek, P., Alkhaldi, G., Slee, A., Hamilton, F. L., & Murray, E. (2018). Quality of publicly available physical activity apps: Review and content analysis. *JMIR Mhealth Uhealth*, 6(3), e53. doi:10.2196/mhealth.9069

Carroll, J. K., Moorhead, A., Bond, R., LeBlanc, W. G., Petrella, R. J., & Fiscella, K. (2017). Who uses mobile phone health apps and does use matter? A secondary data analytics approach. *Journal of Medical Internet Research*, 19(4), e125. https://doi.org/10.2196/jmir.5604

Charnock, D & Shepperd, S. (n.d.). *DISCERN: Quality criteria for consumer health information*. Radcliffe Online. http://www.discern.org.uk/

Cox, D. (2017). *Dr. David Cox*. Headspace. https://www.headspace.com/blog/author/dr-david-cox/

Evolve Medical Systems. (2012). *About Us*. http://www.evolvemedsys.com/about/

Federal Trade Commission [FTC]. (2016). *Lumosity to pay $2 million to settle FTC deceptive advertising charges for its "brain training program"*. https://www.ftc.gov/news-events/press-releases/2016/01/lumosity-pay-2-million-settle-ftc-deceptive-advertising-charges

Fox, S. & Duggan, M. (2012, November 8). *Mobile health 2012*. https://www.pewresearch.org/internet/2012/11/08/mobile-health-2012/

Frahm, N., Hecker, M., & Zettl, U. K. (2019). Polypharmacy in outpatients with relapsing–remitting multiple sclerosis: A single-center study. *PloS one*, 14(1), e0211120. https://doi.org/10.1371/journal.pone.0211120

Fu, H. N. C., Rizvi, R. F., Wyman, J. F., & Adam, T. J. (2020). Usability evaluation of four top-rated commercially available diabetes apps for adults with type 2 diabetes. *Comput Inform Nurs.* doi:10.1097/cin.0000000000000596

Giunti, G., Kool, J., Rivera Romero, O., & Dorronzoro Zubiete, E. (2018). Exploring the specific needs of persons with multiple sclerosis for mHealth solutions for physical activity: Mixed-methods study. *JMIR mHealth and uHealth*, 6(2), e37. https://doi.org/10.2196/mhealth.8996

Headspace. (2017). *Scientific rigor.* https://www.headspace.com/science

Health On the Net Foundation [HON]. (2020). *Health on the Net.* https://www.hon.ch/en/

HIPAA, *Health insurance portability and accountability act of 1996, Pub. L. No. 104–191, 110 Stat. 2548* (1996). https://www.govinfo.gov/app/details/PLAW-104publ191/summary

Höhn, M., von Jan, U., Framke, T., & Albrecht, U. V. (2016). Classification of health related applications. *Studies in Health Technology and Informatics*, 226, 139–142.

Holtz, B., Vasold, K., Cotten, S., Mackert, M., & Zhang, M. (2019). Health care provider perceptions of consumer-grade devices and apps for tracking health: A pilot study. *JMIR mHealth and uHealth*, 7(1), e9929.

Huckvale, K., Prieto, J. T., Tilney, M., Benghozi, P.-J., & Car, J. (2015). Unaddressed privacy risks in accredited health and wellness apps: A cross-sectional systematics assessment. *BMC Med*, 13(214). https://doi.org/10.1186/s12916-015-0444-y

JMIR mHealth and uhealth (n.d.). *E-collections 'quality evaluation and descriptive analysis/reviews of multiple existing mobile apps'.* https://mhealth.jmir.org/themes/217

Joint Commission. (2020). *Accreditation & certification.* https://www.jointcommission.org/accreditation-and-certification/

Kao, C. K., & LIebovitz, D. M. (2017). Consumer mobile health apps: Current state, barriers, and future directions. *Journal of Injury, Function and Rehabilitation*, 9(5S), S106-S115. https://doi.org/10.1016/j.pmrj.2017.02.018

Kim, B. Y., Sharafoddini, A., Tran, N., Wen, E. Y., & Lee, J. (2018). Consumer mobile apps for potential drug–drug interaction check: Systematic review and content analysis using the Mobile App Rating Scale (MARS). *JMIR mHealth and uHealth*, 6(3), e74. https://doi.org/10.2196/mhealth.8613

Manhattan Research. (2014). *Taking the pulse.* https://www.prnewswire.com/news-releases/stethoscopes-and-smartphones-physicians-turn-to-digital-tools-to-boost-patient-outcomes-261089461.html

Marcano Belisario, J.C., Huckvale, K., Greenfield, F., Car, J., Gunn, L.H. (2013). Smartphone and tablet self management apps for asthma. *Cochrane Database of Systematic Reviews*, 11. CD010013. DOI: 10.1002/14651858.CD010013.pub2.

McCabe, C., McCann, M., & Brady, A. M. (2017). Computer and mobile technology interventions for self-management in chronic obstructive pulmonary disease. *Cochrane Database of systematic reviews*, 5(5), CD011425. https://doi.org/10.1002/14651858.CD011425.pub2

Medisafe. (2020). *The company.* https://www.medisafe.com/the-company/

mySugr. (n.d.). *Science and research.* https://mysugr.com/en-us/science-and-research

NHS Digital. (2019). *How we assess health apps and digital tools: All products published on the NHS apps library must meet a set of standards.* https://www.nhs.uk/apps-library/how-we-assess-apps/

Nielsen, J. (2013). *10 usability heuristics for user interface design.* https://www.designprinciplesftw.com/collections/10-usability-heuristics-for-user-interface-design

Office of the National Coordinator for Health Information Technology [ONC]. (2019). *About ONC.* HealthIT.gov, Department of Health and Human Services. https://www.healthit.gov/topic/about-onc

Pagoto, S., & Bennett, G. G. (2013). How behavioral science can advance digital health. *Translational behavioral medicine*, 3(3), 271–276. https://doi.org/10.1007/s13142-013-0234-z

Pagoto, S., Schneider, K., Jojic, M., DeBiasse, M., & Mann, D. (2013). Evidence-based strategies in weight-loss mobile apps. *American Journal of Preventive Medicine*, 45(5), 576–582. https://doi.org/10.1016/j.amepre.2013.04.025

Patient View. (n.d.). *Patient view's team.* http://www.patient-view.com/bull-who-we-are.html

Powell, A. C., Landman, A. B., & Bates, D. W. (2014). In search of a few good apps. *Journal of the American Medical Association*, 311(18), 1851–1852. https://doi.org/10.1001/jama.2014.2564

Read, A.J., & Muza-Moons, M.M. (2017). Patient-focused IBD applications review. *Gastroenterology*, 152(5): 1241–1243.

Stoyanov, S. R., Hides, L., Kavanagh, D. J., Zelenko, O., Tjondronegoro, D., & Mani, M. (2015). Mobile app rating scale: A new tool for assessing the quality of health mobile apps. *JMIR mHealth and uHealth*, 3(1), e27. https://doi.org/10.2196/mhealth.3422

Veazie, S., Winchell, K., Gilbert, J., Paynter, R., Ivlev, I, Eden, K., Nussbaum, K., Weiskopf, N., & Helfand, M. (2018). *Mobile applications for self-management of diabetes. Agency for Healthcare Research and Quality (ARHQ) Comparative Effectiveness Technical Briefs, Publication No. 18-EHCo101-EF.* https://effectivehealthcare.ahrq.gov/products/diabetes-mobile-devices/technical-brief

Viswanathan, P. (2019). *What is a mobile application: Function and fun for every situation.* Lifewire. https://www.lifewire.com/what-is-a-mobile-application-2373354

Welldoc Inc. (n.d.). *Science-based, human designed.* https://www.welldoc.com/product/

West, J. H., Hall, P. C., Arredondo, V., Berrett, B., Guerra, B., & Farrell, J. (2013). Health behavior theories in diet apps. *Journal of Consumer Health on the Internet*, 17(1), 10–24. https://doi.org/10.1080/15398285.2013.756343

West, J. H., Hall, P. C., Hanson, C. L., Barnes, M. D., Giraud-Carrier, C., & Barrett, J. (2012). There's an app for that: content analysis of paid health and fitness apps. *Journal of Medical Internet Research*, 14(3), e72. https://doi.org/10.2196/jmir.1977

Wetter, T. (2015). *Consumer health informatics: New services, roles, and responsibilities.* Cham: Springer International Publishing.

CHAPTER 9

Smart Medical Homes and Their Potential to Support Independent Living

Alla Keselman

T HIS CHAPTER FOCUSES ON smart medical homes and their potential to support independent living for older adults and medically fragile individuals. A smart medical home is a residential environment that uses technology to collect and monitor data related to its residents' health, security, and well-being and responds in ways that protect, support, and promote them. The concept, which grew out of the field of home automation, is a subject of much research, development, and futuristic speculations. The chapter describes independent living needs of populations that are likely to benefit from smart medical home technologies. It also discusses technology and devices that are capable of making homes "smarts" and the flow of information across these devices. Implementing smart medical homes requires establishing three informational operations: (1) acquiring raw data via sensors and trackers, (2) processing, integrating, and analyzing them, and (3) making and implemented data-driven decisions (Ni, García Hernando, & Pau De la Cruz, 2015). When well-implemented, this flow can support activities of daily living. For example, analysis of night-time data collected from a smart bed and various ambient sensors may result in a recommendation to discuss sleep quality with a health professional or an alert to a family member. However, to be effective, smart medical homes technology needs to be developed with user input and careful attention to user feedback, since technology use patterns of developers are typically different from those of users. The chapter also discusses technological challenges of smart medical home technologies, such as energy efficiency, interoperability, and data security, as well as non-technical challenges, such as potential users' trust and privacy concerns. Next, the chapter provides several examples of current technologies that are emerging as part of smart medical homes landscape: voice assistants, web services such as IFTTT (If This Then That), ambient sensors, and home healthcare robots.

The chapter also reviews studies of clinical significance of smart medical homes, an area where more research is needed. Lastly, it considers ethical dilemmas inherent in smart home technologies, such as potential privacy loss, impact on social relationships, impact on users' autonomy, and more.

9.1 WHAT ARE SMART MEDICAL HOMES?

A smart medical home is a residential environment that uses technology to collect and monitor data related to its residents' health, comfort, security, and well-being and responds in ways that protect, support, and promote these characteristics. If you think the notion has a dystopian ring and evokes the image of the omnipresent Big Brother, you are not alone. At the same time, a smart medical home is an environment that can give the gift of independent living to those who would otherwise require care in nursing homes or other residential facilities – older adults and those living with disabilities. Although we already live surrounded by robots and smart devices, the concept of a smart medical home is still in its infancy. Current and future research, development, and policy efforts will determine whether smart medical homes' potential can be realized and their risks curtailed.

9.1.1 Smart Home Concept

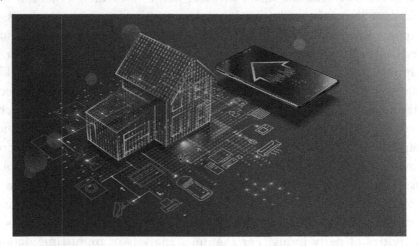

The concept of a smart medical home grew out of earlier concepts of home automation and smart home technology. Smart homes have been defined by Demiris (2016) as follows:

> A "smart home" is a residential setting with embedded technological features that enable passive monitoring of the well-being and activities of their residents aiming to improve primarily overall quality of life, to detect or even prevent emergencies and ultimately increase independence for the involved residents (p. 245).

Smart home technology refers to a connected network of devices and appliances that are equipped with sensors and actuators (controllers) that can be operated remotely. This is related to the concept of the Internet of Things (IoT), or wireless connectivity among traditionally not connected devices. Examples of smart home technologies include lighting, temperature, and entertainment control systems that can be operated via phone, computer, or another device.

More controversially, in addition to devices being remotely operated by residents, the concept includes smart technology that independently responds to users' states, behaviors, and perceived needs. For example, a smart refrigerator may issue an alert when its owner is running out of milk, as well as provide a recommendation to eat more fruit and vegetables.

Adding "medical" to the concept of "smart home" increases both its complexity and potential applications. A smart medical home environment can monitor its resident's health indicators and alert the resident, a family member, or a healthcare provider in case of danger. It can turn a cooking appliance on or off, adjust the temperature of a smart electric blanket, and ring a wakeup alarm during an optimal stage of a sleep cycle. It may remind a resident in an early stage of dementia to take medication or to engage in self-care (e.g., brush teeth). It may also suggest making a video call to a friend or a family member or playing a cheerful movie as a result of assessing the resident's mood.

While no currently existing smart medical home encompasses all of these features, many interesting research and commercial projects implement some of them. The rest of this chapter will review the technologies and functions related to the idea of a smart medical home, describe some existing projects, and analyze technical challenges and ethical implications.

9.2 DO SMART MEDICAL HOMES ACTUALLY EXIST? CONCEPT VERSUS REALITY

Are smart medical homes, or, for that matter, smart homes, science fiction or reality? As you may have guessed from the closing of the previous section, the answer lies somewhere in between. Both smart homes and smart medical homes involve emergent technologies. The concept of a smart home, as described earlier, involves a network of wirelessly connected devices that collaborate to deliver a well-orchestrated system of integrated services. While many components of that concept exist, the integration is a work in progress, so the world of smart homes and smart medical home technology currently operates not like a well-coordinated practiced orchestra, but like a group of musicians performing in the same room without a conductor and wearing noise-canceling headphones that prevent them from hearing one another. While the field is growing rapidly, lack of coordination among multiple players slows down progress. There is no formal definition of how integrated a home needs to be to gain the "smart" designation.

The development is happening on two fronts, commercial and academic. Commercial markets are being rapidly inundated with smart devices, from speakers to doorbells, that connect with other devices or via wireless protocols. These devices typically have a sleek look and a high "wow" factor, as their developers target young, educated, tech-savvy early adopters with disposable income. These users are usually far removed from those who need smart technology to avoid moving into residential care facilities. At the same time, as developers are primarily concerned with improving and marketing their own products, rather than with building the global world of smart homes, different devices often use different communication protocols and do not always work smoothly with one another. As a result, users are on their own when it comes to checking compatibilities, and the outcome, at its best, is homes with individual smart devices and systems, with patchworked communication between some of them. One typically does not buy a smart home, but gradually acquires separate smart appliances that can be linked together. Linking them requires either that the homeowners possess above-average expertise with technology, or that they turn to one of the emerging companies that specialize in smart technology installation. These companies' services, however, typically do not extend to home healthcare devices.

In the world of academic engineering research (e.g., university engineering laboratories), brilliant professors work on smart home components that lie within their interest areas, be they floor sensors or smart grab bars. This results in many captivating projects that ebb and flow with three- to five-year-long academic research funding cycles and often do not translate into commercial products. The technology is often tested in university laboratories, rather than in real living spaces, under conditions that do not resemble the daily life of target users. There are also interesting research projects, some discussed in this chapter, that integrate multiple kinds of smart technologies into lab environments located in real houses or apartments, where volunteers – often, older adults – can experience them in a realistic context for periods of days or weeks. While these projects are much closer to embodying the concept of integrated smart medical homes, they are a lot less common than projects focused on isolated devices, conducted in traditional labs.

In summary, smart medical homes constitute an exciting cutting-edge concept, with many components undergoing various stages of research and development, and a number of interesting devices and system entering commercial markets. Yet, at the present, the field is fragmented and not well-integrated, with many technical and ethical considerations still needed to be addressed before the promise matures into reality.

9.2.1 Who Can Benefit from Smart Medical Homes?

Smart medical homes are most often discussed in the context of prolonging independent living for older adults. Over the last several decades, life expectancy in the developed world has been increasing dramatically, while birthrates have been falling (Majumder et al., 2017), increasing both the number and the proportion of older adults in societies. According to the World Health Organization (World Health Organization, 2018a), by 2050 the number of older adults in the world will reach two billion, bypassing the number of those 14 and younger (see Part I: Chapter 6 for a more detailed review of the needs of older adults).

The ways in which people spend their later years have also been changing. In the past, for most people, a period of good health was followed by a sharp quick decline. Now, the picture in the developed world is that of a longer life, with the late years marked by gradual loss of physical and cognitive functions, as well as independence (Gawande, 2014). This is happening in a social context of high geographic mobility and weakening extended family connections. As a result, while in the past most people could live out their late years at home surrounded by extended family, this period is now often spent in nursing homes and long-term care facilities. Moving to a care facility is often preceded by falls that result in fractures and other injuries.

According to the Centers for Disease Control and Prevention (Centers for Disease Control and Prevention, 2019), over four million Americans are admitted to or live in nursing homes annually, with an additional million living in assisted living facilities. This situation causes distress to individuals and places great financial burden on the healthcare system and the economy. Aging-related loss of independence constitutes a great fear for Americans. A survey conducted by West Health Institute and National Opinion Research Center at the University of Chicago (2017) found that 63% of US adults over 30 worry about eventual loss of independence, and 56% worry about the possibility of having to move into a nursing home.

Aging is not the only condition affecting the quality of independent living. Other conditions that create unique challenges include severe mental (e.g., schizophrenia), cognitive (e.g., Alzheimer's disease), and physical disorders. According to World Health Organization (2018b), 110–190 million people 15 and older worldwide are living with significant functional difficulties that are caused by disability or chronic illness.

Leaving home to move into a residential facility means leaving a familiar environment (which, in combination with a cognitive impairment, may further impair functioning); giving up old habits and favorite things; and abandoning the personal autonomy that stems from the ability to make up one's schedule and choose one's food and activities. Smart medical homes make a promise to support independent living for those who need support, while relieving caregivers and reducing financial burden of healthcare. Another term that you may encounter expressing this concept is ambient assisted living. Ni, García Hernando, and Pau De la Cruz (2015) describe three categories of such systems for the aging. The categories can apply to systems for other fragile population groups. The first category includes examples of "specific health monitoring systems." These are systems that monitor physiological measures or activities in order to detect an onset or a worsening of a health condition, as well as a specific health risk (e.g., a dangerous spike in blood glucose in a person living with diabetes). The second category is "daily activities monitoring, prediction, and reminding" systems that help overcome physical and cognitive barriers to essential daily actions. The third category, "detection of anomalous situations," detects emergencies such as falls and break-ins. As sensing and detection do not always allow prevention, independent living in a smart medical home still entails risks for a fragile individual. Acceptability of that risk for the resident should be evaluated against the value of retaining the autonomy of independent living.

9.3 SMART MEDICAL HOMES' INFORMATION FLOW: IT'S ALL ABOUT THE DATA

Smart medical home implementation involves three stages of data operations: (1) acquiring raw data via sensors and trackers, (2) processing, integrating, and analyzing the data, and (3) making and implementing data-driven decisions (Ni et al., 2015). The outcome, ideally, is a system that constantly monitors the users' external environment and relevant internal states and responds accordingly. Each of the three stages involves technology and processes described below. Specific measures, devices, and components mentioned in this section are theoretical. Examples of actual smart medical homes projects are described in a later section.

9.3.1 Acquiring Raw Data via Sensors and Trackers

9.3.1.1 Trackable Data Types

A number of data types can inform maintaining the smart medical home environment. These include measures of body's basic functions, such as temperature, pulse, respiratory rate, and blood pressure, called vital signs, and other physiological measurements such as blood glucose level, electrocardiogram (ECG), and galvanic skin response. Vital signs are "vital," or essential, because their abnormalities can be strong indicators of serious health problems. For example, blood glucose level and ECG readings provide critical information about diabetes functioning and heart health. Other types of tracked data may include measures of movement (e.g., gait, speed, acceleration, location in space) and activity (e.g., foods taken out of the refrigerator, amount of time spent exercising or watching television, choice of entertainment programming). Yet another relevant data source pertains to communication and social contacts made throughout the day, such as frequency and length of visits from friends and family, phone and video calls, and social media activity. Even appearance can be data, from facial expressions that indicate mood, to clothing choices that indicate ability to engage in self-care. Lastly, the environment can provide much data, particularly related to safety and security (e.g., on and off state of devices, gas leaks, lighting, sound, etc.) or health-related habits and routines. For example, in June 2020, Apple announced launching a new handwashing guide feature for its Apple Watch. The system, which tracks the sound of running water and combines it with hand movement motion sensor data, provides recommended handwashing time count down. Introduced during the COVID-19 pandemic, the feature is being promoted as a prevention measure (Farr, 2020).

9.3.1.2 Data Tracking Devices

Data tracking can be done via a variety of sensors, trackers, recorders, and monitors, which modern technology is making increasingly easier to use. Ni et al. (2015) note that data tracking devices can be divided into two broad categories: (1) audio and video monitors and (2) sensors. Sensors, in turn, can be divided into wearable (carried on the body) and environmental (embedded into objects and the environment).

Audio and video monitors involve cameras and microphones. They can record rich, precise information about actions, conversations, interactions, commands, and environmental sounds and states. At the same time, their potential infringement on privacy is very high, and so is the computational cost of processing the data collected by them (see Ni et al., 2015, for a detailed review).

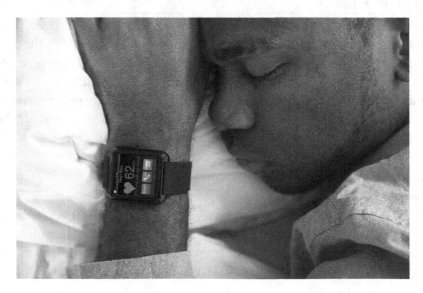

Wearable sensors are most fitting for recording physiological measurements (e.g., vitals) and movement-related data such as acceleration and orientation. They are relatively small, portable, and inexpensive. At the same time, "small" is a relative term, and they can become uncomfortable. These sensors also have the downside of requiring users to remember to wear them. However, as technology keeps advancing, wearable sensors are becoming more and more user-friendly. They can also be incorporated into regular wearable objects such as wristwatches, bracelets, and T-shirts.

Like wearable sensors, environmental sensors embedded in furniture and consumer objects can collect physiological data. For example, a smart bed can be equipped with sensors that measure temperature and heart rate. In addition, object-embedded sensors can also provide data about a user's interaction with that object. A smart refrigerator or a smart cabinet can collect data on when it was opened; a smart toothbrush can collect data on when it was picked up. Many of such sensors are what Ni et al. (2015) call "state-change sensors": simple binary sensors that record changes between two states (an object was picked up or opened; a switch was flipped up or down). Other object- and environmental-embedded sensors are motion detectors, such as infrared sensors or pressure sensors. A pressure sensor can detect changes occurring to beds, chairs, and other surfaces, providing data for making inferences about the resident's location. Still other environmental sensors detect characteristics of the environment: temperature, lighting.

Radio Frequency Identification (RFID) sensors can be either worn by residents or attached to objects and serve as their locators in response to a generated tracking request. These can help residents locate lost objects or, as wearables, assist caregivers in identifying residents' locations.

9.3.2 Processing, Integrating, and Analyzing the Data

The true power of smart medical homes is not in sensing and recording individual data streams, but in the ability to generate knowledge by combining separate streams, drawing powerful inferences about residents' needs, and responding accordingly. Data integration and analysis allow smart medical home technology to identify specific physical or daily life activities in which the resident is engaged (Ni et al., 2015). Examples of physical activities can include walking, sitting, and going up or down the stairs, while examples of daily life activities include eating, cooking, brushing teeth, taking medication, or exercising. Intelligent learning systems can then model and analyze patterns and identify deviations from daily routines (e.g., a resident has not eaten a meal) and react to them. They can also identify anomalous events, such as falls.

9.3.3 Making and Implementing Data-Driven Decisions

Processed data from sensors and trackers trigger activators, which enact a specific response. Responses usually involve sending alerts and reminders to the resident, contacting a family member or a healthcare provider, or adjusting an environmental characteristic. For example, Muse et al. (2017) describe a (hypothetical) scenario where a resident is woken up at by a smart alarm at the lightest phase of her sleep cycle, as determined by motion sensors in her mattress. The same authors give an example of a smart bathroom mirror that displays a morning medication reminder when the resident looks at it. Smart medical home systems can also send a phone alert to a family member if a resident with cognitive problems left her home in the middle of the night or has been out of bed for a specified amount of time. Activators can also turn on and off cooking devices and appliances, turn off the light and entertainment system if the resident is asleep (as sensed by a smart bed), and adjust temperature controls.

9.4 SUPPORTING ESSENTIAL DAILY LIVING ACTIVITIES

The previous section makes it clear that smart home technology is both potentially powerful and potentially intrusive. As with other technologies, in order to improve consumers' well-being, smart homes should focus on what fragile residents need, rather than on what is technologically possible. An effective way to identify these needs is to identify and support activities that residents need to perform at home in order to remain independent.

Aging and disability may complicate independent living by impairing physical functions such as mobility and agility, cognitive function (memory), and perceptual function (e.g., vision, hearing) (Kelly, Fausset, Rogers, & Fisk, 2014). Smart medical home technology may help with these problems by issuing time- and context-sensitive reminders and by reducing perceptual, physical, and cognitive demands of tasks (e.g., via voice-operated commands). In designing technology that helps overcome those challenges, it is important to consider specific daily life activities that happen in the homes, the effect of aging or disability on the ability to carry them out, and the supports that can be put in place.

Developing technological solutions should start with creating meaningful taxonomies of residents' activities and mapping technology (e.g., types of sensors) onto them (Ni et al., 2015). The field of caregiving traditionally distinguishes between activities of daily living (ADLs) and instrumental activities of daily living (IADLs). ADLs include basic self-care activities such as toileting, bathing, dressing, and eating, while IADLs involve more complex tasks such as cooking, cleaning, and managing finances and social schedules. Developing smart supports for these activities requires carefully analyzing them into multiple attributes, such as location, time, duration, sequence of steps, conditions, etc. (Ni et al., 2015). To be effective, technology needs to identify not only individual steps of these activities, but also their place in the broader pattern, types of potential difficulties (e.g., cognitive, perceptual, physical), and places at which supports should be introduced. This requires a significant amount of contextual learning and customization, first by people at the development stage as part of needs assessment, and then by the system itself.

There are other meaningful activity categories that can be used to inform development of smart medical home technologies. For example, Ni et al. (2015) modify the ADL/IADL taxonomy by adding the third category, that of ambulatory (movement-related) activities, which are further separated into stationary (e.g., sitting, lying down), transitional (e.g., moving from a bed to a chair), and dynamic (walking). This category is introduced for two reasons. First, it relates to the very important theme of falls prevention. Second, it provides a foundation for thinking about approaches to solving motion and body position detection problems.

9.5 THE IMPORTANCE OF USER ENGAGEMENT IN IDENTIFYING CHALLENGES OF DAILY LIVING ACTIVITIES

Seeing the world from another person's perspective is always difficult. User engagement, which is always important in developing consumer technology, is absolutely critical in identifying and describing daily living activities to be supported in smart medical homes. If you are a young, able-bodied "digital native," it may be particularly difficult to see home functioning through the eyes of an older person, or a person with a disability. Asking a group of target users about their experiences is much more effective than engaging in a mental walk-through.

Kelly et al. (2014) interviewed 24 individuals aged 65–85 about their daily living activities, rendered difficult by perceptual, physical, and cognitive effects of aging. The findings highlighted difficulties unique to that group. For example, many participants mentioned the impact of perceptual difficulties on domestic activities such as cooking. One person explained that reading cooking instructions on boxes became difficult because of the small font and thus a constant need for glasses. A smart home environment can easily overcome this challenge by providing a function where user reads a product name into an app, which then provides audio-narration of the instructions or displays them on a large screen, for-matted for visibility. However, because perceptual difficulties are often less visible to others than mobility difficulties, designers may overlook them without users' input.

It is also important to remember that life is not a set of isolated activities, and that well-being in one area affects well-being in another. The right level of perspective is essential to understanding users' functioning. For example, a person who is unable to self-groom may be less willing to go out or place a video call to a family member. This, in turn, may affect their emotional state and access to healthy fresh food, which may further exacerbate diffi-culties with self-care and isolation. User engagement at the right level of granularity may help identify such complex networks of related issues. Moreover, with smart technology, the ability to collect information about user needs and preferences needn't be limited to the design phase. Rather, because data can be continuously collected in smart medical homes and integrated with other types of data, they can be used to tailor support.

9.6 TECHNICAL CHALLENGES TO ADDRESS IN SMART MEDICAL HOMES

9.6.1 Energy Efficiency

A number of technical challenges need to be addressed in order for smart homes to become a ubiquitous solution for aging at home and supporting independent living of people with disabilities (Majumder et al., 2017). One challenge has to do with increasing smart homes' energy efficiency. This concern may seem paradoxical, because we are used to hearing of smart technology as an energy-efficient solution. Indeed, smart homes do increase the energy efficiency of lighting, thermostats, and water systems. They may turn off unneces-sary lights in empty rooms, while lighting a resident's path inside the home, and can cus-tomize laundry water usage to the size of the load. However, when the health data layer is added, energy needs increase significantly. Health monitoring generates very large amounts of data that need to be processed in real time. This matters because if energy use is not controlled, residents' utility bills become prohibitively expensive. Energy-efficient solutions, beyond the scope of this chapter, focus on improving computational efficiency of algorithms as well as selection of optimal data types. For example, videos are very informative, but generate very large amounts of data.

9.6.2 Interoperability

Another important consideration is interoperability. Smart medical homes involve a large number of systems and devices, connected via Internet of Things (IoT) networks. For this to work, devices created by different manufacturers need to be able to communicate via wireless protocols and exchange data with one another. At the present time, the market of smart devices and communication technologies is fragmented because of the lack of standards, protocols, and data formats. For example, different standards for connecting devices and systems to the internet can include Wi-Fi, Bluetooth, Z-Wave, and more. Each of these standards is a unique language, and devices are typically developed to speak one of them. Communications from different devices are bridged by hardware hubs that need to understand all these languages. In the absence of interoperability standards, developers often choose to make their products compatible with one big-name hub (e.g., Amazon, Google, Apple, or Microsoft). Consumers, then, need to be cognizant of these compatibilities when choosing devices for their homes. In a later section, we illustrate how interoperability problems limit communication functionality of smart glucose monitors that make blood glucose readings of patients with diabetes available to their caregivers. Lack of standards and limited interoperability make configuring smart technology difficult beyond the comfort level of an average lay user, especially in the target population of smart medical home residents. To be widely accepted, consumer technology needs to be easy and intuitive, operating on "plug-and-play" principle, springing to function on the first use without needing to be configured.

9.6.3 Privacy and Security

In order to be effective, smart medical home technologies need to access large volumes of data pertaining to all aspects of residents' functioning, from their socialization and sleep patterns to eating and toileting. These data – e.g., videos and audios – are detailed and intrusive, and provide insight into users' health status, habits, personality traits, interactions, desires, hopes, and fears. Thus, ensuring both data privacy and data security is of paramount importance. The two concepts – data privacy and data security – are related, but not identical. Privacy refers to laws and policies concerning who has the right to access the data and to what end. The concept of privacy is about regulating access, rather than technical considerations. Security, on the other hand, is about protecting the data from unauthorized access. When data security is compromised in a data breach, privacy is also violated. As more and more IoT devices enter the market, their design increasingly prioritizes innovation and functionality, rather than security. Security breaches occurring via IoT technology have happened in the past, and are likely to happen in the future, with potentially serious consequences.

9.7 ATTEMPTS TO REGULATE PRIVACY AND SECURITY OF SMART HOMES

Protection of smart medical home residents against data breaches and unauthorized use of their data should not be left to the good will of the marketplace. The American Civil Liberties Union (ACLU) has been pointing out surveillance threats inherent in "always on" recording features of smart devices such as voice-activated personal assistants (e.g., Amazon Echo, Google Home, Apple's Siri) and making recommendations for privacy protection measures (Stanley, 2017). In 2015, Electronic Privacy Information Center (EPIC), a public interest research center, wrote a letter to the US Attorney General and Federal Trade Commission (FTC), urging them to conduct a comprehensive investigation and facilitate a joint "Privacy and Law" workshop on potential surveillance concerns surrounding the use of "always on" consumer devices (Rotenberg, Horwitz, & Butler, 2015). The workshop would provide a space to investigate the nuances of "always on" technologies, focusing on whether current practices violate any existing federal and state laws.

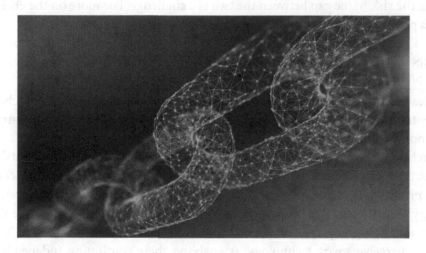

Yet, regulating privacy and security of the IoT data generated by smart medical home technologies is extremely tricky. Smart medical homes data are a special case of electronic personal data, so various general personal data protection laws apply. These laws may specify how personal data should be collected, managed, and protected, what information should be given to users, how consent should be obtained, and what should happen in case of a security breach – the issues that EPIC was urging the Attorney General and the FTC to consider (Rotenberg et al., 2015). Unfortunately, the United States does not have a single comprehensive data protection law. Instead, it has several industry-specific federal laws that govern data protection within specialized sectors (e.g., healthcare, financial services), as well as a patchwork of state laws and regulations. The main US law that regulates privacy of health information is Health Insurance Portability and Accountability Act, or HIPAA, enacted in 1996. Although several later regulations and guidance documents extend HIPAA provisions to address technologies such as cloud computing, HIPAA is not well equipped to regulate evolving technologies that underlie smart medical homes. Additionally, many smart home data transactions draw on data that may not be subject to HIPAA, depending on the status of the entities exchanging data. While FTC has issued a broad set of best practices for businesses that would address privacy and security of consumer IoT devices, those best practices are guidelines, rather than laws.

Unlike the US, the European Union (EU, 2018) has a uniform General Data Protection Regulation (GDPR) that became law in May 2018. GDPR is a very important step in regulating data protection, setting a global example, but applying it to IoT technologies is not straightforward, and many European businesses have difficulty deciding what compliance means for their technology. For example, the regulation requires obtaining users' consent before recording and processing their data, but defining users can be tricky and obtaining permission to record may invalidate the purpose of the device. For example, in the case of a smart doorbell that takes a picture and sends an image of a visitor to the resident's phone, it is not clear whether the visitor should be considered a user. In addition, asking the visitor's permission to record their image may defeat the purpose of the device's security function (Brar, 2018). As is often the case, technologies are evolving faster than legislature, and managing the risk in the gap between the two is a challenge. For more on the ethical complications posed by privacy considerations see Part II: Chapter 11.

9.8 NON-TECHNICAL CHALLENGES TO THE EMERGENCE OF SMART MEDICAL HOMES

The greatest non-technical challenge to proliferation of smart medical homes technology is user acceptance. No matter how potentially useful something is, if users are distrustful of it, it will not spread.

Research suggests that the two biggest factors that negatively affect residents' willingness to accept smart home technology are poor usability and privacy concerns. Yet, although privacy concerns are the most common reason for which older adults reject smart technology (Morris et al., 2013), fear of losing privacy is weighted against the desire for autonomy and aging in place, as opposed to moving to a residential care facility. When individuals perceive smart technology as enabling their continuing independence and view privacy concerns as adequately addressed, they usually welcome the technology.

9.8.1 Making It Specific: Some Examples
9.8.1.1 In the Wild
As mentioned previously, most of the chapter so far has focused on the concept of smart medical homes and their potential. Yet, potential aside, our actual living spaces are now much smarter than they were 10–20 years ago. Many homes have remotely controlled thermostats, motion-sensor-enabled lights, and remotely accessible security systems that will alert an absent resident about a suspected break-in while also notifying a security company.

While all-home-encompassing IoT networks are still rare, many individual devices are connected with smartphones or voice assistants. Smartphones can serve to remotely adjust settings on cooking appliances and operate smart washers and driers, which can then send text notifications when their cycles are over. Voice assistants stream music, set alarms, make calls, and deliver tailored news reports. Moreover, web services such as IFTTT and Stringify allow users to program apps and supported devices to performed sequences linked by conditional if-then statements. For example, one can create a chain of events in which opening a garage door after 6 pm turns on the thermostat in the living room and starts a cooking appliance and a laundry cycle. Another possible chain focusing on older adults could involve turning off cooking appliances when the resident leaves home (as recorded by a security system) and notifying a caregiver if the resident left in the evening and did not return after a specified time.

With regard to technological developments with a more targeted focus on the health domain, chronic disease management at home has been made easier by smart home based or portable medical devices, wirelessly connected to apps that can analyze their data and issue alerts and suggestions. For example, many glucose monitors synch their data with apps and allow sharing results with a doctor.

While interoperability remains a challenge, tech-savvy patients and their families and friends start joining forces in search of creative solutions for overcoming it. A noteworthy example of a grassroots approach is the #WeAreNotWaiting movement by parents of children living with Type 1 Diabetes (HealthLine, 2020). The movement grew out of concerns about the lack of interoperability standards that would allow easy integration and communication of glucose monitoring data. Lack of interoperability prevents the optimal data flow that could connect everyone who needs to be involved. For example, a child's continuous glucose monitor may record a dangerous value in the middle of the night and transmit it to a parent's phone, but flexibly routing the alert to the parent/caregiver of choice is not computationally trivial. To overcome this problem, the community, comprised of diabetes leaders, entrepreneurs, and developers, many of whom are parents of children with Type 1 Diabetes, created an open-source Nightscout project. The project supports uploading continuous glucose measurement data from monitors to the cloud and accessing it in real time via a range of interfaces and devices. Tech-savvy parents can use the technology to add smart features to their homes. For example, one father who works in remote automation and smart homes networking used Nightscout to enable triggering the lights to turn on in the parents' master bedroom if readings became too low. Parents in the #WeAreNotWaiting movement exchange DIY technology tips for using smart technology to make their children's lives safer (Hoskins, 2018).

9.8.1.2 In the Laboratory

In university laboratories, numerous interesting projects in sensors and automation develop and test various technologies for smart medical homes. There are also several academic research testbed facilities that are actual homes or apartments, equipped with multiple sensors and smart medical home features. For example, the Aware Home Research Initiative at Georgia Tech, started in 1998, has several living labs, including a three-story house that simulates a residential home and an apartment at a senior living housing building. These facilities are used by many Georgia Tech research teams, enabling researchers to implement and test their systems in authentic environments, observing how real people from target audience groups interact with them for prolonged periods of time. Smart medical home technologies researched under the umbrella of the Initiative involved supporting many aspects of aging in place and living with disability (Aware Home Research Initiative, n.d.). For example, Digital Family Portrait project used multiple ambient sensors installed throughout the house to collect data on the activity level of an elderly family member living alone and share it with relatives (Do & Jones, 2012). Another project, Cook's Collage, involved video capture of cooking activities that could be reviewed by the resident who got distracted and forgot their place in the cooking process (Do & Jones, 2012). Yet another project involved smart bathrooms that assessed users' level of frailty via ambient sensors (e.g., placed on the floor, grab bars, and the toilet seat) measuring walking speed, stability, and grip strength. It then attempted to adjust height and tilt of bathroom features to accommodate users' needs. Aware Home facilities also served as sites for testing smart robotic assistants able to navigate around the home environment – a topic considered at greater length in the next section (Do & Jones, 2012).

Other noteworthy academic smart medical home testbeds include University of Florida's Gator Tech Smart House (GTSH) and Washington State University's Center for Advanced Studies in Adaptive Systems (Center of Advanced Studies in Adaptive Systems, n.d.) smart apartment (casas.wsu.edu/about). Similarly to Aware Home facilities, these spaces are equipped with multiple sensors (motion, temperature, light, and more) and activators, and have served as labs for testing activity recognition algorithms that could help monitor and manage health of individuals in need of in-home support (e.g., those with diabetes and Alzheimer's disease) (Alberdi et al., 2018; Helal, Cook, & Schmalz, 2009).

Most smart medical homes technology described here is still in the research and development phase, with more work necessary before commercialization is possible. Unfortunately, because university research projects are typically funded for short periods of time, many are short-lived. For example, in a book published in 2016, Wetter compiled a table of various smart home projects worldwide. Writing a book is a lengthy process, so some time certainly had passed between compiling the table and the book's publication. At the time of our researching this chapter in the spring of 2020, we were unable to find evidence of ongoing operation of many of the projects listed in the table (p. 246). Yet, what is currently available, both on the market and in the world of R&D (research and development; e.g., ambient sensors, voice assistants, IFTTT web services, wireless cloud-connected portable homecare devices DIY movements) suggests that the future is near and it holds exciting promise.

9.8.1.3 Home Healthcare Robots

Throughout this chapter, we have mentioned many smart devices, including beds, grab bars, toilets, and kitchen appliances. Another category of devices, which sparks enough promise and controversy to merit a separate subsection, is home healthcare robots. Robots, or automated devices able to carry out complex multi-step tasks, have long been a staple of science fiction. Now they have entered many areas of real 21st-century life, including home healthcare. Home healthcare robots can perform many different functions, which, according to Wilson et al. (2019), can be divided into three categories according to the services they provide: companionship, coaching, and physical assistance.

Social companion robots are typically cute creatures designed to reduce stress and give pleasure by providing simulated social interactions. Currently, Japan, the country with the world's highest proportion of older adults among its population, is the leader in developing these robots, aiming to diminish loneliness and isolation. Two examples of popular social companion robots are Pepper and Paro. Pepper, launched by Japanese SoftBank Robotics in 2014 (SoftBank Robotics, n.d.), is a child-height humanoid robot designed to infer emotions from the tone of voice and facial expressions of its interlocutor and adjust its behavior accordingly. This robot, which interacts with humans via voice and touch screen interface, can sense human presence at a distance and initiate interactions, making eye contact and asking questions. Pepper, which has been used as a greeter/receptionist in Japanese and European banks and hospitals, can also be purchased for home use. There, it can serve to improve a resident's well-being by providing positive social interactions, as well as provide information in response to inquiries.

While humanoid robots like Pepper often serve as information provider and personal assistant, Paro, designed by Taakanori Shibata of a Japanese company called AIST, serves no function other than providing emotional support (see Figure 9.1). This robotic Harper seal pup is covered with antibacterial soft fur and equipped with multiple sensors. Designed to resemble animal therapy animals, Paro makes eye contact and responds to being petted. Paro is classified in the US as a Class 2 medical device. It has been used in nursing homes and dementia care facilities, as well as in homes of older adults (Hung et al., 2019). Clinical benefits and ethical considerations of the use of companion robots are discussed in future sections.

Companion robots elevate mood, while coaching and physical assistance robots help with specific tasks. For example, ROBEAR, developed by RIKEN and Sumitomo Riko

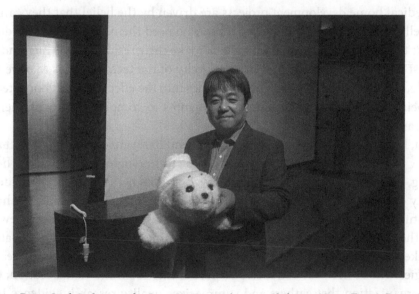

FIGURE 9.1 Paro Seal Robot with Creator, Dr. Takanori Shibata. *Note*: From *Paro (robot)*, by Geraldshields11, 2018, Wikipedia, (https://commons.wikimedia.org/wiki/File:Dr_Takanori_Shibata_and_PARO_2.jpg). CC BY-SA 4.0.

Company Limited, is an experimental nursing care robot that can lift a person from a bed and lower them into a wheelchair, or help them stand up with assistance. Lifting a fragile human without causing discomfort is a different activity from lifting an inanimate object, and the robot is equipped with multiple sensors to handle this delicate task safely. Other robots help with kitchen and household tasks, and even serve as dance exercise partners (Mitzner, Chen, Kemp, & Rogers, 2014). A research challenge in this area is identifying the factors that help human beings *accept* robots (e.g., Chu et al., 2019).

While the robots described above exemplify complex artificial intelligence, they are not part of a "smart" ambient environment. Integrating robots with a smart environment can potentially add a new level of power to smart home capabilities. Wilson et al. (2019) developed and evaluated the Robot Activity Support system (RAS), in which an assistive robot interacts with a smart environment's sensing, object detection, and mapping capabilities. The robot then helps older adults correct errors in everyday activities such as taking medicine with water or food; watering plants; and taking a dog for a walk. Once the system' sensors and analytical processors identify an activity and detect an error, such as an omitted or ineffective step (e.g., opening a medication container without getting food), the robot approaches the resident and asks whether they need help. Depending on the resident's preference, help can be provided as a video or as guided assistance (e.g., leading the resident to the fridge and helping them locate milk). At the present time, robots integrated into ambient environments of smart homes, such as RAS, are not commercialized.

9.9 EVIDENCE OF CLINICAL SIGNIFICANCE OF SMART MEDICAL HOMES TECHNOLOGY

9.9.1 Impact on Health and Well-Being

Smart medical home development projects are driven by the belief that they can improve health, well-being, and quality of life for those who need them. What evidence do we have that smart technologies in the homes, indeed, make their residents healthier and happier? The honest answer, unsurprising given the novelty of the technology, is that we presently know little, because of the lack of rigorous studies into the effect of smart home technology on well-being. Below are some examples of attempts to compile reviews of scientific evidence, arranged chronologically.

Martin, Kelly, Kernohan, McCreight, and Nugent(2008) attempted to conduct a systematic review of studies of the impact of smart home technologies on their users' health and well-being, as well as healthcare cost. However, although these researchers identified a large body of published works about smart home technologies for health, the handful of existing studies that addressed their clinical effectiveness did not meet the review's quality criteria. The authors had to conclude that, at the time of the review's publication, they could make no positive or negative statement about the effectiveness of smart health home technologies. The review was conducted as part of the Cochrane Collaboration, the international organization that gathers and summarizes quality research evidence in healthcare. Cochrane reviews apply stringent quality criteria to evidence evaluation. For example, the inclusion criteria for Martin et al. (2008) review required that studies had control groups, and that residents' health and well-being were assessed at multiple points before and after the introduction of the technology.

In the same year, Demiris and Hensel (2008) did another systematic review that identified 21 smart home projects targeting older adults, and similarly concluded that "evidence for their impact on clinical outcomes is lacking." Morris et al.(2013) reviewed published studies of feasibility (practicality) and effectiveness of smart home technologies aiming to "assist older people to live well at home" (p. 1). Upon narrowing their dataset to 21 studies that met the inclusion criteria – only one of which measured the effectiveness of the technology – these authors concluded that "given the modest number of objective analyses, there is a need for further scientific analysis of a range of smart home technologies to promote community living" (p. 1).

A 2016 systematic review of "smart homes and home health monitoring technologies for older adults" by Liu, Stroulia, Nikolaidis, Miguel-Cruz, and Ríos-Rincón (2016) was the latest effectiveness review that we were able to find when working on this chapter in the spring of 2020. The authors analyzed 48 published studies, 18 of which assessed residents' clinical outcomes. While 12 of 18 reported some positive findings, not all provided high-quality evidence. The highest quality positive evidence came from four studies. One of these showed that, compared with a control group, frail older adults living in homes equipped with multiple smart features showed less decline in their cognitive and physical functions over a period of two years (Tomita, Mann, Stanton, Tomita, & Sundar, 2007). Another showed that, compared with control group participants, older adults living with chronic illness and co-occurring depression who received home health monitoring technology became significantly better at managing their illness (Gellis, Kenaley, & Ten Have, 2014). The third study demonstrated that home health monitoring leads to fewer disease exacerbations and hospital visits in older adults with chronic obstructive pulmonary disease (COPD) (Pedone, Chiurco, Scarlata, & Incalzi, 2013). Finally, one study showed that wireless monitoring improved blood pressure control in older adults living with kidney disease and hypertension (Rifkin et al., 2013). At the same time, there were several moderate- and high-quality studies that showed significantly negative impact of smart home technologies on their users, including in areas of managing living with COPD and heart conditions. The review also found that effectiveness of smart health monitoring technology was, unsurprisingly, related to its level of maturity.

In conclusion, at the present, the field is in acute need of high-quality studies of the impact of smart home technologies on residents' health and well-being. These studies should focus on how technological systems impact specific important physical, emotional, cognitive, and social health outcomes. Other relevant outcome indicators may include frequency of healthcare utilization, reliance on caregivers, ability to perform activities of daily living and age in place, and sense of safety and security. At the present, some evidence suggests that smart technology in older adults' homes contributes to their increased confidence and sense of safety and security, particularly when it comes to alerting caregivers in the event of a fall (Pietrzak, Cotea, & Pullman, 2014)

9.9.2 Special Case: Impact on Ability to Diagnose Depression and Dementia

In addition to improving health and well-being, smart medical home technology can also potentially be used for disease diagnostics. An interesting special case involves some promising pilot research, in which wearable accelerometers and environmentally embedded motion sensors help reliably identify signs of depression and early dementia in independently living older adults (Alberdi et al., 2018; Dawadi, Cook, & Schmitter-Edgecombe, 2016; Galambos, Skubic, Wang, & Rantz, 2013). Some of this research is based on developing classification models that involve processing massive amounts of longitudinal smart homes data. The work is grounded in the knowledge that both dementia and depression decrease activity level and changes sleep patterns. In addition, neurological changes associated with dementia lead to changes in gait and mobility. While at the present smart technology is not yet used for clinical diagnosis of these conditions, the possibility is on the horizon.

9.10 ETHICAL CONSIDERATION OF SMART MEDICAL HOMES DEVELOPMENT

In popular culture, as well as in media discourse of technology-driven social trends, both a utopian and a dystopian view of smart technology are prevalent. For example, Black Mirror, a popular British sci fi TV series about the dark side of modern technology, includes an episode in which a chip implanted into a child's brain allows parents to monitor the child's vital signs and emotions and even see the child's visual field on a computer screen. The technology also allows adults to mute undesirable and disturbing things from the child's vision. Requested by an anxious parent with good intentions, the chip leads to traumatic consequences. At the same time, another episode of the same series depicts futuristic technology that enables bedridden older adults (spoiler alert) to live fuller lives by inhabiting their younger bodies in a virtual world.

The utopian view presents technology as an enabler to overcoming limitations. The dystopian view, exemplified, among other works, in Dave Egger's novel "The Circle" and a children's science fiction animation "WALL-E," includes themes of losses: of privacy, lost to surveillance-enabling technology; of independence; and of relationships with other humans. While we believe that potential benefits of smart medical homes are numerous, to avoid dystopian outcomes in real life, these ethical concerns should be taken very seriously.

9.10.1 Users' Understanding of Privacy and Security Considerations

Thus far, we have discussed ensuring smart medical homes' data privacy and security as a technical challenge. It is also an ethical imperative. One particular ethical concern is about informed consent. How can we help the user to truly understand risks of breaches and unauthorized use and make informed decisions about accepting them?

Older adults usually value autonomy over privacy and will often consent to trade some privacy for an increase in autonomy. However, in the context of smart homes, very complex technology is brought to vulnerable people who can be expected to have limited experience with such technology, and whose understanding may be impaired by cognitive difficulties. As a result, their consent may be less informed than their signatures on informed consent forms suggest.

Moreover, as smart technologies are new and the methods for analyzing the data obtained by them are developing rapidly, even the experts often cannot foretell potential future risks. It is critically important to be thorough in explaining the technology and discussing the risks with potential users and their family members (for more on privacy considerations, see Part II: Chapter 11).

9.10.2 Impact on Social Relationships

Concerns about the negative impact of technology on human relationships have been a persistent theme in societal conversations about technology since the Industrial Revolution. One of the benefits of smart medical technology is alleviating caregivers' burden. A possible downside of this is altering the relationships among family members, sometimes reducing the amount of interactions that older adults or individuals with disabilities have with other people. If an adult daughter knows that her elderly mother's home is equipped with sensors that will activate an alert in case of a perceived emergency, the daughter may visit less frequently, which may make the mother feel lonelier and more isolated.

The ethical quandary of using technology to avoid addressing the social problem of loneliness is often raised in discussions of home healthcare robots like Paro, the charming seal discussed in an earlier section. Equipping seniors' homes with humanlike robots is much easier and cheaper than developing policies and infrastructure that would strengthen social ties – but are those surrogate interactions nearly as fulfilling as the real thing? There is also the question of potential deception when residents with dementia or otherwise impaired cognitive function have difficulty recognizing the artificial nature of their robotic pets or assistants. Is it acceptable to allow fragile individuals to develop emotional attachments to robotic companions they view as alive? While these questions have no easy answers, they certainly merit attention.

9.10.3 Diffusion of Responsibility

Some authors have also raised a concern that smart medical technology in residents' homes potentially diffuses responsibility for the well-being of very fragile residents, shifting that responsibility away from human agents. For example, Stip and Rialle (2005) focused on smart medical homes for individuals living with schizophrenia. These authors point out that smart home technology may lessen the attention of healthcare professionals to individuals living independently with a serious mental illness. They suggest that new organizations and human services may be needed to support technology-enabled independent living.

9.10.4 Impact on Autonomy and Independence

In the best-case scenario, smart medical homes help older adults and individuals with cognitive and physical disabilities retain autonomy by enabling them to live at home. However, smart home features may also reduce autonomy by taking away opportunities for decision-making and choices. Furthermore, automating certain tasks may lead to reduced amount of movement and exercise, with negative consequences. To avoid this, the level of automation should be tailored to the resident's needs and expressed preferences.

9.11 CONCLUSIONS

This chapter shows how smart medical homes can use data from multiple connected environmental and wearable sensors and monitors to inform supporting residents' health, well-being, security, and performance of daily living activities. The technology is promising in supporting autonomy of aging-at-home older adults and individuals living with conditions that pose challenges to independent living. At the same time, the chapter also presents smart medical homes as a concept, full of possibilities, but not yet fully realized. For the concept of smart medical homes to fulfill this promise, several technical, ethical, and legislative challenges need to be addressed. Most importantly, much research is needed for the technology to become truly helpful. Some of this research should focus on assessing nuances of support needs of various groups of potential users. In addition, much remains to be discovered concerning clinical effectiveness of different smart medical technologies. Such work will require collaboration between industry, academia, policymakers, grassroots patient communities, and advocacy groups, as shown throughout this chapter.

WEB RESOURCES

Nightscout Project #WeAreNotWaiting
http://www.nightscout.info/
"Nightscout (CGM in the Cloud) is an open source, DIY project that allows real time access to a CGM [continuous glucose monitoring] data via personal website, smartwatch viewers, or apps and widgets available for smartphones."

Center of Advanced Studies in Adaptive System (CASAS), Washington State University
http://casas.wsu.edu/
This is Washington State University project that focuses on machine learning and computing technologies that "can provide context-aware, automated support in our everyday environments," such as smart homes.

Mobile & Pervasive Computing Laboratory, University of Florida
https://www.cise.ufl.edu/~helal/index.htm
This laboratory, led by Professor Sumi Helal, conducts several research projects in smart homes and assistive technologies.

REFERENCES

Alberdi, A., Weakley, A., Schmitter-Edgecombe, M., Cook, D.J., Aztiria, A., Basarab, A., & Barrenechea, M. (2018). Smart home-based prediction of multi-domain symptoms related to Alzheimer's disease. *IEEE Journal of Biomedical and Health Informatics, 22*(6), 1720–1731. https://doi.org/10.1109/JBHI.2018.2798062

Aware Home Research Initiative. (n.d.). *About AHRI.* Georgia Institute of Technology. Retrieved February 16, 2020, from http://www.awarehome.gatech.edu/

Brar, A. (2018, May 18). *What does the GDPR mean for IoT?* IoT Agenda. https://internetofthingsagenda.techtarget.com/blog/IoT-Agenda/What-does-the-GDPR-mean-for-IoT

Center of Advanced Studies in Adaptive Systems. (n.d.). *About.* http://casas.wsu.edu/

Centers for Disease Control and Prevention. (2019). *Nursing homes and assisted living (long-term care facilities [LCTFs]).* Retrieved February 16, 2020 from https://www.cdc.gov/longtermcare/

Chu, L., Chen, H. W., Cheng, P. Y., Ho, P., Weng, I. T., Yang, P. L., … Yeh, S. L. (2019). Identifying features that enhance older adults' acceptance of robots: A mixed methods study. *Gerontology*, 65(4), 441–450. doi: 10.1159/000494881

Dawadi, P. N., Cook, D. J., & Schmitter-Edgecombe, M. (2016). Automated cognitive health assessment from smart home-based behavior data. *IEEE Journal of Biomedical and Health Informatics*, 20(4), 1188–1194. https://doi.org/10.1109/JBHI.2015.2445754

Demiris, G. (2016). Smart homes: Empowering the patient till the end. In T. Wetter (Ed.,) *Consumer health informatics: New services, roles and responsibilities* (pp. 245–254). Springer.

Demiris G., & Hensel B. K. (2008). Technologies for an aging society: A systematic review of "smart home" applications. *Yearbook of Medical Informatics*, 33–40.

Do, E. Y., Jones, B.D. (2012). Happy Healthy Home. In J.C. Augusto, M. Huch, A. Kameas, J. Maitland, P. McCullagh, J. Roberts, A. Sixsmith, & R. Wichert. (Eds.). *Handbook of ambient assisted living: Technology for healthcare, rehabilitation and well-being.* (Vol. 11, pp. 195–210). IOS Press.

Farr C. (2020). *Apple introduces new COVID-19 features: Hand washing guides and a mask-wearing emoji.* CNBC. https://www.cnbc.com/2020/06/22/apple-introduces-apple-watch-handwashing-reminders.html#:~:text=The%20new%20feature%20includes%20a,as%20to%20wash%20their%20hands.

Galambos, C., Skubic, M., Wang, S., & Rantz, M. (2013). Management of dementia and depression utilizing in- home passive sensor data. *Geron* 2013;11(3):457–468. doi:10.4017/gt.2013.11.3.004.00

Gawande, A. (2014). *Being mortal: Medicine and what matters in the end.* New York: Metropolitan books; Henry Holt and Company.

Gellis, Z. D., Kenaley, B. L., & Ten Have, T. (2014). Integrated telehealth care for chronic illness and depression in geriatric home care patients: the Integrated Telehealth Education and Activation of Mood (I-TEAM) study. *Journal of the American Geriatrics Society*, 62(5), 889–895. https://doi.org/10.1111/jgs.12776

Healthline. (2020). *The #wearenotwaiting diabetes DIY movement.* https://www.healthline.com/health/diabetesmine/innovation/we-are-not-waiting#2

Helal, A., Cook, D. J., & Schmalz, M. (2009). Smart home-based health platform for behavioral monitoring and alteration of diabetes patients. *Journal of Diabetes Science and Technology*, 3(1), 141–148. https://doi.org/10.1177/193229680900300115

Hoskins, M. (2018, September 25). *D-dad automates home for diabetes safety.* Healthline. Retrieved February 16, 2020, from https://www.healthline.com/diabetesmine/automating-home-monitor-diabetes#2

Hung, L., Liu, C., Woldum, E., Au-Yeung, A., Berndt, A., Wallsworth, C., Horne, N., Gregorio, M., Mann, J., & Chaudhury, H. (2019). The benefits of and barriers to using a social robot PARO in care settings: a scoping review. *BMC Geriatrics*, 19, 232. https://doi.org/10.1186/s12877-019-1244-6

Kelly, A. J., Fausset, C. B., Rogers, W., Fisk, A. D. (2014). Responding to home maintenance challenge scenarios: The role of selection, optimization, and compensation in aging-in-place. *Journal of Applied Gerontology*, 33(8), 1018–1042. https://doi.org/10.1177/0733464812456631

Liu, L., Stroulia, E., Nikolaidis, I., Miguel-Cruz, A., Ríos-Rincón, A. (2016). Smart homes and home health monitoring technologies for older adults: A systematic review. *International Journal of Medical Informatics*, 91, 44–59.

Majumder, S., Aghayi, E., Noferesti, M., Memarzadeh-Tehran, H., Mondal, T., Pang, Z., & Deen, M. J. (2017). Smart homes for elderly healthcare-Recent advances and research challenges. *Sensors (Basel)*, 17(11). https://doi.org/10.3390/s17112496

Martin, S., Kelly G., Kernohan, W. G., McCreight, B., & Nugent C. (2008). Smart home technologies for health and social care support. *Cochrane Database of Systematic Reviews*. https://doi.org/10.1002/14651858.CD006412.pub2

Mitzner, T. L., Chen, T. L., Kemp, C. C., & Rogers, W. A. (2014). Identifying the potential for robotics to assist older adults in different living environments. *International Journal of Social Robotics*, 6(2), 213–227. https://doi.org/10.1007/s12369-013-0218-7

Morris M.E., Adair, B., Miller, K., Ozanne, E., Hansen R., et al. (2013) Smart-home technologies to assist older people to live well at home. *Journal of Aging Science* 1: 101. doi:10.4172/jasc.1000101

Muse, E. D., Barrett, P. M., Steinhubl, S. R., & Topol, E. J. (2017). Towards a smart medical home. *Lancet (London, England)*, 389(10067), 358. https://doi.org/10.1016/S0140-6736(17)30154-X

Ni, Q., García Hernando, A. B., Pau De la Cruz, I. (2015). The elderly's independent living in smart homes: A characterization of activities and sensing infrastructure survey to facilitate services development. *Sensors (Basel)*, 15(5), 11,312–11,362. https://doi.org/10.3390/s150511312

Pedone, C., Chiurco, D., Scarlata, S., & Incalzi, R. A. (2013). Efficacy of multiparametric telemonitoring on respiratory outcomes in elderly people with COPD: A randomized controlled trial. *BMC Health Services Research*, 13, 82. https://doi.org/10.1186/1472-6963-13-82

Pietrzak, E., Cotea, C., Pullman, S. (2014) Does smart home technology prevent falls in community-dwelling older adults: a literature review. *Journal of Innovation in Health Informatics*, 21(3):105–112.

Rifkin, D. E., Abdelmalek, J. A., Miracle, C. M., Low, C., Barsotti, R., Rios, P., Stepnowsky, C., & Agha, Z. (2013). Linking clinic and home: a randomized, controlled clinical effectiveness trial of real-time, wireless blood pressure monitoring for older patients with kidney disease and hypertension. *Blood pressure monitoring*, 18(1), 8–15. https://doi.org/10.1097/MBP.0b013e32835d126c

Rotenberg, M., Horwitz, J., & Butler, A. (2015, July 10). EPIC letter to the attorney general and the FTC chairwoman: Request for workshop and investigation of "always on" consumer devices. *Electronic Privacy Information Center [EPIC]*. Retrieved February 16, 2020, from https://epic.org/privacy/internet/ftc/EPIC-Letter-FTC-AG-Always-On.pdf

SoftBank Robotics. (n.d.). *Pepper press kit*. Retrieved February 16, 2020, from https://www.softbank-robotics.com/emea/sites/default/files/press-kit/Pepper-press-kit_0.pdf

Stanley, J. (2017, January 13). *The privacy threat from always-on microphones like the amazon echo*. American Civil Liberties Union. https://www.aclu.org/blog/privacy-technology/privacy-threat-always-microphones-amazon-echo

Stip, E., & Rialle, V. (2005). Environmental cognitive remediation in schizophrenia: Ethical implications of "smart home" technology. *The Canadian Journal of Psychiatry*, 50(5), 281–291. https://doi.org/10.1177/070674370505000509

Tomita, M., Mann, W.C., Stanton, K., Tomita, A., & Sundar, V. (2007). Use of currently available smart home technology by frail elders: process and outcomes. *Topics in Geriatric Rehabilitation*, 23(1), 23–24. Doi: 10.1097/00013614-200701000-00005

West Health Institute & National Opinion Research Center at the University of Chicago. (2017, March 22). *Worries about aging loom large for Americans over 30, survey finds*. https://www.westhealth.org/press-release/worries-about-aging-loom-large-for-americans-over-30-survey-finds/

Wetter, T. (2016). Chapter 11: Smart Homes: Empowering the patient till the end. In Wetter T, *Consumer health informatics: New services, roles and responsibilities*. (pp. 245–252). Springer International Publishing. https://doi.org/10.1007/978-3-319-19590-2

Wilson, G., Pereyda, C., Raghunath, N., de la Cruz, G., Goel, S., Nesaei, S., Minor, B., Schmitter-Edgecombe, M., Taylor, M. E., & Cook, D. J. (2019). Robot-enabled support of daily activities in smart home environments. *Cognitive Systems Research*, 54, 258–272. https://doi.org/10.1016/j.cogsys.2018.10.032

World Health Organization. (2018a, February 8). *Aging and health*. Retrieved February 16, 2020, from https://www.who.int/news-room/fact-sheets/detail/ageing-and-health

World Health Organization. (2018b, January 16). *Disability and health*. Retrieved February 16, 2020, from https://www.who.int/en/news-room/fact-sheets/detail/disability-and-health

CHAPTER 10

Patient Communities

Catherine Arnott Smith

10.1 INTRODUCTION

In this chapter, we discuss the importance of online patient communities and forums as sites for both information and data exchange. The need for peer support is older than the Web, but the Web has made it very easy for patient-to-patient connections to take place. These communities can be standalone websites (e.g., PatientsLikeMe) or components of larger social networks (e.g., Facebook). This environment presents both challenges and opportunities for consumer and patient support around healthcare.

The search for health information is one of the most common human activities there is. The National Cancer Institute's Health Information National Trends Survey (or HINTS) has been polling US citizens about their information seeking in the healthcare domain since 2003. The motivation for the survey's development: a Harris poll revealing that 70% of respondents had searched for health information – 15% for cancer information (Rice, 2001).

The 2018 HINTS survey found that 79% of adults polled had looked for health or medical information in *any* source (National Cancer Institute, 2018). Ninety percent of US adults are now online, a proportion that has remained unchanged since at least 2015 (Anderson et al., 2019). So it is not surprising that "the internet" was the most popular of all those sources, used by 75% of respondents (with "doctor or health care provider" a distant second at 14%). Slightly more than half (56%) of these respondents were looking for health information for themselves, with another 24% helping someone else as well. Closely related to health information seeking is the activity of *sharing* personal health information with other people. This online activity remains less common. Fourteen percent of respondents drawn from the general public indicated that they had shared health information on social media (National Cancer Institute, 2018). And the difference between the 79% who seek, and the 14% who share, may be the difference between *consumers* – who may or may not be living with a health condition – and *patients* – who are living with health conditions for which they may be seeking support from people like them.

A recent survey of 930 consumers drawn from an online vendor panel was called "fairly representative of the US population." Fifty-one percent were female; 67% were Caucasian,

12% African-American, and 13% Hispanic, 42% had an associate's or bachelor's degree, and 41% had annual incomes less than $50,000. These consumers were asked about the importance of 27 different social media and networking variables to their preventive health care. The need "to connect with a support group of persons with health conditions like your own" was ranked the second most important, 35.3 of respondents calling it "Very important" (Cangelosi et al., 2017).

Their family members, partners, and spouses may also be in need of support because of caregiving concerns that center on the same diagnosis. Patients and the people who love and care for them increasingly rely on the internet not just as a source of health information, but as a platform promoting emotional strength and coping strategies (see Part I: Chapter 6 for detailed discussion of caregivers in this context).

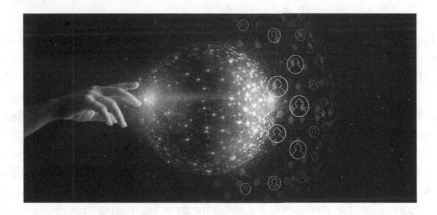

10.2 BRIEF HISTORY

Patient communities are a particular kind of virtual community, something defined by one researcher as "social networks formed or facilitated by electronic media" (Eysenbach et al., 2004). The literature focusing on *patient* virtual communities calls them many things, including online patient meetings (Feenberg et al., 1996), online self-help groups (Madara, 1999), online forums (Tanis, 2008), social networking sites (or SNS) (Boyd & Ellison, 2008), and computer-mediated support groups (Rains & Young, 2009). The term "peer-to-peer," which first appeared in the medical literature in 1997 (Gupta et al., 1997), has become increasingly popular in the twenty-first century.

Patient communities are a phenomenon that predates the Web, since the desire of consumers and patients to seek support from each other is a very old one. The nineteenth and early twentieth-century physician Joseph Hersey Pratt is credited as originating the patient self-help group into medical practice. It began when he prescribed bed rest and fresh-air tent camping at home to tuberculosis patients who were unable to live in sanitariums because their families were dependent on their weekly salaries – or whose TB was too advanced for sanitarium care. Pratt's response was called "the Home Sanatorium Method," and part of the treatment involved weekly class meetings in which individual patients met with other patients. Pratt changed its name to the "Class Method" when he realized how important the group dynamics were to homebound patients' recovery (Ambrose, 2011). Over time, the practice of group work expanded from the domain of tuberculosis to conditions that people were living with longer and longer, with improvements in public health and healthcare: diabetes and heart disease, for example. And in time, patient groups moved out of the clinic. Peer support is now an evidence-based strategy integrated into treatment modalities in many diagnostic settings.

After World War II, the first diagnosis-specific groups were organizations founded by parents of child patients – a group of stakeholders that continues to be a powerful force in consumer health informatics today (for discussion of the role of parents as caregivers in the CHI context, see Part I: Chapter 6). For example, the March of Dimes was created in 1938 as the National Foundation for Infantile Paralysis. When its funded research into vaccine resulted in the eradication of polio, the foundation shifted its attention to "disabilities and disorders appearing in infancy and childhood" (Rose, 2010). Today, organizations like the March of Dimes are called "voluntary health agencies," defined as "any nonprofit, nongovernmental agency, governed by lay or professional individuals and organized on a national, state or local level, whose primary purpose is health related" (Voluntary Health Agency, 2009).

One important function of voluntary health agencies is to direct interested people – including patients – to support groups meeting in various media, as for example, the American Syringomelia and Chiari Alliance Project features groups that meet face-to-face, online, and even via telephone (American Syringomelia & Chiari Alliance Project, 2013). The National Library of Medicine's MEDLINEPlus consumer health information website lists hundreds of similar agencies on its Organizations page (for a discussion of MEDLINEPlus, see Part I: Chapter 5: Trusted Sources) [https://MEDLINEplus.gov/organizations/all_organizations.html].

Patient virtual communities were among the earliest such communities online, and predated the World Wide Web, being a feature of newsgroups from the early internet era. But it was clear from the start that some patients relied on these groups more than others (Jadad et al., 2006). One of the earliest references in print to an online support group focusing on a particular diagnosis appears in Feenberg et al. (1996). These authors describe internet-facilitated support groups for people living with Amyotrophic Lateral Sclerosis (ALS; also known as Lou Gehrig's or Motor Neuron Disease) in the early years of the internet. A weekly magazine called the *ALS Digest* featured email messages from participants – "patients, caregivers, and physicians" – that were published online; a separate, unmoderated chat group for patients and caregivers, with about 500 subscribers, was held via the Prodigy Medical Support Bulletin Board. The non-profit portal ACOR – Association of Cancer Online Resources – was founded in 1996 as "a loose confederation of more than 150 publicly accessible mailing lists" with from less than ten to more than 2000 subscribers. ACOR still survives today, although many of its lists have migrated to the online community SmartPatients (Association of Cancer Online Resources, n.d.) www.acor.org. Madara (1999) too describes the origins of patient communities in BBS (Bulletin Board Systems). By 2001, almost 30 million internet users were estimated to be members of medically themed online groups (Horrigan et al., 2001). In 2004, Meier et al. reported that Yahoo! hosted 33,000 distinct communities (2007) and stated that most online group lists were hosted in the United States. However, only 9% of "health seekers" – defined at this early date as "Internet users who have gone online for health or medical information" had participated in a health-related support group. A few years earlier, Rainie and Fox had seen a similarly small number and speculated that this low participation was due to health seekers being "more protective of their privacy" than the general population (2000). By 2009, the Pew researchers found that 39% of the people they were now calling "e-patients" used social networks, particularly but not surprisingly when they were between the ages of 18 and 29. However, they were not using those networks for health-related reasons – except for lurking. While 41% had read about others' health experiences in places like online news groups or websites, only 6% had posted their own stories in similar places, so apparently privacy concerns had not diminished with time (Fox & Jones, 2009). And in 2011, 18% of that general population reported that they had gone online because they were actively *looking* for people like them, and more so if they were living with chronic illnesses such as diabetes, cancer, or lung conditions (23%). People living with rare diseases utilized peer-to-peer support even more than those with chronic illnesses, "online by necessity, since they are unlikely to live near to the people who share their conditions" (Fox, 2011).

Frustrated by a lack of attention to the teen and young adult population, in 2018 researchers at Hopelab and the Well Being Trust conducted a survey of young people aged 14–22 and their "digital health practices." This study revealed a much higher level of engagement with "patients like me" as respondents aged out of their teens. Sixty-nine percent of young adults and 52% of teens had watched or read about the health experiences of other people; 51% of young adults and 25% of teens reported trying to find people online who had similar health issues to their own. And 20% of those young adults shared those health issues online (in social media, blogs, or videos) compared to 8% of teens. Youth who identified as LGBTQ were more than twice as likely as straight peers to have shared narratives about their health in an online context (28% vs. 13%), and Blacks were more likely (24%) than either Whites or Latinos (13% each). Females were more likely than males (44% vs. 33%) to say that they had tried to find people online with similar health issues (Hopelab, 2018).

10.3 EXAMPLES OF PATIENT COMMUNITIES

CHESS – the University of Wisconsin's Comprehensive Health Enhancement Support System – has been called one of the most studied virtual communities in the medical literature (Winkelman & Choo, 2003). This early computer-based system served the needs of patients and families in domains including breast cancer, HIV/AIDS, and alcoholism. Not only did the system assist users in decisionmaking and provide access to both patient narratives and clinical experts, but it provided "detailed articles, tutorials about services, and brief answers to many questions" (Gustafson et al., 2008). Gustafson et al. described the contents of CHESS' AIDS module in 1999:

- Questions & Answers
- Instant Library

- Getting Help/Support

- Referral Directory

- Assessment

- Decision Aid

- Action Plan

- Discussion Groups

- Ask an Expert

- Personal Stories

Early studies found not only improvement in quality of life among CHESS community members, but "significant" decreases in utilization of healthcare services (Gustafson et al., 1999). One 2013 randomized trial found that caregivers assigned to the CHESS arm reported reduced physical symptom distress in patients compared to a control group (Gustafson et al., 2013). The CHESS lab is still an active center for research collaboration today. In May 2020, CHESS and the University of Wisconsin-Madison journalism school collaborated on producing a free website and mobile app dedicated to COVID-19 resources, including not only discussion forums but meditation exercises, a fact checker and symptom-tracking logs (Kim, 2020).

The PatientsLikeMe (PLM) community – self-described as a "health learning system" – offers similar benefits to its members in terms of information and support – but in a crowd-sourcing era, the information flow is not from physician to patient, as in CHESS, but from patient to patient, and even from patient to researcher. PLM was founded by brothers of a young man diagnosed with ALS. It began with three diagnostic subcommunities focusing on ALS, Parkinson Disease, and MS, but expanded to cover more and more non-neurological conditions before merging its separate communities into one overarching platform. Today, over 650,000 members report living with more than 2,900 distinct conditions (PatientsLikeMe, 2019a). Moderated discussion forums activate personal connections between members. However, PLM was noted early for its provision of clinical tools on the site, so that community members can report not only symptoms of their conditions, but both treatments and side effects of medications. A "PEHR" (Personal Electronic Health Record) facilitates tracking and visualization of personal health data. One controversial aspect of this particular patient community: Members' self-reported data is deidentified, aggregated, and sold to partners ("companies that are developing or selling products to patients … [including] drugs, devices, equipment, insurance, and medical services.") (PatientsLikeMe, 2019b). Ferguson (2012) points out that on PatientsLikeMe, patients are not only members of their own community, but brokers of their own data, from which more than 100 research studies have now been published (PatientsLikeMe, 2019a). For a discussion of PatientsLikeMe in the context of participatory medicine, see Part I, Chapter 1 of this book.

10.4 BENEFITS OF PATIENT COMMUNITIES AS INFORMATION SOURCES

"Support" is a frequently cited benefit of participation in patient communities. But there are different kinds of support. Evans et al. identified three principal types: *Emotional* ("concern, affection, comforting, and encouragement"); *Informational* ("advice giving, information sharing, and personal knowledge development"); and *instrumental* ("tangible assistance such as practical help with daily living") (Evans et al., 2012, p. 406). Hartzler and Pratt focused on recommendations only and found four principal kinds: *action strategies* ("things to do"), *knowledge* ("things to know"), *perspectives* ("ways of believing or approaching situations"), and *information resources* ("things to obtain and use") (Hartzler & Pratt, 2011).

10.4.1 Patients Supporting Each Other

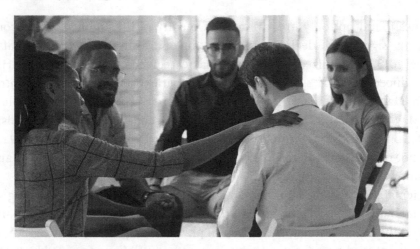

One 22-year-old White man in the Hopelab study described above related his own sharing experience in a way that illustrates how patients use information to simultaneously give and receive support:

> I told others how I experienced depression. How it developed, what it did to me and how it affected those around me. I also told of what helped me cope and get through it in the end. The other people either congratulated me or asked me for advice on the topic.
>
> (Hopelab, 2018)

One recent integrative review of 26 research studies published between 2009 and 2016 (Laukka et al., 2019) considered patient communities as information *sources*, together with other expressions of online participation like review and rating websites, and found the greatest impacts on consumers' feeling of empowerment; their health literacy; well-being (physical, mental, and emotional); their relationship with their healthcare organizations; management of their illness; and peer support. The evidence base is accumulating for the utility of information and communication technology (ICT) for disease prevention and health promotion (Veinot et al., 2013). Thus it becomes increasingly important to understand information flows within communities and how they benefit the individual.

It is critically important to understand that in patient communities, information is provided by *patients*. This means that it is never simple question asking and answering that drives the community; rather, it is the presentation of information *in context* by people with the authority of lived experience: "socially contextualized knowledge .. explicit knowledge ... in tandem with a vibrant social support system" (Winkelman & Choo, 2003). Entwisle et al. (2011) call this "personal experiences" information, which is different from "general facts."

A patient community story from the very early days of the World Wide Web illustrates how difficult it can be to disentangle the three kinds of support: emotional, informational, and instrumental. In 1995, the author of this chapter was a medical librarian working for a large reinsurance company in Fort Wayne, Indiana, when she happened to see a message on a medical librarians' listserv™ from two college students in Italy named Cris and Jo. That message read:

> Alice, our friend, has a very bad disease ... We are trying to connect with a hospital in Michigan ... because we know that in that hospital there is the other person who has the same bad disease. We know only the Italian name: dysautonomia familiar del II tipo.

The students had posted this message to every internet bulletin board they could find that referenced Michigan, genetic, disease, or health, which even in 1995, according to the *Washington Post,* meant "it must have appeared in hundreds of sites." They were looking for help for a family friend in Venice, a child suffering from a rare disease closely related to Familial Dysautonomia, or FD. After corresponding with Cris and Jo – whose English was much better than the author's non-existent Italian – the author was able to find an internet-based support group of parents living with FD – a listserv™ called FD Net. This community had been established by an FD parent who happened to be a professor of telecommunications at the University of Wisconsin-Madison – just the year before. Cris and Jo were able to connect their young friend's parents with the members of FD Net. Alice's father wrote to the group a few months later: "You all have done in a few weeks more than the doctors {in Italy} have done in eight years." A freelance journalist who saw one of the students' posts in a newsgroup interviewed the author, the Italian students, the child patient, and her parents for a story that ran in the Washington Post in 1995 – an early example of consumer health informatics gone viral (Rovner, 1995). Patient communities seem to satisfy social, emotional, and informational needs at the same time.

It matters *who* is providing the answer. Hartzler and Pratt (2011) examined patient expertise versus clinician expertise in a context of breast cancer, looking at patient-centric sources like online communities and books, as well as clinician-centric sources like books and online forums run by physicians ("Ask-A-Doctor"). These researchers found a statistically significant difference in the kind of content patient-generated sources discussed, as opposed to clinician-generated. Patient expertise relied on the personal; clinical expertise, unsurprisingly, on the medical. One medical topic appeared across the board, from patient forums to physicians. That one: "understanding biomedical concepts and processes," which hints at the crucial interaction of informational support and health literacy. If the patient with the question does not understand the nature of her illness, no answer will completely meet her needs – regardless of whether emotional, informational, or instrumental advice is what she seeks.

The pediatrician Wendy Sue Swanson, Chief of Digital Innovation at Seattle Children's Hospital, explains why peer-to-peer knowledge complements physician expertise:

> As a doctor, I can help you sort through the evidence on a test or a treatment, but I haven't actually had diabetes or the conditions I help families understand and treat. If you can find somebody like you who has been there, who understands the nuances and is willing to share, this can be a huge advantage for informing your choices. Many health decisions are not right or wrong – just what's right for you. … Talking with a peer who has been down similar paths may illuminate something absolutely new that I never would have been able to suggest. In my work as pediatrician and as a doctor using digital tools, I know peers bring wisdom and evidence of all kinds that clinicians cannot always uncover.
>
> (Fox, 2020)

The knowledge generated by patient communities is useful to non-patients – which, of course, includes physicians. "I had no idea that 'brain fog' was one of the commonest symptoms for people with multiple sclerosis until I saw how patients were ranking their symptoms on PatientsLikeMe," commented one family doctor (Hodgkin et al., 2018).

The patient's search for information from people like them means that even social media platforms without explicitly medical themes can become sites of information sharing. The social media site Reddit, with more than 232 health forums, hosts a subreddit called r/STD devoted to discussion of sexually transmitted diseases. Analysis of 500 random posts to r/STD revealed that 58% of posters were looking for a crowd-diagnosis – that is, a diagnosis obtained through crowdsourcing – asking questions like "Help! What is this… " and quoting healthcare providers: "My doc told me that guys have nothing to worry about and everyone has it. But, the internet says it gives women cancer. Do I need to tell future partners?" r/STD has almost 11,000 members as of January 1, 2020. Eighty-seven percent of these posts received a reply, 79% in less than a day (Nobles et al., 2019).

Contrast this with the typical physician office visit, which occurs out of the patient's daily life context and is extremely limited in duration: the patient is not situated in a social network, but rather engages in "a 'point interaction' because it is discrete, discontinuous, and takes place at a point in time and space" (Johnson & Ambrose, 2006).

Over the years, many researchers have attempted to quantify the benefit of patient communities by exploring their impact on health outcomes. A systematic review by Eysenbach et al. analyzed 45 articles about 38 research studies published between 1986 and 2003. Those 38 studies reported on seven specific health outcomes: depression; social support;

healthcare utilization; eating disorders; weight loss; diabetes control; and smoking. Depression and social support were the most frequently investigated outcomes in those 17 years (accounting for 12 studies each). The conclusion of Eysenbach et al.: Because very few controlled studies evaluated the effect of peer-to-peer groups on a "standalone" basis – most built-in "psychoeducational programmes or one to one communication with health-care professionals" – there was no "robust" evidence on the effects of these communities on these specific outcomes. The benefits of virtual patient communities remained unclear in large part because no researchers had *focused on the communities as interventions on their own*. Instead, the communities were investigated at the same time as other treatment modalities, for example, educational or cognitive behavior therapy components offered to community members (Eysenbach et al., 2004).

This article, published in 2004, represents not only the first but the only publication assessing an association of clinical outcomes with patient communities in which research-ers looked at more than one health outcome at a time. The trend ever since has been to investigate effects of patient community membership in groups of people living with the same diagnosis. This has resulted, of course, in a voluminous literature. A search of PubMed MEDLINE on January 1, 2020, reveals 907 studies of patient communities published since 1998, focusing on diagnoses from hidradenitis suppurativa to breast cancer. A collection of 186 such studies, published in a leading open-access medical informatics journal, can be found at https://www.jmir.org/themes/76 [the *Journal of Medical Internet Research*'s E-Collection: 'Peer-to-Peer Support and Online Communities'].

A few years after Eysenbach et al.'s systematic review, researchers at PatientsLikeMe sur-veyed members of six distinct subcommunities within PLM (ALS, MS, Parkinson Disease, HIV/AIDS, fibromyalgia, and mood disorders) who self-reported the site's perceived effects on their treatment decisions, symptom management, and clinical management as well as outcomes. Among the findings: 41% of patients in the HIV/AIDS community reduced risky behaviors; 42% of all respondents reported that PatientsLikeMe had helped them find another patient who helped them "understand what it was like to take a specific treatment for their condition." Forty-two percent said they were moderately or a lot more involved in their treat-ment decisions because of the site. Seventy-two percent of respondents found the site moder-ately or very helpful in understanding their symptoms (Wicks et al., 2010). In 2017 WEGO Health, which coordinates a network of over 100,000 "Patient Leaders" in hundreds of diag-nosis community contexts, surveyed 433 patient participants in seven communities: advanced melanoma; rheumatoid arthritis; epilepsy; COPD; bipolar depression; multiple sclerosis; and parenting/family health. Ninety-one percent of respondents reported that online communi-ties hosted on Facebook, Twitter, blogs, and other platforms play a role in their decisionmak-ing, and 93% ask their physicians about health information they hear about from an influential person in their patient community (WEGO Health Solutions, 2017).

Caregivers have an important role to play in patient communities, too. April Starr is the widow of Lucas Daniel. Daniel died of neuroendocrine cancer; he and his wife met at the Institute of Design at the Illinois Institute of Technology, and one of Ms. Starr's responses to her loss was to create useful worksheets for other patients to use. She got feedback from her widow's support group – the Hot Young Widow's Club – in designing this patient-centered system. The worksheets help patients (and caregivers) to articulate questions as well as answers in the domains of diagnosis, treatment, medications, and symptom monitoring (Starr, 2018).

10.5 CHALLENGES OF PATIENT COMMUNITIES

While virtual communities are very popular with many patients for the reasons outlined above, healthcare providers have been concerned from the beginning about potential negative consequences from participation.

Entwisle et al. (2011) distinguished general facts from "personal experience information." The latter type of information, they argue, can help patients in decisionmaking situations to "recognize decisions.. identify possible options ... appraise options and make a selection ..and support coping – including living with decisions made" (e296). The challenge in patient communities is to understand the difference between questions that require this context-based assistance – informational support – and questions that require fact-based answers.

The concern that patients will receive and act on health *mis*information is much older than the World Wide Web (in Part I of this book, both Chapter 1 and Chapter 5 go into detail on the problem). One 19th-century physician wrote about the need to screen information on library shelves to protect the "poor silly community, hypnotized by ignorance and befouled by quackery" (Gould, 1898). This old problem has been considerably accelerated by the popularity of social media, which helps people spread false facts along with the true. There is a spectrum of misinformation – while some websites are "deliberately deceitful," others make claims that have no scientific credibility (Keselman et al., 2019). Patient communities are not immune from the risks of sharing inaccuracies along with the facts. In fact, the "patient influencer" can in some cases serve as Patient Zero for bad information – "Patient Zero" being the public health term for the first identified carrier of a disease. Misinformation seems to spread more easily than the truth (Chou et al., 2018).

Healthcare professionals' typical concerns about online patient communities, voiced from the earliest days of the internet, were summarized by Gilles Frydman, the founder first of the Association of Cancer Online Resources and later of SmartPatients.com, this way:

> the communities would become a source of constant misinformation ... force people to make bad decisions and put them in opposition to their doctors .. [and] create an army of patients bringing reams of irrelevant printouts to each medical encounter.
>
> (Smart Patients Team, 2014)

These fears were, and are, not entirely groundless. A 2015 editorial piece in a patient safety journal argued that the combination of patient needs and internet access made for a "perfect storm" combining information access and social media:

> [T]he major initial use of the internet for healthcare by patients was simply to seek health information ... But, in many ways, the reference information function of the internet was just the beginning. It is increasingly clear that social

media represents a strong force. ... Facebook has become a significant source of healthcare information.

(Rozenblum & Bates, 2013)

Patient communities have responded by using strategies of information sharing and community rules. According to one study, Facebook is now the dominant platform for patients sharing health information: 87% through public posts (WEGO Health, 2017). Tory Aquino moderates a Facebook group of more than 5,000 parents, supporters and young patients living with an unusual type of juvenile arthritis. Ms. Aquino comments:

> Sometimes fake news can seem innocent ... but there are questions that are intentionally misleading my community, like 'has anyone else's kid experienced seizures with this drug?' I know it's fake, and I share medical research to counter it – because a parent might stop a critical medication.
>
> (Barrette, 2017)

Ronny Allan is a patient in the UK, active as a patient advocate, speaker, social media influencer, and moderator of his own Facebook support group devoted to provision of information about his rare cancer type, neuroendocrine tumor. This, like many rare and incurable diseases, is usually misdiagnosed until it has reached its late stages. Raising awareness is thus an important part of reducing mortality from this unpreventable cancer. With over 2.45 billion monthly active users in November 2019, 66% of which log on daily (Noyes, 2019), Facebook drives 50% of Allan's blog traffic. He writes: "I can tell you now, I will not allow ... fake news and peddling of 'snake oil' on any of my sites. My sites are targeted weekly by those who wish to sell their wares... They are quickly blocked" (Allan, 2019).

Jackie Zimmerman, the founder of Girls with Guts – a Facebook group for girls and women living with inflammatory bowel disease – runs a private parallel group which screens people interested in becoming members. "We have to be selective in who we 'let in'," comments Kathy Reagan Young, leader of a Facebook group for MS patients. "We have to be discerning in what we believe and do our own-fact-checking" (Barrette, 2018).

Community moderators, no matter what the community platform, have a thin line to walk between quality control and open communication – as cancer patient advocate Ronny Allan puts it,

> It's worrying that people are taken in by such drivel but we mustn't forget that people with cancer can often be in a distressed and anxious state and may look to other sources of therapy if they felt the conventional treatment was not working, not available in their healthcare system, or not within their budget/insurance cover (in insurance based health systems). Of course this is not helped by the well-intentioned friends and family who get carried away by what they read on the internet and pass it on to their loved ones.
>
> (Allan, 2019)

Allowing free and open dialog within patient communities means allowing space for the accurate information to be shared. WEGO Health patient advocates offer these guidelines for constructive communication that reinforce the importance of health information to the conversation:

* "Do the research, share the research" – that is, "credible medical journals and expert quotes"

* "Post the rules, enforce the rules" – and offer members a chance to correct the information they've posted

* "Partner with your physician" – and reiterate "the golden rule of patient conversation: 'Ask your doctor.'" (Barrette, 2017)

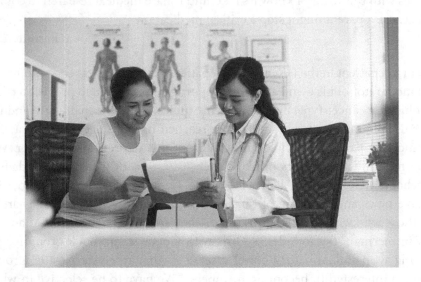

Another response to "misinformation, misbehavior, and safety in online patient communities" (Young, 2018) is illustrated by the case of the Mayo Clinic. This internationally renowned US medical center with headquarters in Rochester, Minnesota, built and maintains its own patient community, Mayo Clinic Connect. This community consists, as of January 2020, of 63 distinct subcommunities, ranging from "Addiction & Recovery" to "Women's Health." Groups can be specific to participants in one clinical trial, one phase of healthcare delivery (Intensive Care Unit), or focused on diagnosis (cancer), prevention (skin health, sleep health, healthy living). Members are patients, caregivers, or partners of and there are groups for adults, children, or teens.

Connect's forums are public; the Connect Network has designated Moderators, who are Mayo staff, work with volunteer Mentors in each group to ensure that posts meet community guidelines. Volunteer mentors themselves have to meet specific criteria, including "personal experience to contribute to the discussions," although mentors can be patients, caregivers, or family members (About Connect, n.d.). The volunteer mentors themselves are "the secret ingredient" that enable the online community to succeed. One of their functions is to watch for incorrect information. Mayo policies spell out Terms of Use for the Connect communities, and content moderators can warn or remove members that violate these terms. Members are asked *not* to tell other members what to do; volunteer mentors use language to center their expertise appropriately, such as "in my experience…" (Young, 2018) Community Guidelines (listed below) act as guardrails to prevent misinformation sharing and other bad behaviors:

- "Be careful about giving out medical advice."
- "Remain respectful at all times."
- "Be polite."
- "No commercial postings, advertisements, or solicitations."
- "No illegal activity."
- "No copyrighted postings."
- "Be yourself."
- "Follow the rules."
- "Report misuse" (Mayo Clinic, n.d.).

While the need for community guidelines in patient communities – many developed by the patients and moderators themselves – speaks to the potential pitfalls of this particular consumer health information technology, the popularity of these groups over the decades means that their continued existence is assured. Consumer health informatics developers, researchers, and healthcare professionals need to continue to collaborate to make the patient community space of the highest quality available – focusing not only on human problems such as content moderation, but also on aspects of design, such as usability.

WEB RESOURCES

Susannah Fox
Extensive resources on peer-to-peer research from a longtime advocate for health information seeking in digital spaces; video "Peer to Peer Health Advice" intended for patients and caregivers
https://susannahfox.com/

Peers for Progress: Peer Support Around the World
Advocacy and research organization presenting information about peer group tools, training and resources for doing effective peer support, as well as a collection of published papers with scientific evidence for peer support in numerous conditions, including diabetes and mental health.
www.peersforprogress.org

e-collection: "Peer-to-Peer Support and Online Communities"
Collected articles on this theme in a leading peer-reviewed medical informatics journal.
https://www.jmir.org/themes/76

Patient Communities: A Starter List
Maintained by patient advocate e-Patient Dave, this list illustrates the variety of general and specific support groups available. Dave notes: "There are many, many more communities than the few listed below."
https://www.epatientdave.com/communities/

REFERENCES

About Connect: Who, What & Why. (n.d.) https://connect.mayoclinic.org/page/about-connect/tab/volunteer-mentors/

Allan, R. (2019, July 21). Cancer kills but so can fake cures. https://ronnyallan.net/2019/07/21/cancer-kills-but-so-can-fake-cures/

Ambrose, C. T. (2011). Joseph Hersey Pratt, M.D.: The man who would be Osler. Microbiology, Immunology, and Molecular Genetics Faculty Publications. 44. Retrieved December 12, 2019, from https://uknowledge.uky.edu/microbio_facpub/44

American Syringomelia & Chiari Alliance Project. (2013). https://asap.org/index.php/resources/find-support/

Anderson, M., Perrin, A., Jiang, J., & Kumar, M. (2019, April 22). 10% of Americans don't use the Internet. Who are they? https://www.pewresearch.org/fact-tank/2019/04/22/some-americans-dont-use-the-internet-who-are-they/

Barrette, J. (2017, June 12). Fake news in healthcare can be quite dangerous in Facebook's health communities. https://www.wegohealth.com/2017/06/12/fake-news-in-healthcare/

Barrette, J. (2018, March 28). For health communities, Facebook is too important to delete. https://www.wegohealth.com/2018/03/28/facebook-is-too-important-to-delete/

Boyd, D., & Ellison, N. B. (2008). Social network sites: Definition, history and scholarship. *Journal of Computer Mediated Communication, 13*, 210–230.

Cangelosi, J., Kim, D., Griffin, K., & Ranelli, E. (2017). The role of social media and social networking as marketing delivery systems for preventive health care information. [Unpublished manuscript.] https://www.researchgate.net/publication/319851560_The_Role_of_Social_Media_and_Social_Networking_as_Marketing_Delivery_Systems_for_Preventive_Health_Care_Information

Chou, W.-Y. S., Oh, A., & Klein, W. M. P. (2018). Addressing health-related misinformation on social media. *JAMA, 320*(23), 2417–2418.

Entwisle, V. A., France, E. F., Wyke, S., Jepson, R., Hunt, K., Ziebland, S., & Thompson, A. (2011). How information about other people's personal experiences can help with healthcare decision-making: A qualitative study. *Patient Education and Counseling, 85*, e291–e298.

Evans, M., Donelle, L., & Hume-Loveland, L. (2012). Social support and online postpartum depression discussion groups: A content analysis. *Patient Education and Counseling, 87*, 405–410.

Eysenbach, G., Powell, J., Englesakis, M., Rizo, C., & Stern, A. (2004). Health related virtual electronic support groups: Systematic review of the effects of online peer to peer interactions. *BMJ: British Medical Journal, 328*(7449), 1166–1170.

Feenberg, A. L., Licht, J. M., Kane, K. P., Moran, K., & Smith, R. A. (1996). The online patient meeting. *Journal of the Neurological Sciences, 139*(Supp), 129–131.

Ferguson, R. D. (2012). Crowdsourcing health information: An ethnographic exploration of public and private health information on PatientsLikeMe.com (Unpublished master's thesis). York University, Toronto, Canada.

Fox, S. (2011, February 28). Peer-to-peer healthcare. https://www.pewresearch.org/internet/2011/02/28/peer-to-peer-health/

Fox, S. (2020). Video: Peer health advice. https://susannahfox.com/video-peer-health-advice/

Fox, S., & Jones, S. (2009, June 11). The social life of health information. Pew Internet and American Life Project. https://www.pewresearch.org/internet/2009/06/11/the-social-life-of-health-information/

Gould, G. M. (1898, July 30). The union of public and medical libraries. *Philadelphia Medical Journal*, 237.

Gupta, S. C., Klein, S. A., Mehl, D. C., & Finger, P. E. (1997). Using the World-Wide Web for peer-to-peer patient support. *Studies in Health Technology & Informatics*, 39, 307–318.

Gustafson, D. H., DuBenske, L. L., Namkoong, K., Hawkins, R., Chih, M. Y., Atwood, A. K., Johnson, R., Bhattacharya, A., Carmack, C. L., Traynor, A. M., Campbell, T. C., Buss, M. K., Govindan, R., Schiller, J. H., & Cleary, J. F. (2013). An eHealth system supporting palliative care for patients with non-small cell lung cancer: A randomized trial. *Cancer*, 119(9), 1744–1751.

Gustafson, D. H., Hawkins, R., Boberg, E., Pingree, S., Serlin, R. E., Graziano, F., & Chan, C. L. (1999). Impact of a patient-centered, computer-based health information/support system. *American Journal of Preventive Medicine*, 16(1), 1–9.

Gustafson, D. H., McTavish, F., Hawkins R., Pingree, S., Arora, N., Mendenhall, J., & Simmons, G. S. (2008). Computer support for elderly women with breast cancer. *JAMA*, 280(15), 1305.

Hartzler, A., & Pratt, W. (2011). Managing the personal side of health: How patient expertise differs from the expertise of clinicians. *Journal of Medical Internet Research*, 13(3), e62. https://doi.org/10.2196/jmir.1728

Hodgkin, P., Horsley, L., & Metz, B. (2018, April 10). The emerging world of online health communities. https://ssir.org/articles/entry/the_emerging_world_of_online_health_communities#

Hopelab/Well Being Trust Teens and Young Adults Survey. (2018, February/March). https://hopelab.org/report/a-national-survey-by-hopelab-and-well-being-trust-2018/digital-health-practices/demographic-differences-in-digital-health-use/

Hopelab/Well Being. (2018, February/March). https://hopelab.org/report/a-national-survey-by-hopelab-and-well-being-trust-2018/appendix/

Horrigan, J. B., Rainie, L., & Fox, S. (2001). Online communities: Networks that nurture long distance relationships and local ties. Pew Internet & American Life Project. https://www.pewresearch.org/internet/2001/10/31/online-communities/

Jadad, A. R., Enkin, M. W., Glouberman, S., Groff, P., & Stern, A. (2006). Are virtual communities good for our health? *BMJ*, 332(7547): 925–926.

Johnson, G. J., & Ambrose, P. J. (2006). Neo-tribes: The power and potential of online communities in health care. *Communications of the ACM*, 49(1), 107–113.

Katz, A. H., & Bender, E. I. (1976). Self-help groups in Western society: History and prospects. *The Journal of Applied Behavioral Science*, 12(3), 265–282.

Keselman, A., Smith, C. A., Murcko, A. C., & Kaufman, D. R. (2019). Evaluating the quality of health information in a changing digital ecosystem. *Journal of Medical Internet Research*, 21(2). https://www.jmir.org/2019/2/e11129/

Kim, Y. (2020, May 4). UW team launches website, app with COVID-19 resources. *Capital Times*. https://madison.com/ct/news/local/education/uw-team-launches-website-app-with-COVID-19-resources/article_c74090c2-4a3f-5374-812c-597ee90a4be1.html

Laukka, E., Rantakokko, P., & Suhonen, M. (2019). Consumer-led health-related online sources and their impact on consumers: An integrative review of the literature. *Health Informatics Journal*, 25(2), 247–266.

Madara, E. J. (1999). From church basements to world wide web sites: The growth of self-help support groups online. *International Journal of Self Help & Self Care*, 1(1), 37–48.

Mayo Clinic. (n.d.) Community Guidelines. https://connect.mayoclinic.org/page/about-connect/tab/community-guidelines/

Meier, A., Lyons, E. J., Frydman, G., Forlenza, M., & Rimer, B. K. (2007). How cancer survivors provide support on cancer-related internet mailing lists. *Journal of Medical Internet Research*, 9(2), e12. https://doi.org/10.2196/jmir.9.2.e12

National Cancer Institute. (2018). Health Information National Trends Survey 5 (HINTS 5): Cycle 2. https://hints.cancer.gov/view-questions-topics/question-details.aspx?PK_Cycle=11&qid=687

Nobles, A. L., Leas, E. C., Althouse, B. M., Dredze, M., Longhurst, C. A., Smith, D. M., & Ayers, J. W. (2019). Requests for diagnoses of sexually transmitted diseases on a social media platform. *JAMA*, 322(17), 1712–1713.

Noyes, D. (2019). The top 20 valuable Facebook statistics: Updated November 2019. https://zephoria.com/top-15-valuable-facebook-statistics/

PatientsLikeMe. (2019a). About us. Retrieved December 31, 2019, from https://www.patientslikeme.com/about

PatientsLikeMe. (2019b). How does PatientsLikeMe make money? https://support.patientslikeme.com/hc/en-us/articles/201245750-How-does-PatientsLikeMe-make-money-

Rainie, L., & Fox, S. (2000, November 26). The online health care revolution. https://www.pewresearch.org/internet/2000/11/26/acknowledgement/

Rains, S. A., & Young, V. (2009). A meta-analysis of research on formal computer-mediated support groups: Examining group characteristics and health outcomes. *Human Communication Research*, 35(3), 309–336.

Rice, R. E. (2001). The Internet and health communication: A framework of experiences. In R. Rice & J. E. Katz (Eds.) *The Internet and Health Communication: Experiences and Expectations*. Thousand Oaks, CA: Sage Publications.

Rose, D. (2010, August 26). A history of the March of Dimes. https://www.marchofdimes.org/mission/a-history-of-the-march-of-dimes.aspx

Rovner, S. (1995, October 10). Internet offers a world of information. *The Washington Post*. https://www.washingtonpost.com/archive/lifestyle/wellness/1995/10/10/internet-offers-a-world-of-information/980e623a-b499-4c1b-9227-68f8b1c4ed21/

Rozenblum, R., & Bates, D. W. (2013). Patient-centred healthcare, social media and the internet: The perfect storm? *BMJ Quality & Safety*, 22(3), 183–186.

Smart Patients Team. (2014, November 21). Online communities for sarcoma. https://www.smartpatients.com/stories/online-communities-for-sarcoma/

Starr, A. (2018). Cancer diagnosis and treatment worksheets. www.Cancerworksheets.com

Tanis, M. (2008). Health-related on-line forums: What's the big attraction? *Journal of Health Communication*, 13(7), 698–714.

Veinot, T. C., Meadowbrooke, C. C., Loveluck, J., Hickok, A., & Bauermeister, J. A. (2013). How "community" matters for how people interact with information: Mixed methods study of young men who have sex with other men. *Journal of Medical Internet Research*, 15(2), e33.

Voluntary Health Agency. (2009). https://medical-dictionary.thefreedictionary.com/voluntary+8health+agency

WEGO Health Solutions. (2017). Role of Patient Influencers: Do online patient communities drive doctor conversations? https://www.wegohealth.com/wp-content/uploads/2017/03/WEGO-Health-Solutions_BIS_behavior.pdf?utm_source=BIS&utm_medium=Email&utm_campaign=Core

Wicks, P., Massagli, M., Frost, J., Brownstein, C., Okun, S., Vaughan, T., Bradley, R., & Heywood, J. (2010). Sharing health data for better outcomes on PatientsLikeMe. *Journal of Medical Internet Research*, 12(2), e19.

Winkelman, W. J., & Choo, C. W. (2003). Provider-sponsored virtual communities for chronic patients: Improving health outcomes through organizational patient-centered knowledge management. *Health Expectations*, 6(4), 352–358.

Young, C. (2018, September 13). Don't let these 3 common fears stop you from creating a vibrant patient community. *Social Media Network*. https://socialmedia.mayoclinic.org

CHAPTER 11

The Ethics of Consumer Health Informatics

Catherine Arnott Smith and Alla Keselman

T HE CHAPTER, LAST IN THE BOOK, discusses ethical considerations surrounding consumer health information technology (CHIT) and their impact on consumer health informatics research and development. To illustrate how these considerations play out in a real-life context, the chapter draws on examples from the domain of direct-to-consumer genetic (DTC-G) testing. The chapter opens with an overview of widely recognized core biomedical ethical principles of respect for the patient's autonomy, non-maleficence, beneficence, and justice. In describing them, the chapter provides examples of their relevance to the field of consumer health informatics. The chapter also discusses how these principles are expressed in the ethical codes of computer and health information science professions. The rest of the chapter is written with a focus on DTC-G testing, showing how conflict among ethical principles creates ethical dilemmas in the cutting-edge CHIT domain of DTC-G. The chapter provides a brief history of DTC-G and discusses motivations for testing, accuracy concerns, implications of health literacy and other consumer competencies for people's ability to interpret test results, and DTC-G testing clients' reactions to receiving and interpreting test results alone. The chapter also discusses privacy issues surrounding CHIT and, specifically, DTC-G, presenting ethical dilemmas related to use of DTC-G data in law enforcement and biomedical research.

11.1 FOUNDATIONS OF ETHICS IN CHIT

Core biomedical ethical principles have long been articulated in a widely used, widely translated, and very influential text authored by prominent ethicists Tom L. Beauchamp and James F. Childress (2013). Currently in its seventh edition, Beauchamp & Childress' was the first biomedical ethics book ever published by Oxford University Press. Today, it is read all over the world, not only by future doctors, nurses, dentists, and biomedical informaticists, but also by the people in the trenches, at the bedsides, and in the consult rooms of the world's healthcare systems. The core principles these authors describe are thus principles that affect many practitioners and patients outside these systems as well as inside.

For this reason, future researchers and practitioners of consumer health informatics need to be aware of what these principles mean in the real world of biomedicine.

Biomedical ethics, as an academic field of its own, did not exist when Beauchamp and Childress met, at Yale University, in the mid-1960s (Beauchamp & Childress, 2019). And, like medical informatics, biomedical ethics was multi- and interdisciplinary. Beauchamp's doctoral training was in Philosophy, and Childress' in Religious Studies. They became colleagues at Georgetown University in 1975. That year Georgetown's Kennedy Institute – the "center for practically engaged ethics" and one of the oldest such centers in the world (Kennedy Institute of Ethics, n.d.) launched its Intensive Bioethics course – the first in the world (Beauchamp & Childress, 2019). One motivation, for both the Institute and the book, was a dawning recognition that ethical issues in healthcare had been only little discussed, and dialogue about them limited to voices within the healthcare professions (Beauchamp, 2010). The new Georgetown course was just as interdisciplinary too: targeting "scientists, physicians, nurses, public policy experts, journalists, and others." Out of these diverse origins arose a need first to articulate, and then to share, certain core teachings, "a common set of ethical principles for bioethical discourse and practice" connecting ethical theory to practical problems (Beauchamp & Childress, 2019, p. 9).

Beauchamp defines "principle" as "an essential norm in a system of moral thought and one that is basic for moral reasoning" (Beauchamp, 2010, p. 36). The classic Beauchamp & Childress text articulates, through seven editions to date, that common set of principles.

These four core principles are Respect for Autonomy, Non-Maleficence, Beneficence, and Justice. Beauchamp & Childress refer to them as both "framework" and "core" because they are central to the structure of ethical decision-making in healthcare. These four principles are defined below, and CHI examples are provided to illustrate why they are so important.

11.1.1 Respect for Autonomy

> Respecting autonomy means asserting that individuals have the right to "hold views, to make choices, and to take actions based on their personal values and beliefs" (Beauchamp & Childress, 2019, p. 103). To have these capacities, individuals need to be acting free from "external constraint" and have the mental understanding needed to take said actions.
>
> (Beauchamp, 2010, p. 37)

> Respect, on this account, involves acknowledging the value and decision-making rights of persons and enabling them to act autonomously, whereas disrespect of autonomy involves attitudes and actions that ignore, insult, demean, or are inattentive to others' rights of autonomy.
>
> (Beauchamp, 2010, p. 37)

Under this principle, a person's right to their own desires is of paramount importance; "no other person or social institution ought to intervene" to counter those desires, "whether or not those desires are right from any external perspective" (Furrow, 2009).

Healthcare example: A patient's right to refuse a medical intervention, such as life-sustaining treatment in the shadow of an incurable disease. That right to refuse is contingent upon the patient's ability to make a medical decision.

(Cooper, 2010)

Consumer health informatics example: Decisions about the end of life require surrogates – perhaps the patient's family members, friends, or other loved ones – to consider "the decision a patient would have made if they had mental capacity." Bioethicists are beginning to discuss the use of personal information exchanged via social networking services (SNS; e.g., Facebook) as a substitute for an individual's advance directive or otherwise legally expressed opinion. By considering the wishes expressed in discussion forum posts, evaluating them carefully, and discussing them with caregivers, it might be possible to arrive at a decision about what the patient would have wanted to express verbally in the moment if they could.

(Siddiqui & Chan, 2018)

11.1.2 Non-Maleficence

Trainee physicians are taught a Latin saying: *Primum non nocere* ("First do no harm"). Beauchamp and Childress note that this medical education concept is "closely associated" with the principle of non-maleficence, which "imposes an obligation not to inflict harm on others" (Beauchamp & Childress, 2019, p. 149). Non-maleficence also requires that we do not even pose a *risk* of harm. Adhering to the principle of non-maleficence may mean a conflict with respecting a patient's autonomy. If a patient does not want treatment in the moment, but that treatment may prevent them from serious complications in the future, the treatment will cause less harm, in the long term, than the patient's exercise of autonomy will. Weighing one against the other, autonomy is the worse choice! "Sometimes harmful action is necessary, but it should never be automatic," cautions one author (Morrison, 2006).

Healthcare example: Beauchamp comments about this principle that:

Numerous problems of non-maleficence are found in health care ethics today … blatant examples … are found in the use of physicians to classify political dissidents as mentally ill, thereby treating them with harmful drugs and incarcerating them with insane and violent persons..[or] medications for the treatment of aggressive and destructive patients.

(Beauchamp, 2010, p. 39)

Consumer health informatics example: Edzard Ernst, MD, PhD, etc., is a retired physician in the United Kingdom. For several decades, he directed a center of research into complementary and alternative medicine (CAM); he became the first-ever Chair of CAM in an academic medical center in 1993, at the University of Exeter. He founded three medical journals focusing on CAM and publishes widely in the mainstream medical press. His specialty: critical evaluation of CAM therapies and their evidence base. "This ambition does not endear him to many believers in SCAM [sic], including Prince Charles," he notes of himself on his website [edzardernst.com].

(Ernst, 2020)

In 2009, Ernst wrote that the problem of advice offered by CAM practitioners online presented "an important ethical issue" because of its scientific unreliability and the failure of these practitioners to give patients evidence that their therapies worked. For this reason, the principle of non-maleficence – doing no harm – was violated by these practitioners (Ernst, 2009, p. 335).

11.1.3 Beneficence

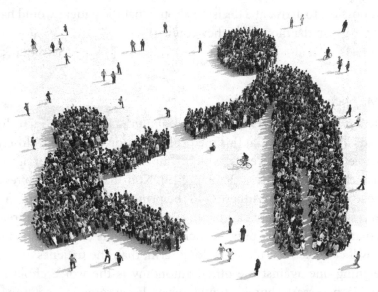

The principle of beneficence "includes all forms of action intended to benefit other persons" (Beauchamp, 2010, p. 197) and has been called "*the* foundational value in health care ethics." [Italics original] (Beauchamp, 2010, p. 40). Beneficence does not consist simply of personally avoiding non-maleficence but requires conscious attention to the interests of other people besides yourself:

> Many duties in medicine, nursing, public health and research are expressed in terms of a positive obligation to come to the assistance of those in need of treatment or in danger of injury. The harms to be prevented, removed, or minimized are the pain, suffering, and disability of injury and disease.
>
> (Beauchamp, 2010, p. 40)

Healthcare example: It may be necessary, in medicine, to cause a small amount of harm in order to effect a cure. Beauchamp gives the example of "saving a person's life by a blood transfusion [which] clearly justifies the inflicted harm of venipuncture on the blood donor".

(Beauchamp, 2010, p. 40)

Consumer health informatics example: The physicians interviewed by Moerenhout (2020) expressed their feelings about the changes in their relationship with their patients due to technological interventions in medical recordkeeping. These doctors felt a tension between patient access to their electronic medical records, perceived as an action respecting autonomy, and causing confusion through access to information these patients might not understand fully, perceived as an action violating the principle of beneficence. "I think there would be a lot of emotions involved that would have to be overcome for [one patient] to appreciate the benefits of the documentation," commented one physician (Moerenhout et al., 2020, p. 111) (for more on patient portals and patient access, see Part II: Chapter 7).

11.1.4 Justice

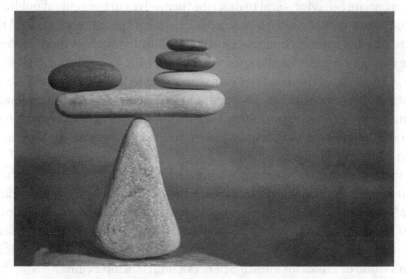

Justice, in biomedical ethics, has been defined generally as "fair, equitable and appropriate treatment in light of what is due or owed to persons" (Beauchamp, 2010, p. 241). The difficult and controversial part, of course, is the "what is due or owed." In medical research, the principle of justice is articulated through the Belmont Report – the statement which specifies human subject protections in research studies – and requires researchers to "ascertain that the risks of the study do not outweigh the benefits" (Cassel & Bindman, 2019).

Healthcare example: A timely and serious issue in the United States is the question of which citizens are entitled to healthcare: "the demands of the principle of justice must apply at the bedside of individual patients but also systematically in the laws and policies of society that govern the access of a population to healthcare."

(McCormic, 2018)

Consumer health informatics example: Researchers, policymakers, educators, and citizens are concerned about long-term effects of the digital divide – that is, "the gap between those who have and do not have access to computers and the Internet" (van Dijk, 2006) – both inside and outside of the field of CHI. Adhering to the ethical principle of justice requires attention not just to reducing unequal access to beneficial technologies, but teaching and reaching potential stakeholders to level the playing field. For example, Nebeker et al. (2017) investigated *barriers* to wearable technologies such as the Fitbit in minority communities – Latino, Somali, and Native Hawaiian Pacific Islanders – in order to understand challenges to implementing wearable health solutions in these populations.

11.2 ETHICAL CODES OF THE PROFESSIONS

Professional codes of ethics exist because members of the professions want simultaneously to explain themselves to each other – welcoming new practitioners and setting expectations for appropriate behavior – and to describe themselves to the general public who is the audience and client base. By setting out codes of ethical "norms and values," the professions "assure persons entering into relationships with individuals in these professions that they will be ethically competent and trustworthy" (Byrd & Winkelstein, 2014).

In Part I, Chapter 2, of this book, we introduced you to the diversity of fields that make up consumer health informatics: fields operating in academia, government, and industry. It may or may not surprise you to learn that the biomedical ethical principles outlined above are found not only in the codes of health professions, but also in the computer and information science professions.

Two organizations that represent key information/informatics professions that incorporate work in consumer health informatics are the Medical Library Association and the American Medical Informatics Association (AMIA) (for more information on professional associations relevant to CHI, see Part I: Chapter 2). Unsurprisingly, each of the codes relies on information as central to its profession's ethical behavior. The Medical Library Association's Code of Ethics for Health Sciences Librarianship begins:

> The health sciences librarian believes that knowledge is the sine qua non of informed decisions in health care, education, and research, and the health sciences librarian serves society, clients, and the institution by working to ensure that informed decisions can be made.
>
> (Medical Library Association, 2010)

Because AMIA is multi-professional as well as multi-disciplinary, its code of ethics is explained as "organized around the common roles of AMIA members and the constituents they serve, including patients, caregivers, clinicians, researchers, students, agencies, hospitals and practices, medical organizations, vendors, insurance companies, and others with whom they interact" (Petersen et al., 2018). Like MLA, AMIA leads with a discussion of information, but unlike MLA, the *handling* of information, as well as the *devices used to access* information, are equally important to the ethical code:

Recognize that patients and their loved ones and caregivers have the right to know about the existence and use of electronic records containing their personal healthcare information, and have the right to create and maintain their own personal health records and manage personal health information using a variety of platforms including mobile devices.

(Petersen et al., 2018)

The AMIA code goes on to specify how medical informatics professionals should intermediate in the relationship between patients and their data: AMIA members should:

Not mislead patients about the collection, use, or communication of their healthcare information.

Enable and – as appropriate, within reason and the scope of their position and in accord with independent ethical and legal standards – facilitate patients' rights and ability to access, review, and correct their electronic health information.

(Petersen et al., 2018)

And finally, the code makes a tenet of consumer health informatics explicit in directing members to:

Recognize that patient-provided/generated health data, such as those collected on mobile devices, deserve the same diligence and protection as biomedical and health data gathered in the process of providing health care.

(Petersen et al., 2018)

In other words, data generated in the process of health care monitoring – by professionals *or* the consumers themselves – is considered equally ethically "valuable."

Byrd and Winkelstein (2014) examined statements from eight other associations' ethical codes to determine resemblances between MLA, AMIA, and the rest. Two of these codes were taken from general librarianship: the American Library Association, a key association representing many academic (college and university) libraries as well as public librarians; and the Special Libraries Association, whose members serve clients in specific occupational settings from corporations to museums to zoos. Another code pertains to health information management (the American Health Information Management Association); and three from the health professions, the American Medical Association, the American Nurses Association, and American Public Health Association. Among these eight ethical codes, at least one of the four moral principles is specified at least once, and usually more than once, from Beneficence (mentioned 4–13 times) to Autonomy (3–6 times) to Justice (1–5 times). The MLA and AMIA codes show the most agreement between any two codes, which probably derives from their joint origins in the intersection of medical information and the practice of medicine.

Many of the ethical considerations inherent in CHI are similar to those found in the field of medicine generally. However, the public's unique role, very different from the patient's role, in consumer health information transactions produces some distinctive concerns. Direct-to-consumer genetics provides a useful example.

11.3 EXEMPLAR: DTC GENETIC TESTING

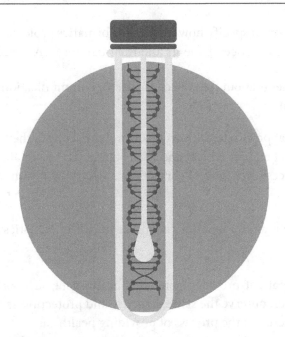

DTC, or Direct-to-Consumer, genetics companies include 23andMe, Ancestry.com, and MyHeritage. They market their products directly to consumers, who can purchase the product online or in physical stores. The absence of clinically trained intermediators in the process is important, as will become clear below.

Other names for DTC genetic testing include "direct-access genetic testing, at-home genetic testing, and home DNA testing" – as well as "recreational genomics" and "boutique genetics" (Evans, 2008). We will use the acronym DTC-G in this chapter for consistency.

It is important to understand the difference between DTC-G testing for health reasons, and DTC-G testing for other reasons. Some of these same companies also perform ancestry, or genealogy, testing, in which the consumer's motivation is to obtain information about their ethnicity from their genes (Genetics Home Reference, 2020a). In this chapter, we will focus on the health motivations, and the health-related products, alone, as an example of biomedical ethics in play in the consumer health informatics domain. We will focus on 23andMe as a case study.

One of the oldest such companies, launched in 2007, today 23andMe is "a genomic and biotechnology research company that provides health and ancestry services." Based in Mountain View, CA, 23andMe has 500 employees as of February 2020 and reported revenue as 113.4 million USD (GlobalData, 2020). It received a rating of "Also great" from one product review site, the *New York Times'* Wirecutter, out of a lineup of 15 distinct DNA testing kits. Wirecutter's top pick for "Great" was 23andMe's competitor AncestryDNA, which began as a genealogy service but recently added a health component (Molteni, 2019).

All genetic tests assess human DNA, which are the building blocks of genes – the information that determines human attributes such as eye color or height, and also our risk of acquiring particular diseases (Federal Trade Commission, nd). A consumer who engages in home DNA testing begins with the relatively simple process of spitting into a tube provided to them in a kit they ordered online: as 23andMe puts it, "Order → Spit → Discover." To enable discovery to happen, the consumer must send the sample to a company for processing. Results arrive via a secure portal set up at the time the order was placed. What happens next is discussed below.

11.3.1 DTC-G: A Brief Timeline

2002: A review of such products available for purchase via the internet found 105 websites, but most were not focusing on the health market; of the 14 that did, available tests ranged from drug metabolism (Genelex.com) to nutrition lifestyle advice (Sciona.com) to carrier screening (cystic fibrosis, sickle cell anemia, Tay-Sachs, and fragile X syndrome; Datagene.com). The price of testing ranged from $25 to $275 (Gollust et al., 2003).

2007: 23andMe kicks off its business with 14 available reports on specific traits. These traits included late-onset Alzheimer's Disease, Parkinson's, celiac, and a specific type of hemophilia (Curnutte, 2017). Cost: $999 each, not cheap, but less expensive than the competition, Navigenics and deCODE Genetics of Iceland, which reached prices as high as $2500 (Kaiser, 2007). A "spit party" was held during New York Fashion Week in 2008, "less noteworthy for being at the cutting edge of democratized science than for its combination of opulence and decadence"(Hughes, 2013), although the attendees were somewhat un-opulently given a 40% discount on the kits (Salkin, 2008); backers included Harvey Weinstein and Wendi (Mrs. Rupert) Murdoch.

April 2008: A survey (McGuire et al., 2009) asks 1,080 respondents acquired from a standing panel to answer questions about DTC-G companies. 47% had heard of such companies; only 6% had actually used one, but 64% were interested in using one in the future, 74% for health-related reasons.

June 2008: California Department of Public health follows lead of New York. These states have notified genetic testing companies that they need to cease and desist; that marketing them to consumers puts them in the "medical advice" territory. Early criticism of the DTC-G industry coming from state health departments and then from the FDA stressed the need for a line between genetic information and medical information: "We think if you're telling people you have increased risk of adverse health effects, that's medical advice," according to Ann Willey of the NY State Department of Health (Pollack, 2008). DTC-G was named the 2008 Invention of the Year by *Time* magazine (Hamilton, 2008).

2009: 23andMe lays off staff this year, falling to less than 40 employees. Competitor Navigenics retools and pivots away from the consumer market to focus on physicians and corporations. DeCode, in Iceland, goes into bankruptcy and also turns to physicians as customers.

March 2010: *New York Times* coverage (Pollack, 2010a) refers to 35,000 23andMe customers, with fewer at Navigenics and DeCode. 23andMe's service has a price tag of $999 (Roberts & Ostergren, 2013) – during a recession.

May 2010: Pathway Genomics publicizes a deal with Walgreens – to sell its tests in Walgreens stores nationwide. Walgreens will sell the kit – "Discover Your DNA" – and the specific tests will be ordered through Pathway Genomics' website (Dealbook, 2010). This proposed arrangement with Walgreens motivates the FDA to send cautionary letters to "almost all" providers of DTC-G testing, including 23andMe (Gollust et al., 2017, p. 293). One result: the deal between Pathway Genomics and Walgreens is killed (Hercher, 2018).

June 10, 2010: FDA notifies 23andMe President that the FDA "does not consider your device to be a laboratory developed test because the 23andMe Personal Genome Service™ is not developed by and used in a single laboratory." The letter also notes that 23andMe has started distributing through Amazon – a third party (Gutierrez, 2010). The FDA's letter is viewable online here:

https://www.fda.gov/media/79205/download

This characterization of DTC-G tests as "medical devices" was meant as a warning to DTC-G companies that their "devices" required approval.

September to November 2012: FDA requests evidence that 23andMe has addressed issues they identified and states that the company has left requests for additional information unanswered (Quelch & Rodriguez, 2016).

July 2013: 23andMe files for premarket authorization of the product – the only DTC-G company to do so (Gollust et al., 2017).

November 25, 2013: FDA accuses 23andMe of failing to provide necessary evidence of accuracy; the agency stresses that it is "concerned about the public health consequences" of users taking serious action, such as surgery or medication changes, based on the consumer's interpretation of possibly inaccurate results. There are also accusations of false advertising, poor protections of, and misuse of consumer data (Update to 'Direct-to-Consumer…', 2015). The company is ordered to stop selling its "medical device," in the sense that the FDA orders 23andMe to withhold health-related results from its customers, while still permitting genealogy data to be released (Edwards & Huang, 2014).

"About half a million people" are customers at the time of the FDA crackdown (Pollack, 2013, November 25). Goal had been a million (Miller, 2013). The price of 23andMe test has plummeted to $99 (Roberts & Ostergren, 2013). This tussle makes things awkward for consumers: Kira Peikoff writes in the *New York Times* that after she signed up with 23andMe, she discovered that the state in which she lived did not legally permit 23andMe to accept her samples because it was not a credentialed lab (Peikoff, 2013). It also makes things awkward for 23andMe: although the FDA restricted only the health aspect of 23andMe's DNA testing, not the genealogy aspect, the restriction itself has a downward effect on sales. This is itself evidence of what demand had been created for what kind of service: "Evidently, people care much more about their chances of getting Alzheimer's than about how much Neanderthal DNA they have," as one commentator puts it (Hof, 2014).

February 19, 2015: 23andMe having resolved things with the FDA, the first FDA authorization is announced for the marketing of a DTC-G test – for a marker of carrier status for a condition called Bloom Syndrome. The taker of this genetic test will know if they could pass on that condition to offsprings (Curnutte, 2017). It is now also permitted for 23andMe to tell consumers if they have a copy of a mutated gene (e.g., cystic fibrosis).

April 2017: Several significant events occur: the FDA, in a change of tone from its 2013 crackdown, announces that it will permit marketing of genetic tests for ten diseases/conditions directly to consumers. 23andMe is on the top five best-seller list for Amazon.com's Black Friday weekend.

Summer of 2018: A Harris Poll asks 4,038 respondents aged over 18 about the likelihood of their taking a DTC-G test. 25% report that they have actually taken one for *any* reason, but health markers were not the dominant reason: 15% did it for family history reasons, 9% to understand cancer risk, and 7% to understand risks for other conditions. Asked about the possibility that they would take it in the future, 36% call it somewhat or very likely; 35% called it not likely at all (American Society of Clinical Oncology/Harris, 2018). This is roughly similar to results of a Mintel survey the same month. In that survey of 2000 internet users aged over 18, researchers found that 15% had taken a DTC-G test; 36% had no interest in doing so; and the other 49% had not, but were interested. In specific age ranges, the highest proportion reporting that they have done such a test are found in the age 25–34 category (Mintel, 2019).

October 2018: 23andMe receives FDA approval for testing and reporting on the relationship between individual genetic markers, including several in the BRCA1 and BRCA2 genes implicated in breast cancer, as well as and some pertaining to response to medications.

November 2018: the FDA announces that 23andMe is allowed, with other such services, to skip premarket review for some tests for health risks: "usher[ing] in a rapid expansion of the consumer genetics industry" (Hercher, 2018).

January 22, 2019: FDA approval is announced for specific gene testing in hereditary colorectal cancer (Brown, 2019). Type 2 diabetes is added to the list in March (Ducharme, 2019).

January 2020: With sales slumping, 23andMe announces it is laying off 15% of staff. Only about 20% of growth occurred in 2019–2020 (Regalado, 2020).

February 2020: Both 23andMe and Ancestry.com report further reductions in the workforce, which one commentary blames on factors including "market saturation, privacy concerns, and limited usefulness" (Molla, 2020).

11.3.2 Motivation For Use

Why do consumers engage with this particular technology? People express different motivations for doing DTC-G testing. Through January 2019, more than 25 million people had been tested by any genetics company, nine million by 23andMe (Regalado, 2019). In August 2019, the Pew Internet Research Project reported that 15% of all adults surveyed (N = 9,834) had ever used such a service, and 36% of those did it for health reasons (Graf, 2019). A 2018 Harris Poll of 1,459 adults in the U.S. found that the two most common reasons were either a family history of a particular cancer (18%) or a general fear of cancer (also 18%). These cancer-related reasons were closely followed by social ones: a friend or family member who had done genetic testing was the reason given by 17%. The least cited reason? "A public figure/celebrity who has gotten a genetic/DNA test" (5%) (American Society of Clinical Oncology/Harris, 2018).

11.3.3 Concerns about Inaccuracy and Incompleteness of Test Results

The FDA's early tussle with 23andMe centered on the question of accuracy as well as devices. The FDA 2013 warning letter to 23andMe says that harmful actions could result from access to genetic information, using testing for BRCA mutations as an example: "If the BRCA-related risk assessment for breast or ovarian cancer reports a false positive, it could lead a patient to undergo prophylactic surgery, chemoprevention, intensive screening, or other morbidity-inducing actions …" (Edwards & Huang, 2014, p. 17). The FDA's FAQ on DTC-G states that inaccuracies can happen for two reasons: "Some tests may be wrong due to an error in the test, and some results may be wrong due to an incorrect interpretation of the meaning of the result"(Food & Drug Administration, 2019). One concern is with the quality control of the laboratories where samples are processed. Clinical laboratories used by healthcare providers are subject to the Clinical Laboratory Improvement Amendments (CLIA) accreditation. The amendments cover quality control in labs, as well as laboratory personnel credentials. However, in the domain of DTC-G testing, neither clinical validity nor clinical utility is addressed by the CLIA standards (Spencer & Topol, 2019).

In addition to accuracy of specific tests, there is a concern over the scope of DTC-G testing and the consumer's understanding of that scope. No DTC-G test screens for all possible mutations. For example, the three best-known BRCA mutations, detected by 23andMe, are not the only mutations implicated in breast cancer. A non-peer-reviewed study presented at a geneticists' conference in 2019 suggested that the 23andMe's test would have missed 90% of all BRCA mutations (Murphy, 2019). A similar concern has been voiced about

Alzheimer's Disease testing; one gene, APOE, is assessed in 23andMe's DTC-G test, but NIH cautions that it doesn't tell the whole story:

> Certain variations in this gene are associated with the likelihood of developing late-onset Alzheimer disease (the most common form of the condition, which begins after age 65). Specifically, the test allows you to find out how many copies (zero, one, or two) you have of a version of the gene called the e4 allele. People who have zero copies of the e4 allele have the same risk of late-onset Alzheimer disease as the general population. The risk increases with the number of copies of the e4 allele, so people with one copy have an increased chance of developing the disease, and people with two copies have an even greater risk. However, many people who have one or two copies of the e4 allele never develop Alzheimer disease, and many people with no copies of this allele ultimately get the disease.
>
> Variations in the APOE gene are among many factors that influence a person's overall risk of developing Alzheimer disease. Variations in many other genes, which are not reported in the FDA-approved direct-to-consumer genetic test, also contribute to disease risk. Additionally, there are risk factors for Alzheimer disease that have yet to be discovered. Therefore the APOE e4 allele represents only one piece of your overall Alzheimer disease risk.
>
> (Genetics Home Reference, 2020a)

> Based in part on inaccuracy and incompleteness concerns, the Pentagon has recommended to all members of the U.S. Armed Services that they refrain from taking DTC-G tests: "they create security risks, are unreliable, and could negatively affect service members' careers."
>
> (Murphy & Zeveri, 2019)

There has been pushback from 23andMe about accuracy criticisms. Anne Wojcicki, the CEO of 23andMe, quoted an "over 99%" accuracy rate for the Genetic Health Risk Reports (Wojcicki, 2019). Even at that rate, however, a staff geneticist pointed out to the *New York Times* that since the service checks 600,000 variants, an almost perfect accuracy rate of 99.9% would mean about 600 errors per person (Hercher, 2018). Kira Peikoff, who received her results during the period of DTC consumer limbo imposed by the FDA's initial crackdown, heard from 23andMe that she had elevated risk for two autoimmune conditions, but a different DTC lab told her she had low risk for those identical conditions. As a journalist and (in 2013) a graduate student in bioethics, Peikoff was unusually well-equipped to grapple with these results – and to write about them (Peikoff, 2013). But was she typical of the DTC-genetics customer?

Pushback also comes from some bioethicists. In an essay about regulation of the DTC-G market, Edwards and Huang counter the FDA concern about potential harm by responding that "the willing participation of a doctor" would be required for any actual harm to result, first, through the physician's ordering a follow-up genetic test to confirm 23andMe's findings, and next, through integration of those genetic results, if confirmed, with the medical history of the patient and her family. "Information provided by DTC-G testing companies, even if it has medical implications, is still just information" (Edwards & Huang, 2014, p. 17).

On its part, 23andMe is careful to present consumers with copious warnings and recommendations to work with medical professionals in their terms of service agreements:

> You understand that information you learn from 23andMe is not designed to independently diagnose, prevent, or treat any condition or disease or to ascertain the state of your health in the absence of medical and clinical information. You understand that the 23andMe Services are intended for research, informational, and educational purposes only, and that while 23andMe information might point to a diagnosis or to a possible treatment, it should always be confirmed and supplemented by additional medical and clinical testing and information. You acknowledge that 23andMe urges you to seek the advice of your physician or other health care provider if you have questions or concerns arising from your Genetic Information.
>
> (23andMe, 2019)

The FDA uses similar language on its DTC-G FAQ page, stressing that results from a test cannot replace the value of visiting a healthcare professional. It does this while acknowledging the positive outcomes from consumer empowerment:

> While direct-to-consumer tests can lead to consumers becoming more engaged in their overall health and lifestyle decisions, results from direct-to-consumer tests should not be the sole basis of any type of medical decision making as these tests provide only one layer of a bigger picture. Therefore, results from direct-to-consumer tests should always be discussed with your health care provider. In addition, these tests are not a substitute for visits to a health care provider for recommended screenings or appropriate follow-up and should not be used to determine any treatments.
>
> (Food and Drug Administration, 2019)

While worry about accuracy and completeness of the results, as well as consumers' ability to deal with them (discussed further), are valid concerns, the debate of patients' and consumers' health information access has long history. Two leading bioethicists, Annas and Elias, sum up the DTC-G problem this way: "To oversimplify, the debate has been framed as a struggle between medical (or government) paternalism and individuals' right to information about ourselves" (Annas & Elias, 2014). Annas and Elias analogize the DTC-G problem to the much older argument over patient access to their own clinical information in medical records, a dialogue that continues in the debate over just how much information to release to patients via patient portals. The primary care physicians interviewed in a recent study saw, in the use of patient portals, a conflict between respecting patient autonomy and adhering to the principle of beneficence. A patient who misunderstands what she reads in the portal could, like the DTC-G consumer, be not only confused but made more anxious by encountering this information in the absence of a person to answer her questions:

> People see their labs before I've replied to them and they get very nervous about some … very stupid lab abnormality that is … completely irrelevant … then they're … emailing me or calling me … I saw this, what does this mean, and they're freaking out.
>
> (Moerenhout et al., 2020, p. 109)

The Open Notes movement, discussed in Part II: Chapter 7, relies on patient portal technology to deliver medical record content to the patients. The movement takes as a given that "health information transparency can empower patients and families" (Bourgeois et al., 2017). But what if the patient is 13 years old, and there is potentially sensitive content in that record that the patient should not see? What if the patient is 16 years old, considering contraceptive use, and does not want her parent to see her record? Should there be "two sets of books", one for a parent and one for the teenage patient? Consider the DTC-G parallel described here:

> What happens when a toddler's exome [a piece of a person's DNA; (Genetics Home Reference, 2020b)] is sequenced to determine the cause of a developmental delay and the lab discovers that the child has the BRCA1 mutation? Should the lab withhold that information? What about the pediatrician?
>
> (Cottle, 2013)

Tension among biomedical ethical principles, specifically, respect for patient autonomy and beneficence, is inherent in every healthcare situation. The right to self-determination requires that patients – and, by extension, consumers, have access to the knowable. Yet, it is important for the information, made available as a right, to be as complete, accurate, and unbiased as possible. As previewed in this section, in addition to the issue of accuracy and completeness of the results, there is also one of consumers' understanding of them. This understanding relates to the fundamental concepts of consumer health literacy and other information competencies. The following sections discusses ethical implications of health literacy and competencies concerns in the context of DTC-G.

11.3.4 Ethical Implications of Literacies' Requirements

Honoring the patient's right to autonomy involves helping her to make decisions that are truly informed. This refers to the professional's ethical behavioral norm of veracity: "the professional duty to provide accurate, timely, objective, and comprehensive transmission of information" (Byrd & Winkelstein, 2014). Adhering to this norm can be a challenge, however, because the success of an information transaction is not a function of the information alone. Rather, it is determined by the interaction among: 1) the information provider, 2) the message; 3) the delivery channel, and 4) various competencies and characteristics of the person on the receiving end.

Part I: Chapter 3 of this text outlines six knowledge-related competencies that determine one's ability to deal with digital health information (Norman & Skinner, 2006). These include:

- Traditional literacy: the ability to read and understand texts
- Information literacy: knowledge how to search for information
- Media literacy: the ability to understand social and political context behind messages
- Health literacy: the ability to deal with health information, from understanding medical terms to interpreting risks in the health context
- Computer literacy: the ability to use computers (and other digital information devices) effectively
- Science literacy: the ability to understand scientific foundations of health information

In addition to these competencies, there are other characteristics that affect information access, including money, time, health, and emotional state. This section will focus on the six literacies, drawing on DTC-G testing as an exemplary domain.

People vary with regards to their levels of the above competencies. For example, in Part I, Chapter 3, we state that, according to an authoritative assessment study, only about 12% of American adults have a "Proficient" level of health literacy, defined by that study as "the ability to understand medical terms and information" (US Department of Education, 2006). According to the same study, 14% have the level that is "Below Basic." There are also differences with regard to computer and internet use competencies. For example, according to Anderson et al. (2019), 10% of Americans reported not using the internet in 2019. Those less likely to be comfortable with internet technologies are more likely to be older (over 65), poorer, non-White, and living in rural areas (Anderson & Kumar, 2019; Perrin, 2019; Perrin & Turner, 2019). This discrepancy in information access and use, as noted earlier in this chapter, is often referred to as the "digital divide" (van Dijk, 2006).

When seen from one angle, the digital divide is closing. More and more people, from more and more diverse population groups, go online, and their motivation often includes searching for health information. Ubiquity of smartphones is also playing a role in closing the divide, as more people come to rely on them as their primary tool for going online (Perrin & Turner, 2019). At the same time, as new exciting devices appear, their relatively faster spread in the younger, healthier, and more well-off segment of the market contributes to broadening the divide at the cutting edge of technology access. Thus, pioneering cutting-edge technology has ethical implications. When introducing new features, designers and developers of resources should ask themselves the uncomfortable question: what population segment is this choice most likely to leave behind? The next question should be pragmatic: what information formats and tools should be provided to level the playing field for those unlikely to benefit from the shiniest option?

When it comes to DTC-G testing, the access differential is significant, in large part due to the cost of testing, which has ranged from under a hundred to several thousand dollars for. In addition, the impact of one's social environment and health and scientific literacy determine one's perception of the test's utility and the interpretation of the results.

11.3.5 Science Literacy and Understanding Risk

When people wish to obtain DTC-G tests for health-motivated reasons, it is usually to learn their risk of acquiring various diseases and conditions in the future. Interpreting quantitative risk information is notoriously difficult for people, as it represents one of the most challenging health literacy tasks. One particularly difficult situation is the proportionally large increase of a small risk. As Cottle (2013) puts it: "Many people do not understand, for instance, that having a 50 percent greater risk for a disease that the average person has a 0.25 percent chance of developing is not cause for alarm" (para 11). Let's unwrap this example. Let's say, without added genetic knowledge about the individual, a person's risk of getting Disease A is 0.25%. That number may be based on that disease's prevalence in the general population, or it may be additionally adjusted to the person's demographic and behavioral characteristics (e.g., ethnicity, age, activity level). To obtain 50% of 0.25%, we need to divide 0.25% in half. The result of that division is 0.125%. This is the amount of risk increase, with the risk then rising from 0.25% to 0.375%. In many people's minds, a 50% risk increase sounds like a very disturbing number, a cause for alarm and a call to action – but the increase from 0.25% to 0.375% risk, not so much.

Providing an explanation like the one in the above paragraph, or, even better, supplementing it with a good dynamic infographic, is not particularly daunting. Yet interpreting risk information, in the specific context of DTC-G testing, and in general, requires a much more nuanced approach. Rogers and Walker (2016) point out that, despite people's hopes, numbers obtained as a result of medical tests often increase, rather than reduce uncertainty. While risk is a number representing the probability of an event, a wish to reduce uncertainty is a wish to know what to do. What am I to do, if my risk of a Disease A is 0.375%, 5%, 25%, 50%? There is a lot I need to know in order to make that decision, or, rather, those decisions. (There are many decisions. Do I change my diet? Inform potential romantic partners? Undergo a preventive surgery while healthy?) In many cases, probabilistic information generates more questions than it answers, creating anxiety and posing difficult dilemmas.

Many challenges related to interpreting results of genetic testing have to do with science literacy. One such challenge has to do with understanding how reliable or unreliable the findings are. Consider the story of Sarah Hartz (2015), a physician and a genetics researcher, who wrote a fascinating and very personal story of her experience as a consumer of DTC-G testing. Out of pure curiosity, Hartz sent her sample to four DTC-G testing companies and was shocked to discover that she had an elevated risk for macular degeneration, an eye disorder that is the leading cause of severe age-related vision loss. Most shockingly, although the results from all four companies showed elevated risk, the degree of risk was remarkably different among the tests.

This is how Hartz describes her attempt to understand the discrepancy:

> I first looked to confirm that they genotyped the same genetic markers. This was the easiest thing to do because ... the specific genotypes were in all of my reports. Then I looked to see if they used the same medical studies to compute the risk. These were also essentially the same. It turned out that the difference is the methods they used for calculation of risk. I had assumed that was the easy part because it's just a matter of multiplying numbers together, including baseline risk of macular degeneration, the joint impact of the genetic variants on this risk. It turns out that the problem is that we actually don't know the baseline risk of macular degeneration for people who don't have the genetic variants, and we don't know how the genetic variants interact with each other and the environment to lead to the development of macular degeneration. ...Prior to engaging in this exercise, I didn't realize how difficult and imprecise it is to calculate risk of disease that includes genetic information.
>
> (Hartz, 2015)

Hartz's experience is noteworthy, because discrepancies in risk predictions issued by different DTC-G testing companies are common (Covolo et al., 2015). Yet, the vast majority of tested individuals have no training in genetics. The vignette highlights the impressive array of skills required of Hartz to reach her conclusion. She first needed to understand how the scientific method works (what is baseline risk? why is it important?). Then she needed to know how science uses mathematics (not everyone will agree that this is "the easy part"). Finally, she needed to be well-versed in genetics terms and concepts (e.g., what, exactly, are "genetic markers"? What does it mean, to "genotype" them?). The conclusion that Hartz reaches on the basis of this complex knowledge is that the results of her testing are not clinically useful – something that is true of the vast majority of DTC-G test results. She points out that information derived from testing may lead people to unnecessary medical procedures. And she closes her article without yielding to temptation to draw a conclusion about what should be done regarding DTC-G testing. She acknowledges feeling "confused" about everything related to the issue: from the relevance of her tests' findings to her health, to the allowance that the public's access to DTC-G testing should be limited by regulations.

11.3.6 Supporting Consumer Experience: The Current State of Affairs

Supporting people's understanding of DTC-G testing and their test results requires a thoughtful approach, tailored to the specific needs and skills of the individuals. As with other types of health information, it is important that genetic testing information is delivered in plain language and that both the process and the possible implications of testing are thoroughly explained.

There are also some ethical dilemmas unique to DTC-G. For example, consumers need to understand how their data will be protected from misuse. This is challenging, because, as the field develops, the amount of information that can be gleaned from the data keeps growing; something that does not appear significant today may prove to contain highly sensitive information tomorrow (see Part II, Chapter 9 on smart homes for a similar situation with data from embedded sensors). There is also the unique dilemma of determining just what information is relevant in the face of uncertainty. 23andMe states in almost poetic terms that "Once you obtain your Genetic Information, the knowledge is irrevocable" (23andMe, 2019). About which potential findings and implications should people know prior to deciding whether to undergo testing? As there are no clear-cut answers, it is particularly important to help people think through the possibility of dealing with irrevocable knowledge, as well as to assist them in connecting with professionals who can help interpret that knowledge (Messner, 2011).

The ethical ideal of proper support of people's autonomy in the realm of DTC-G testing is somewhat vague in execution. Covolo et al. (2015) conducted a systematic review of studies of websites offering DTC-G testing, published before October 2014. Studies generally agreed that most DTC-G testing companies did not provide sufficient essential information about the testing. For example, the websites provide very little scientific information about the test's clinical validity, or "how well the genetic variant being analyzed is related to the presence, absence, or risk of a specific disease" (Genetics Home Reference, 2020c). This lack of information is significant because the clinical validity of these tests, and, consequently, their clinical usefulness, is low, and discrepancies and inconsistencies among test results are common, as described in an earlier section. According to Covolo et al. (2015), "A total of 14 papers, including two reports from the US Government Accountability Office (GAO) [11,129], question the scientific quality, clinical validity, and utility of DTC-GT." According to Hennen et al. (2010), a majority of DTC-G testing providers' websites do not tell individuals what actions to take given positive or negative results. Some studies found that the majority of DTC-G testing websites they analyzed recommended dietary supplements (Lewis et al., 2011; Singleton et al., 2012), while very few sites recommend discussing the results with a doctor. On the positive note, most sites surveyed in two reviews recommend talking to a genetic counselor (Covolo, Martignone, & Orizio, 2010; Geransar & Einsiedel, 2008), even if DTC-G companies do not provide such consultations themselves (Covolo et al., 2015). Studies reviewed by Covolo et al. (2015) also suggest that DTC-G testing sites do not adequately explain risks of testing, privacy, and confidentiality concerns, the possibility of genetic discrimination on the basis of the results, and potential emotional impact of information that cannot be unlearned. In a later study, Hall et al. (2017) gauged consumer information provided by DTC-G testing companies against "good practice principles" developed by the UK Human Genetics Commission (HGC). The authors concluded that "no provider complied with all the HGC principles, and overall levels of compliance varied considerably."

Suboptimal presentation of DTC-G testing information is a cause for concern. How big of a concern it is depends on how people react to that information. While the literature is full of hypothetical scenarios regarding the detrimental effects of DTC-G testing on customers, not many studies address this question. Of those that do, many are case studies. Some of these, indeed, are disconcerting. For example, Moscarello (2019) describes the case of a 22-year-old man whose DTC-G test indicated a genetic mutation associated with hypertrophic cardiomyopathy (HCM), a condition that involves abnormal thickening of the heart muscle. Sometime after receiving the test result, the young man came for an evaluation to an HCM clinic. According to Moscarello:

> During the clinical intake, the patient had significant anxiety about this result: he had taken medical leave from his PhD program after learning of his results "to focus on [my] HCM and risk of sudden death." He was an avid cyclist, but gave it up after learning that vigorous exercise is not recommended for people with HCM. He had looked into joining a support group, but did not feel ready to discuss the possibility of myectomy or transplant "yet."
>
> (Moscarello, 2015, p. 540)

The evaluation at the HCM clinic showed that the young man did not have HCM. Moreover, confirmatory genetic testing did not detect the previously flagged mutation.

This case study dramatically illustrates how DTC-G testing without proper support can do harm, a finding echoed in several other case studies. However, as powerful as they are, case studies cannot replace comprehensive quantitative data. In their review, Covolo et al. (2015) identified 29 studies that addressed the impact of DTC-G testing on users: 20 of these studies were quantitative, and nine qualitative. The studies typically aimed to evaluate "psychological reactions, behavioral effects, and perception risk" (p. 5). Most involved small samples of participants, and some focused on potential users rather than actual test consumers. Covolo et al. concluded that the percentage of individuals worried about results of their genetic testing is low. The majority showed no test-related change in their anxiety levels, and when change did occur, it was more likely to be positive – that is, reduced anxiety (Egglestone et al., 2013). Strikingly, in people receiving news that they were carriers of BRCA mutations – meaning a very significant increase of breast and ovarian cancer risks – the increase in anxiety was moderate and temporary (Francke et al., 2013). Importantly, most women in Francke et al.'s study went on to share their findings with a doctor, and both men and women shared the information with female relatives, knowing now that their relatives had a potentially increased risk of having the mutation. One woman's encounter with BRCA through 23andMe is detailed in the next section. The next section also contains a more detailed discussion of the psychological impact of DTC-G.

Studies of this type typically do not focus on users' competencies (health literacy, numeracy, etc.) and their impact on comprehension. One exception is a study by Kaufman et al. (2012), which shows that difficulty comparing hypothetical absolute risk numbers (is a 25% risk greater or smaller than 30% risk?) correlates with difficulty interpreting actual genetic testing reports.

Proponents of stricter regulation of DTC-G testing market point to the variable quality of consumer information by test providers, as well as cases of emotional anguish caused by test results, as a justification for stricter control. At the same time, many point out that paternalistic regulations limit people's autonomy. Finally, once the proverbial cat is out of the bag, it is impossible to put back. As a field, consumer health informatics can support consumers by studying and developing ways to enhance comprehension, thus lowering the bar for competencies required to become an informed consumer.

11.3.7 Receiving Bad News Alone

In general, Americans see a lot of value in receiving professional support in interpreting their test results. In 2011, 2,100 adults in the U.S. were asked to "imagine they were at increased risk" for heart disease, colon cancer, or Alzheimer's Disease. This was a representative sample of consumers: 75% called their health "good" or "excellent"; 53% were female, 75% White, 10% African American, and 8% Latino/a; the sample was also roughly split in terms of political identification between Democrats, Republicans and Independents. Less than 1% of the respondents were DTC-G customers, which means these consumers' decisions were extremely hypothetical for more than 99% of this sample. But of these, a "strong majority" of 65% agreed that "medical professionals should be involved in explaining genetic test results" (Almeling & Gadarian, 2014).

In 2017, Gollust et al. did a similar study but with a different population. They solicited opinions from 941 23andMe and Pathway (another DTC-G testing company) actual customers. These people were very supportive (90% affirmative) that all consumers should have access to DTC-G testing. But those customers who had more confidence in *their own ability to apply and use the genetic information they received* – perhaps unsurprisingly – were more in favor of access to testing without a medical professional's involvement. And customers who reported "feeling upset" about the results they had received were less likely to support such access (Gollust et al., 2017).

From the very beginning of DTC-G, the presence or absence of a clinical specialist in the process was noted as an important piece of the equation. In a 2003 review of genetic tests online, Gollust, Wilfond, and Chandros Hull (2003) found only 14 health-related tests on the market, of which seven allowed the consumer to bypass their personal physician, requesting that the results are sent directly to the consumer; four allowed consumers to order directly, but sent results only to physicians, thus necessitating a conversation; and three required that consumers requested test-ordering information (Gollust, Wilford, & Chandros Hull, 2003). Of the seven companies that sent the results directly to the consumer, four advertised consultation services by a physician or a genetics counselor on their websites. Gollust et al., wrote:

> For consumers to have the greatest likelihood of understanding the implications of a health-related genetic test, clinicians with appropriate genetics knowledge and experience should be involved in this process.
>
> (Gollust et al., 2017, p. 5)

Journalist Dorothy Pomerantz has written eloquently about what it's like to receive bad news from a DTC-G test alone. She had learned about DTC-G tests from their repeated presence in her social media feeds. "Any concerns I had were around privacy," Pomerantz related: "Privacy, it turned out, was the least of my worries" (Pomerantz, 2019). The results showed that she had a mutation in BRCA1, the gene implicated in breast and ovarian cancer.

With breast cancer in her family history, facing this result, Pomerantz "immediately turned to Google ... After 20 minutes of Googling, I felt like I couldn't breathe anymore. My husband wisely suggested I step away from the computer and call my gynecologist."

CHI technology was implicated at every step of the process of this consumer's bad news. The social media that connected her to other people served to create a need for a genetic testing service, as a consumer – not a patient – she was then empowered to engage with by herself, through the mail. And because she had been so empowered, she was not a *patient* in the sense of having medical supervision or assistance when she received the resulting data. A cancer patient in a genetics clinic attached to a cancer center is not left alone to interpret the results. She is given counseling. But in Pomerantz' case, as a consumer, she had to read the data without any experienced intermediary to cushion the blow: "Talking to someone about the results versus reading them in an online report – even after wading through a long tutorial – was the difference between day and night" (Pomerantz, 2019).

Pomerantz later commented on her experience: "I needed more than a tutorial. I needed a genetic counselor – a human being to hear my questions and give me guidance based on deep knowledge." That counselor was found within a few days, and the 23andMe result was confirmed. Pomerantz did have the genetic mutation. Unfortunately, in this case 23andMe was all too accurate.

While she was fortunate in being able to meet with such a counselor a few days after her 23andme results were revealed, Pomerantz writes that not everyone receiving bad news is in this position:

> For most people, there's a large gap between access to at-home genetic tests and access to genetic counseling. Anyone with a few extra dollars can order a test online and get their results fairly quickly. But finding someone to help interpret those results can be expensive when insurance doesn't cover counseling. It can also take weeks to get an appointment and, in some communities, it may be impossible.
>
> (Pomerantz, 2020)

Part of the impossibility is a function of high demand in a context of low supply. As of February 19, 2020, the National Society of Genetic Counselors reports a membership of just under 5,000 – or one for every 66,000 people in the United States (United States Census, 2020). The Bureau of Labor Statistics forecasts a 27% increase in the number of jobs for genetic counselors by 2028, considerably more than average for all jobs and a threefold increase over other healthcare practitioners; the entry-level degree for this profession is a master's degree (Bureau of Labor Statistics, 2019). But in the fall of 2018, Jill Goldman, a genetics counselor at Columbia University Medical Center, could say of the oncoming flood of potential business: "People are going to need help… And we are not ready to handle it" (Hercher, 2018).

Given the gulf that exists between available counselors and consumer demand for assistance, second-hand companies have sprung up to assist DTC-G customers in interpreting their results. Promethease is one example. This company bills itself as a "literature retrieval system" and the reports it sells integrate data from commercial platforms – Ancestry.com, 23andMe, deCODEme, Navigenics, FamilyTreeDNA, and NatGeo – with published scientific literature connected via SNPedia and representing 565 distinct medical conditions (SNPedia, 2019).

The "empowering" act of providing information directly to consumers has figured in arguments in favor of DTC pharmaceutical advertising for decades. The idea is that when consumers encounter information in the marketplace, it spurs conversation with physicians about whether the medication is appropriate for them. Note the elision of "patient" with "consumer" in this quote from 2001:

> Patients, framed as autonomous consumers of health care, have a right to be informed about breakthrough technologies and products so they can be active participants in managing their health care.
>
> (Rubin, 2001)

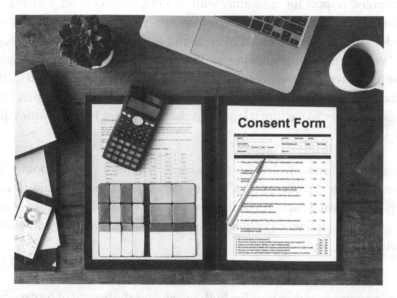

23andMe's CEO Anne Wojcicki has invoked the "patient empowerment" argument several times. The *American Journal of Bioethics* published an editorial defending 23andMe's stance in 2009. The piece was authored by four 23andMe staffers, including Wojcicki itself. Positioning selective release of genetic information, including risk information, as a reduction in access, the writers stressed that such "paternalism could hinder education and active participation in one's own health. Preventing all risk information from reaching consumers can be impractical" (Hsu et al., 2009). Howard and Borry, writing about clinical geneticists' attitudes toward DTC-G, point to companies like 23andMe as "emphasiz[ing] a form of 'active consumerism'" due to the information-access strain of the argument (Howard & Borry, 2012).

Ten years later, in a response to criticism of DTC-G, Wojcicki continued to maintain that consumer access to genetic information was necessary to enable "more equitable healthcare … access without a medical professional barrier…We believe that consumers can learn about genetic information without the help of a medical professional" (Wojcicki, 2019). In an earlier interview with Claire Miller of the *New York Times*, Wojcicki made her desired connection between consumer empowerment, consumer *responsibility* for health, and access to personal genetic data extremely clear:

> Genetics is going to be a ubiquitous part of health care. ... At some point, health care is going to reimburse for it ... There's a big societal shift where we're putting the onus of your health onto you, the individual. One of the best aspects of health care reform is it starts to emphasize prevention.
>
> (Miller, 2013)

One of 23andMe's directors, venture capitalist Esther Dyson, commented in a separate interview that it was "appallingly paternalistic" to assume a doctor was required to interpret 23andMe's results (Pollack, 2010b).

Delaney and Christman (2016) object to presenting the dilemma as a choice between two opposite poles, respect for autonomy with "unfettered access for patients to data, but with uncertain and even misleading conclusions" vs. "paternalism and denial" on the part of the provider" (p. 146). What needs to be found is the place in the middle. Maybe the question is: "What genetic information should a patient have access to? Raw genomic data is of little use to the average consumer" (p. 147). Opponents counter, of course, that the raw genomic data – the information – already belongs to the average consumer, whether they can understand it or not. An editorial in the impactful science journal *Nature* put the conflict this way:

> The simplest and most restrictive approach is to inform people about findings only once they are discovered ... A better solution would be withholding data by default, but releasing them if participants request it. Ideally, that release should occur only with guidance on how to interpret the information and alongside counseling on its significance.
>
> (Editorial, 2015, p. 5)

As mentioned previously, public opinion both recognizes the benefit of professional support and values independent access. A large minority of McGuire et al.'s early survey respondents in 2009 didn't think they needed professional interpretation: 40% reported they *would* use direct-to-consumer testing without consulting with a physician (McGuire et al., 2009). However, 65% of the 64% who said they would use a DTC-G service felt it would give them information that "would influence their future healthcare decisions." Caulfield (2009) points to this as indicating "they view it as valuable health information" (p. 48).

The consumer's understanding of the *value* of genetic information – with or without the interpretive assistance of the right clinician – is part of the ethical consideration:

> The patient [Caulfield's term—Authors] is left to interpret the data on his/her own, or with a varying degree of help from the company that sold the service. Since the data is of only marginal health value, little or no health benefit has been achieved. But the interaction with the physician costs the system both time and money.
>
> (Caulfield, 2009, p. 48)

A consumer triggered to request follow-up testing based on genetic results they cannot understand "is an unjustified use of healthcare resources and constitutes a raid on the medical commons" (McGuire & Burke, 2008).

Dorothy Pomerantz's story above gives one person's experience. How does that generalize to the larger population of consumers interacting with their own genetic information for the first time and – as noted – on their own? Is Pomerantz typical or atypical?

One argument is that healthcare professionals need to prepare patients for the impact of receiving results (Delaney & Christman, 2016). The problem of inducing stress and anxiety through revealing of test results has been an important question for more time than DTC-G has been a viable technology. Studies of effects of genetic testing for such hereditary conditions as Tay-Sachs or Huntington's Disease on mental health and overall well-being have found short-term impacts, but the evidence of long-term impact is more mixed. In an early Canadian study of the impact of carrier status testing, high school students who were told they were carriers of Tay-Sachs – with serious implications for reproductive choices, but no clinical consequence to the carrier – were "more upset" than non-carriers after getting their results, but when followed up 6-weeks to 17 months later, had clearly adjusted (Clow & Scriver, 1977).

Another early study looked at the effect on patients of receiving results of genetic testing for Huntington's Disease. Multiple tests measuring distress, depression and well-being were administered to 135 Canadian patients before testing occurred, and then at three points up to a year after the patients had received their test results. The conclusion: that such testing "may maintain or even improve the psychological well-being of many people at risk" (Wiggins et al., 1992).

Finally, a study of 162 adult children of parents diagnosed with Alzheimer's Disease assessed anxiety, depression and distress at similar intervals to the Huntington's study referred to above (Green et al., 2009). These adults were randomized to either a disclosure group, which was given genetic test results for a marker for Alzheimer's, or a non-disclosure group, which was not given results. At six weeks post-reveal, those who tested positive for the gene did have "significant but not clinically meaningful differences" on the test-related distress measure. But overall, the investigators found no greater levels of anxiety, depression, or distress in the disclosure group than in the non-disclosure group.

The critical difference between those *patients* and *family members of patients* who had been investigated in studies like this, and the *consumers* who purchase DTC-G test kits today, is that the former group of people were dealing with the news in the context of healthcare – and the latter, without a net.

Roberts and Ostergren (2013) conducted an extensive review of the literature on DTC-G and found differences in response depending on the actuality of the genetic test. If people were given hypothetical scenarios and hypothetical genetic risk profiles and test results, 40% *anticipated* worry and anxiety over seeing those results – before they saw them (Bansback et al., 2012). The same finding held when other investigators performed a deceptive study – in which, with IRB approval, the researcher deceives participants in order to test particular hypotheses. 160 undergraduate students contributed real saliva to the "spit test" but got back fake results indicating (or not) that they had a genetic marker predisposing them to alcoholism. Students who thought they had this marker experienced a drop in positive emotions (Dar-Nimrod et al., 2013).

However, when test results were real, multiple researchers found little impact on recipients of the results. Researchers at the Scripps Translational Science studied DTC-G customers, and the findings, while limited, shed some light on the difficulty of investigating this problem. The participants were recruited from health and tech companies including Microsoft, Qualcomm, and Scripps Research (Bloss et al., 2010) and received subsidized rates on DTC-G, specifically a product called Navigenics Health Compass (Bloss et al., 2011). The 2,024 participants in this study were provided with 90-page reports detailing their genetic risks for diagnoses ranging from obesity to Alzheimer's. The 27% who shared their DTC-G results with their healthcare providers were typically older, higher-income, more likely to be married, and more religious, when compared with non-sharing consumers. However, these results must be interpreted with caution because the cohort from which these participants were drawn was itself "well-educated, generally healthy, and [had] a high socio-economic status." They were also people who exercised more and whose diets – on self-report – were lower-fat. The researchers for this reason cautioned readers that DTC-G data sharers might be "more proactive about their health" to begin with. However, it was "somewhat surprising" that the risk estimates these consumers shared were not statistically associated with being a sharer or not. Exactly one medical condition – Lupus – was "even nominally associated with sharing behavior" (Darst et al., 2014). And those consumers who did share their results did not change their behaviors accordingly: "We had theorized there would be an improvement in lifestyle, but we saw no sign whatsoever," according to one author.

11.4 PRIVACY AND ETHICS

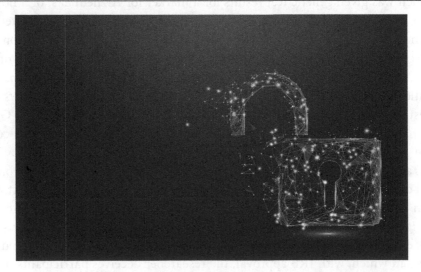

In any conversation about healthcare and medical ethics, the individual's privacy is a paramount concern. The concept of privacy has to do with rights to information access, which refers to laws and policies governing who has the right to access an individual's data and for what purpose. It is distinct from technical considerations of guarding data against breaches and unauthorized access, which is referred to as data security. The two concepts are related, because a security breach violates privacy.

Privacy is an ethical concept because it relates to autonomy, non-maleficence, and justice. If an individual's information falls into unauthorized hands (or unauthorized servers), this mishap may limit their ability to make autonomous decisions. For example, a person living with a chronic illness may decide to make her condition known at work, obtaining reasonable accommodations, such as flexible work hours. Another individual may choose not to disclose her diagnosis to co-workers, out of concern for possible discrimination. Whatever the decision, it is the individual's to make, and the diagnosis should be protected from access by employers. Sensitive health information in the wrong hands can do harm, violating the non-maleficence principle, and, thus, causing injustice. For example, the Smart Homes chapter (Part II: Chapter 9) explains that data collected in order to support older individuals' independent living at home can, in the wrong hands, be used for surveillance. Below, we also discuss potentially dangerous unauthorized uses of individuals' genetic data.

While consumer health informatics privacy considerations are largely similar to privacy considerations in healthcare and medical research, one important unique characteristic sets it aside. The main US law that protects privacy of personal health information is the Health Insurance Portability and Accountability Act (HIPAA) Privacy Rule, which took effect in April of 2003 (Office of Civil Rights, 2013). However, HIPAA Privacy Rule generally does not apply to consumer health applications, because their data transactions usually occur outside "covered entities," such as healthcare organizations. In the absence of governing laws, privacy of consumer health applications can be guarded by best practices and non-binding guidelines created by governmental or non-governmental organizations.

Other important considerations, mirroring those in some areas of medicine and medical research, are the unfolding relationship between data – and the resulting information – and individuals' understanding of the implications of sharing those data. Many consumer health informatics tools collect large volumes of cutting-edge data that may not provide valuable insights today. However, in the future, the same data may yield sensitive diagnostic information. Individuals' understanding of the informational *potential* of novel data is a subject of much discussion, especially when the individuals belong to vulnerable populations: the elderly, the medically fragile, those with less education or lower health literacy. In Part II: Chapter 9, we address this in depth in the context of smart medical homes and ambient (located in the environment) and wearable sensors. Here, we consider privacy considerations as they apply to the example of DTC-G testing.

11.4.1 Privacy Considerations in DTC-G Testing

DTC-G testing companies are not covered by HIPAA Privacy Rule. In the absence of this coverage, individuals are protected against some potential misuses of their genetic information by the Genetic Information Nondiscrimination Act (GINA). GINA, which went into effect in 2009, applies to all genetic testing done in the US, including DTC-G testing. GINA prohibits health insurance providers from obtaining genetic information and using it for establishing individual insurance eligibility or cost of premiums. It also prohibits employers from obtaining genetic information and using it in employment-related decisions (National Research Council and Institute of Medicine, 2010).

These prohibitions are important but limited in scope. For example, GINA does not prohibit life, long-term care, and disability insurers from obtaining and using genetic information. Aside from GINA, consumers' rights are defined by individual DTC-G testing companies' privacy policies. In lieu of specific regulations, the Federal Trade Commission issues the following recommendation to those considering DTC-G testing:

> Protect your privacy. Before you do business with any company online, read the privacy policy: It should specify how the company secures the information it collects, how it will use your information, and whether it will share your information with third parties.
>
> (Federal Trade Commission, N.D.)

In other words, aside from health insurance and employment discrimination, the weight of due diligence in ensuring data privacy is on consumers. Too often, individuals sign privacy policy agreements without reading them, scrolling through an online form and clicking "I agree." Even with the best intentions, doing due diligence is not easy. Hendricks-Sturrup and Lu (2019) point out that some DTC-G testing privacy policies are written at a college reading level, despite the National Library of Medicine's recommendation that consumer health materials be written at the 7th- to 8th-grade reading level (for a discussion of reading levels as they relate to health literacy in CHI, see Part I, Chapter 3).

In the meantime, privacy policies of DTC-G companies may contain things that violate the implicit assumptions of their customers. For example, in a criticism directed at Ancestry.com's Terms of Service and Privacy Policy, Winston (2017) points out:

> There are three significant provisions in the AncestryDNA Privacy Policy and Terms of Service to consider on behalf of yourself and your genetic relatives: (1) the perpetual, royalty-free, world-wide license to use your DNA; (2) the warning that DNA information may be used against "you or a genetic relative"; (3) your waiver of legal rights.

To date, two specific uses of DTC-G testing data, in law enforcement and in research, have sparked public debates pertaining to privacy. The law enforcement instance is best illustrated by the case of Joseph James DeAngelo, the Golden State Killer, "suspected of more than a dozen murders and 50 rapes in California," committed in the 1970s and 1980s (Ram et al., 2018). DeAngelo was finally arrested in April 2018, after investigators determined a match between DNA collected from crime scenes and DNA profiles in a free genealogical database called GEDmatch.

Capture of a serial killer is certainly a good outcome of genetic testing progress. However, it highlights a situation where a person's genetic data can be easily accessed without their consent or even awareness of their existence. While the US has a national forensic database that includes DNA profiles of convicted offenders, obtained via compulsory DNA sampling, GEDmatch is not a forensic database. Rather, it is a free genealogical database to which individuals voluntarily submit their genetic data, sequenced by various genetic testing companies, for amateur genealogical research. DeAngelo never uploaded his DNA profile to GEDmatch; he was identified on the basis of a profile uploaded by a distant relative. Because relatives share genetic material, your relative's decision to contribute their DNA profile to a public database makes your genetic information publicly searchable, quite possibly, without your awareness.

While DeAngelo's case was the one to attract public attention, it was not the first case of law enforcement's use of a non-forensic database. In a thought-provoking piece in Science Magazine, Ram et al. (2018) point out that there are not many legal protections against this, as the Fourth Amendment, which protects people from "unreasonable searches and seizures by the government" (US Courts, n.d.) does not apply to information that was voluntarily shared with an intermediary, such as a genetic testing company or a database.

After DeAngelo's case, GEDmatch updated its privacy policy. Now, users have to choose whether they wish to allow their data to be shared with law enforcement, with "no" as the default option (Takano, 2019). The American public, in the meantime, seems conflicted in its beliefs about whether DTC-G testing data should be protected from access by law enforcement (Hendricks-Sturrup & Lu, 2019). In one survey, 74% of respondents say that it is important and 15% somewhat important for it to be illegal for law enforcement to access such data (Bollinger et al., 2013). However, a more recent survey suggests that the public largely supports law enforcement access to such data in order to solve violent crimes and crimes against children (Guerrini et al., 2018).

Concerns about DTC-G testing data privacy protection in research arise from the fact that genetic companies collaborate and share data with commercial research entities, such as pharmaceutical companies. For example, in July 2018, the major pharmaceutical company GlaxoSmithKline paid 23andMe $300 million, in exchange for exclusive access to 23andMe customer data for drug development research (Ducharme, 2018). 23andMe spokespeople stress that participation in research is voluntary, with customers signing consent forms and having an opportunity to change their mind, and that the data used in research are de-identified (23andMe, 2019). Opponents counter that the consent process as implemented by DTC-G testing companies may be inadequate, and not on a par with consent obtained in academic research (Ducharme, 2018; Howard, Knoppers, & Borry, 2010). Individuals "signing" the click-through consent form may not understand to what they are consenting, and the forms do not explain how genetic materials may be used in the future and by whom. Additionally, as in the case of serial killer DeAngelo, consenting participants' genetic information is shared by their non-consenting relatives. As in case with any electronic data, there is also a risk to privacy stemming from the risk of a security breach, potentially inherent in any third-party data transfer. While researchers and medical ethicists discuss concerns of potential privacy threats, the public may be less aware of those risks. Surveying over a thousand DTC-G testing consumers, Bollinger et al. (2013) found that 96% of them agreed or strongly agreed with the statement "In thinking about [the company's] service, I am confident my privacy has been protected" (p. 426). Of the respondents, 36% thought that their DTC-G data were better protected than the data in their medical records, 38% thought it was similarly protected, 23% were not sure, and only 4% thought the protection was weaker than for medical records data.

11.5 CONCLUSIONS

This chapter highlights complex ethical dilemmas inherent in consumer health information provision, drawing on DTC-G testing as an example. As a field, consumer health informatics upholds the same core ethical principles as biomedicine: respect for the user's autonomy, non-maleficence, beneficence, and justice. As in biomedicine, the dilemmas lie in balancing the core principles against one another. This balancing is especially challenging in cutting edge areas, where information is characterized by high levels of uncertainty. In this regard, DTC-G testing is an illustrative, though not unique, example. One serious concern, brought on by uncertainty, is difficulty assessing the potential for maleficence. When it comes to genetic testing – like ambient sensor data collection in smart homes, and data sharing by individuals via online platforms like PatientsLikeMe (see Part I: Chapter 1 and Part II: Chapter 9), knowledge that can be gleaned from the data is not static. What can be inferred from the data tomorrow may be more informative and sensitive than what can be inferred from it today.

As was discussed in examples throughout the chapter, this makes privacy requirements both essential and, at times, difficult to define. The difficulty of ensuring data privacy also stems from the fact that developers of health information tools, such as DTC-G tests or health-related apps, are usually not covered by the laws that govern healthcare data transactions in the US. In addition to privacy concerns, there are concerns about accuracy of test results and the ethics of leaving people on their own as they transition from being just people to, suddenly, needing to become patients; or wondering whether they need to become patients.

Removing paternalistic barriers to people learning about their genetic predisposition to serious diseases serves their right to autonomy. Yet, it also leads to potential trauma of interpreting bad news and deciding what to do next alone. Respecting a user's autonomy while doing no harm (non-maleficence), and, moreover, actively doing good (beneficence) requires a lot of thoughtful planning.

The chapter also stresses how people's health literacy and other information seeking and information management competencies are essential requirements for true exercise of autonomy. A health-related decision that is not grounded in true understanding of the issue is not an expression of its maker's values, priorities, and preferences. We saw in this chapter how such decision may be cause for regret. Unfortunately, both the decision to participate in DTC-G testing and the decision regarding how to interpret the results require high levels of health and science literacy. The tasks of interpreting information and making decisions are further complicated by unreliability and/or low clinical significance of many genetic test results. Developers of consumer health informatics tools have an ethical responsibility to provide assistance, but their ability and eagerness to do so may be affected by a number of factors, such as lack of time and experience, competing commercial interests, and a limited evidence base as to how this should be done.

Yet another ethical dilemma has to do with the tension between rapid progress of technological innovations that drives consumer health information technologies and justice. The digital divide between those with and without information access has been a concern since the early days of the internet. Some parts of the divide are closing, as more and more people from all demographics acquire mobile phones and get online. Yet, other aspects of the divide are growing. While the wealthier segment of the population increasingly makes use of voice assistants, activity trackers, vitals monitors, ambient sensors, and DTC-G tests, which have the potential to make them healthier, others are left behind.

This book is written from a position that, despite all the challenges to upholding respect for autonomy and exercising autonomy effectively, equitably, and toward improved health outcomes, individuals have a basic right to participate in their care. We also hold that professionals in consumer health informatics and related fields (healthcare, library and information science, education) have an important ethical responsibility, as well as exciting opportunities to help them find, evaluate, develop, share, and use information in ways that restrict harm and lead to better health.

WEB RESOURCES

National Association of Genetic Counselors
Clearinghouse for all kinds of genetics-related information, including privacy FAQs and counselor directories, from the principal professional association for genetic counseling in the US.
http://aboutgeneticcounselors.com/FAQs-Resources/GINA-Resources

FDA on Direct-to-Consumer Testing
FAQ from the Food and Drug Association relating to DTC-G.
https://www.fda.gov/medical-devices/vitro-diagnostics/direct-consumer-tests#faq

Genetics 101
Khan Academy
Videos produced by 23andMe on genes and genetics.
https://www.youtube.com/watch?reload=9&v=ubq4eu_TDFc&list=PLF9969C74FAAD2BF9

REFERENCES

23andMe. (2019, September 30). *Terms of service*. https://www.23andme.com/about/tos/

Almeling, R., & Gadarian, S. (2014). Public opinion on policy issues in genetics and genomics. *Genetics in Medicine* 16, 491–494.

American Society of Clinical Oncology/Harris Poll. (2018, October). *ASCO 2018 Cancer Opinions Survey*, p. 29. https://www.statista.com/statistics/944250/influences-for-likely-future-genetic-testing-by-test-type/

Anderson, M., & Kumar, M. (2019). Digital divide persists even as lower-income Americans make gains in tech adoption. https://www.pewresearch.org/fact-tank/2019/05/07/digital-divide-persists-even-as-lower-income-americans-make-gains-in-tech-adoption/

Anderson, M., Perrin, A., Jiang, J., & Kumar, M. (2019). 10% of Americans don't use the Internet. *Who are they?* https://www.pewresearch.org/fact-tank/2019/04/22/some-americans-dont-use-the-internet-who-are-they/

Annas, G. J., & Elias, S. (2014). 23andMe and the FDA. *New England Journal of Medicine*, 370(11), 985–988.

Bansback, N., Sizto, S., Guh, D., & Anis, A. H. (2012). The effect of direct-to-consumer genetic tests on anticipated affect and health-seeking behaviors: a pilot survey. *Genetic Testing and Molecular Biomarkers*, 16(10), 1165–1171.

Beauchamp, T. L. (2010). *Standing on principles: Collected essays* Oxford University Press.

Beauchamp, T. L., & Childress, J. F. (2013). *Principles of biomedical ethics* (7th ed.). New York: Oxford University Press.

Beauchamp, T. L., & Childress, J. F. (2019). Principles of biomedical ethics: Marking its fortieth anniversary. *American Journal of Bioethics*, 19(11), 9–12.

Bloss, C. S., Ornowski, L., Silver E., Cargill, M., Vanier, V., Schork, N. J., & Topol, E. J. (2010). Consumer perceptions of direct-to-consumer personalized genomic risk assessments. *Genetics in Medicine*, 12, 556–566.

Bloss, C. S., Schork, N. J., & Topol, E. J. (2011). Effect of direct-to-consumer genomewide profiling to assess disease risk. *New England Journal of Medicine*, 364(6), 524–534.

Bollinger, J. M., Green, R. C., & Kaufman, D. (2013). Attitudes about regulation among direct-to-consumer genetic testing customers. *Genetic Testing and Molecular Biomarkers*, 17(5), 424–428.http://doi.org/10.1089/gtmb.2012.0453

Bourgeois, F. C., DesRoches, C. M., & Bell, S. K. (2017). Ethical challenges raised by OpenNotes for pediatric and adolescent patients. *Pediatrics*, 141(6), e20172745.

Brown, K. V. (2019). 23andMe just got FDA approval for a DNA cancer test. *Time*.

Bureau of Labor Statistics, U.S. Department of Labor. (2019). *Occupational Outlook Handbook, Genetic Counselors*. www.bls.gov/ooh/healthcare/genetic-counselors.htm

Byrd, G. D., & Winkelstein, P. (2014). A comparative analysis of moral principles and behavioral norms in eight ethical codes relevant to health sciences librarianship, medical informatics, and the health professions. *Journal of the Medical Library Association: JMLA*, 102(4), 247–256. https://doi.org/10.3163/1536-5050.102.4.006

Cassel, C., & Bindman, A. (2019). Risk, benefit, and fairness in a big data world. *JAMA*, 322(2), 105–106. https://doi.org/10.1001/jama.2019.9523

Caulfield, T. (2009). Direct-to-consumer genetics and health policy: A worst-case scenario? *American Journal of Bioethics*, 9(6–7), 48–50.

Clow, C. L., & Scriver, C. R. (1977). Knowledge about and attitudes toward genetic screening among high-school students: The Tay-Sachs experience. *Pediatrics*, 59(1), 86–90.

Cooper, S. (2010). Taking no for an answer: Refusal of life-sustaining treatment. *Virtual Mentor*, 12(6), 444–449. https://doi.org/10.1001/virtualmentor.2010.12.6.ccas2-1006

Cottle, M. (2013, June 5). The morality test. *Newsweek Global*. https://www.newsweek.com/2013/06/05/why-your-doctor-afraid-your-dna-237480.html

Covolo, L., Martignone, G., & Orizio, G. (2010). Online direct-to-consumer genetic testing: Analysis of the websites. *IADIS International Conference e-Health*: 264–268.

Covolo, L., Rubinelli, S., Ceretti, E., & Gelatti, U. (2015). Internet-based direct-to-consumer genetic testing: A systematic review. *Journal of Medical Internet Research*, 17(12), e279. https://doi.org/10.2196/jmir.4378

Curnutte, M. (2017) Regulatory controls for direct-to-consumer genetic tests: A case study on how the FDA exercised its authority. *New Genetics and Society*, 36(3), 209–226. https://doi.org/10.1080/14636778.2017.1354690

Dar-Nimrod, I., Zuckerman, M., & Duberstein, P. R. (2013). The effects of learning about one's own genetic susceptibility to alcoholism: A randomized experiment. *Genetics in Medicine*, 15, 132–138.

Darst, B. F., Madlensky, L., Schork, N. J., Topol, E. J., & Bloss, C. S. (2014). Characteristics of genomic test consumers who spontaneously share results with their health care provider. *Health Communications*, 29(1), 105–108. https://doi.org/10.1080/10410236.2012.717216

Dealbook. (2010). Start-up may sell genetic tests in stores. *The New York Times*.

Delaney, S. K., & Christman, M. F. (2016). Direct-to-consumer genetic testing: Perspectives on its value in healthcare. *Clinical Pharmacology & Therapeutics*, 99(2), 146–148.

Ducharme, J. (2018). A major drug company now has access to 23andMe's genetic data. Should you be concerned? https://time.com/5349896/23andme-glaxo-smith-kline/.

Ducharme, J. (2019). 23andMe has a new Type 2 Diabetes risk report. Here's what to know. *Time*. https://time.com/5549014/23andme-diabetes-test/

[Editorial.] (2015). Personal responsibility. *Nature*, 525, 5.

Edwards, K. T., & Huang, C. J. (2014). Bridging the consumer-medical divide: How to regulate direct-to-consumer genetic testing. *Hastings Center Report*, 3, 17–19.

Egglestone, C., Morris, A., & O'Brien, A. (2013). Effect of direct-to-consumer genetic tests on health behaviour and anxiety: A survey of consumers and potential consumers. *Journal of Genetic Counseling*, 22(5). https://doi.org/10.1007/s10897-013-9582-6

Ernst, E. (2009). Advice offered by practitioners of complementary/alternative medicine: An important ethical issue. *Evaluation & the Health Professions*, 32(4), 335–342.

Ernst, E. (2020). About Edzard Ernst. https://edzardernst.com/about/

Evans, J. P. (2008). Recreational genomics; what's in it for you? *Genetics in Medicine: Official Journal of the American College of Medical Genetics*, 10(10), 709–710. https://doi.org/10.1097/GIM.0b013e3181859959

Federal Trade Commission. (n.d.) Direct-to-consumer genetic tests. https://www.consumer.ftc.gov/articles/0166-direct-consumer-genetic-tests

Food and Drug Administration. (2019, December 12). Frequently asked questions about Direct-To-Consumer tests. https://www.fda.gov/medical-devices/vitro-diagnostics/direct-consumer-tests#faq

Francke, U., Dijamco, C., Kiefer, A. K., Eriksson, N., Moiseff, B., Tung, J. Y., & Mountain, J. L. (2013). Dealing with the unexpected: Consumer responses to direct-access BRCA mutation testing. *PeerJ*, 1, e8. https://doi.org/10.7717/peerj.8

Furrow, B. R. (2009). Health law and bioethics. In V. Ravitsky (Eds.), *The Penn Center Guide to Bioethics*. Springer Publishing Company. Accessed via Credo Reference

Genetics Home Reference. (2020a, February 11). Your guide to understanding genetic conditions. https://ghr.nlm.nih.gov/primer/dtcgenetictesting/directtoconsumer

Genetics Home Reference. (2020b, February 11). What are whole exome sequencing and whole genome sequencing? https://ghr.nlm.nih.gov/primer/testing/sequencig

Genetics Home Reference. (2020c, February 11). How can consumers be sure a genetic test is valid and useful? https://ghr.nlm.nih.gov/primer/testing/validtest

Geransar, R., & Einsiedel, E. (2008). Evaluating online direct-to-consumer marketing of genetic tests: Informed choices or buyers beware? *Genetic Testing*, 12(1), 13–23.

GlobalData. (2020, January 16). *23andMe Inc.* New York: Dun & Bradstreet. [D&B Business Browser].

Gollust, S. E., Gray, S. W., Carere, D. E., Koenig, B. A., Lehmann, L. S., McGuire, A. L., Sharp, R. R., Spector-Bagdady, K., Wang, N., Green, R. C., & Roberts, J. S. (2017). Consumer perspectives on access to direct-to-consumer genetic testing: Role of demographic factors and the testing experience. *Milbank Quarterly*, 95(2), 291–318.

Gollust, S. E., Wilfond, B. S., & Hull, S. C. (2003). Direct-to-consumer sales of genetic services on the Internet. *Genetics in Medicine: Official Journal of the American College of Medical Genetics*, 5(4), 332–337.

Graf, N. (2019, August 6). Mail-in DNA test results bring surprises about family history for many users. https://pewrsr.ch/31lVe46

Green, R. C., Roberts, J. S., Cupples, L. A., Relkin, N. R., Whitehouse, P. J., Brown, T., Eckert, S. L., Butson, M., Sadovnick, A. D., Quaid, K. A., Chen, C., Cook-Deegan, R., Farrer, L. A., REVEAL Study Group. (2009). Disclosure of *APOE* genotype for risk of Alzheimer's disease. *The New England Journal of Medicine*, 361(3), 245–254.

Guerrini, C. J., Robinson, J. O., Petersen, D., & McGuire, A. L. (2018). Should police have access to genetic genealogy databases? Capturing the Golden State Killer and other criminals using a controversial new forensic technique. *PLoS Biology*, 16(10), e2006906. https://doi.org/10.1371/journal.pbio.2006906

Gutierrez, A. (2010, June 10). [Letter to Anne Wojcicki/23andME]. https://www.fda.gov/media/79205/download

Hall, J. A., Gertz, R., Amato, J., & Pagliari, C. (2017). Transparency of genetic testing services for 'health, wellness and lifestyle': analysis of online prepurchase information for UK consumers. *European journal of human genetics: EJHG*, 25(8), 908–917. https://doi.org/10.1038/ejhg.2017.75

Hamilton, A. (2008, October 29). Best inventions of 2008. *Time*.

Hartz, S. M. (2015). My experience with direct to consumer genetic testing. *Narrative Inquiry in Bioethics*, 5(3), 208–210.

Hendricks-Sturrup, R. M., & Lu, C. Y. (2019). Direct-to-consumer genetic testing data privacy: Key concerns and recommendations based on consumer perspectives. *Journal of Personalized Medicine*, 9(2), 25. https://doi.org/10.3390/jpm9020025

Hennen, L., Sauter, A., & Van Den Cruyce, E. (2010) Direct to consumer genetic testing: Insights from an internet scan. *New Genetics and Society*, 29(2), 167–186. https://doi.org/10.1080/14636778.2010.484232

Hercher, L. (2018, September 15). 23andMe said he would lose his mind. Ancestry said the opposite. Which was right? *The New York Times*.

Hof, R. D. (2014). 23andMe tries to woo the FDA. *MIT Technology Review*, 117(5), 70–71.

Howard, H. C., & Borry, P. (2012). To ban or not to ban? Clinical geneticists' views on the regulation of direct-to-consumer genetic testing. *EMBO Reports*, 13(9), 791–794.

Howard, H.C., Knoppers, B.M., & Borry, P. (2010). Blurring lines. *EMBO Reports*, 11(8): 579–582.

Hsu, A. R., Mountain, J.L., Wojcicki, A., & Avey, L. (2009). A pragmatic consideration of ethical issues relating to personal genomics. *The American Journal of Bioethics*, 9(6–7), 1–2.

Hughes, A. L. (2013, Fall). Me, my genome, and 23andMe. *The New Atlantis*, 40, 3–18.

Kaiser, J. (2007, December 21). It's all about me. *Science*, 318, 1843.

Kaufman, D. J., Bollinger, J. M., Dvoskin, R. L., & Scott, J. A. (2012). Risky business: risk perception and the use of medical services among customers of DTC personal genetic testing. *Journal of genetic counseling*, 21(3), 413–422. https://doi.org/10.1007/s10897-012-9483-0

Kennedy Institute of Ethics. (n.d.) About. https://kennedyinstitute.georgetown.edu/about

Lewis, N. P., Treise, D., Hsu, S. I., Allen, W. L., & Kang, H. (2011). DTC genetic testing companies fail transparency prescriptions. *New Genetics and Society*, 30(4), 291–307.

McCormic, T. R. (2018). Principles of bioethics. https://depts.washington.edu/bhdept/ethics-medicine/bioethics-topics/articles/principles-bioethics

McGuire, A. L., & Burke, W. (2008, December 10). An unwelcome side effect of direct-to-consumer personal genome testing: Raiding the medical commons. *JAMA*, 300(22), 2669–2671.

McGuire, A. L., Diaz, C. M., Wang, T., & Hilsenbeck, S. G. (2009). Social networkers' attitudes toward direct-to-consumer personal genome testing. *The American Journal of Bioethics: AJOB*, 9(6–7), 3–10. https://doi.org/10.1080/15265160902928209

Medical Library Association. (2010, June). Code of ethics for health sciences librarianship. https://www.mlanet.org/p/cm/ld/fid=160

Messner, D. A. (2011). Informed choice in direct-to-consumer genetic testing for Alzheimer and other diseases: Lessons from two cases. *New Genetics and Society*, 30(1), 59–72. https://doi.org/10.1080/14636778.2011.552300

Miller, C. C. (2013, November 11). For $99, eliminating the mystery of Pandora's genetic box. *The New York Times*.

Mintel. (2019, January). *Health Management Trends - US - January 2019*. From Mintel Academic database.

Moerenhout, T., Fischer, G. S., Saelaert, M., De Sutter, A., Provoost, V., & Devisch, I. (2020). Primary care physicians' perspectives on the ethical impact of the electronic medical record. *Journal of the American Board of Family Medicine*, 33(1), 106–117. https://doi.org/10.3122/jabfm.2020.01.190154

Molla, R. (2020, February 13). Why DNA tests are suddenly unpopular. *Vox*. https://www.vox.com/recode/2020/2/13/21129177/consumer-dna-tests-23andme-ancestry-sales-decline

Molteni, M. (2019, October 15). Ancestry branches out into genetic health screening. https://www.wired.com/story/ancestry-branches-out-into-genetic-health-screening/

Morrison, E. E. (2006). *Ethics in health administration: A practical approach for decision makers* (p. 46). Sudbury, MA: Jones Bartlett.

Moscarello, T., Murray, B., Reuter, C.M., & Demo, E. (2019). Direct-to-consumer raw genetic data and third-party interpretation services: More burden than bargain? *Genetics in Medicine*, 21:539-541

Murphy, H. (2019, April 16). Don't count on 23andMe to detect most breast cancer risks, study warns. *The New York Times*.

Murphy, H., & Zeveri, M., (2019, December 24). Pentagon warns military personnel against at-home DNA tests. *The New York Times*.

National Research Council (US) and Institute of Medicine (US) Roundtable on translating genomic-based research for health. (2010). Direct-to-consumer genetic testing: Summary of a workshop. National Academies Press. (US) https://www.ncbi.nlm.nih.gov/books/NBK209632/

Nebeker, C., Murray, K., Holub, C., Haughton, J., & Arredondo, E. M. (2017). Acceptance of mobile health in communities underrepresented in biomedical research: Barriers and ethical considerations for scientists. *JMIR Mhealth and UHealth*, 5(6), e87. https://doi.org/https://mhealth.jmir.org/2017/6/e87/

Norman, C. D., & Skinner, H. A. (2006). eHEALS: The eHealth Literacy Scale. *Journal of Medical Internet Research*, 8(4), e27

Office of Civil Rights. (2013, July 26). What does the HIPAA Privacy Rule do? https://www.hhs.gov/hipaa/for-individuals/faq/187/what-does-the-hipaa-privacy-rule-do/index.html

Peikoff, K. (2013, December 30). I had my DNA picture taken, with varying results. *The New York Times*.

Perrin, A. (2019, May 31). Digital gap between rural and nonrural America persists. https://www.pewresearch.org/fact-tank/2019/05/31/digital-gap-between-rural-and-nonrural-america-persists/

Perrin, A., & Turner, E. (2019, August 20). Smartphones help blacks, Hispanics bridge some – but not all – digital gaps with whites. https://www.pewresearch.org/fact-tank/2019/08/20/smartphones-help-blacks-hispanics-bridge-some-but-not-all-digital-gaps-with-whites/

Petersen, C., Berner, E. S., Embi, P. J., Hollis, K. F., Goodman, K. W., Koppel, R., Lehmann, C. U., Lehmann, H., Maulden, S. A., McGregor, K. A., Solomonides, A., Subbian, V., Terrazas, E., & Winkelstein, P. (2018). AMIA's code of professional and ethical conduct. *Journal of the American Medical Informatics Association*, 25(11), 1579–1582. https://doi.org/10.1093/jamia/ocy092

Pollack, A. (2008, June 26). Gene testing questioned by regulators. *The New York Times*. https://www.nytimes.com/2008/06/26/business/26gene.html

Pollack, A. (2010a, March 19). Consumers slow to embrace the age of genomics. *The New York Times*. https://www.nytimes.com/2010/03/20/business/20consumergene.html

Pollack, A. (2010b, March 19). Is a DNA scan a medical test or just informational? Views differ. *The New York Times*. https://www.nytimes.com/2010/03/20/business/20consumergenebar.html

Pollack, A. (2013, November 25). F.D.A. orders genetic testing firm to stop selling DNA analysis service. *The New York Times*. https://www.nytimes.com/2013/11/26/business/fda-demands-a-halt-to-a-dna-test-kits-marketing.html

Pomerantz, D. (2019, August 8). 23andMe had devastating news about my health. I wish a person had delivered it. *Stat*. https://www.statnews.com/2019/08/08/23andme-genetic-test-revealed-high-cancer-risk/

Pomerantz, D. (2020, February 7). I was fortunate to get post-23andMe genetic counseling. Everyone should have that option. *STAT*. https://www.statnews.com/2020/02/07/genetic-counseling-after-home-genetic-testing/

Quelch, J. A., & Rodriguez, M. L. (2016). 23andMe: Genetic testing for consumers (A). In J. A. Quelch (Ed.), *Consumers, corporations, and public health: A case-based approach to sustainable business*. New York: Oxford University Press.

Ram, N., Guerrini, C. J., & McGuire, A. L. (2018, June 8). Genealogy databases and the future of criminal investigation. *Science*, 360(6393), 1078–1079.

Regalado, A. (2019, February 11). More than 26 million people have taken an at-home ancestry test: The genetic genie is out of the bottle. And it's not going back. *MIT Technology Review*. https://www.technologyreview.com/s/612880/more-than-26-million-people-have-taken-an-at-home-ancestry-test/

Regalado, A (2020, January 23). Is the consumer genetics fad over? https://www.technologyreview.com/f/615088/is-the-consumer-genetics-fad-over/

Roberts, J. S., & Ostergren, J. (2013). Direct-to-consumer genetic testing and personal genomics services: A review of recent empirical studies. *Current Genetic Medicine Reports*, 1(3), 182–200.

Rubin, P. H. (2001). Pharmaceutical advertising as a consumer empowerment device. *Journal of Biolaw and Business*, 4(4), 59–65.

Salkin, A. (2008, September 12). When in doubt, spit it out. *The New York Times*. https://www.nytimes.com/2008/09/14/fashion/14spit.html

Siddiqui, S., & Chan, V. T. (2018). In the patient's best interest: Appraising social network site information for surrogate decisionmaking. *Journal of Medical Ethics*, 44, 851–856.

Singleton, A., Erby, L. H., Foisie, K. V., & Kaphingst, K. A. (2012). Informed choice in direct-to-consumer genetic testing (DTCGT) websites: A content analysis of benefits, risks, and limitations. *Journal of Genetic Counseling*, 21(3), 433–439.

SNPedia:FAQ. (2019, July 2). https://www.snpedia.com/index.php/SNPedia:FAQ

Spencer, E. G., & Topol, E. J. (2019). Direct to consumer fitness DNA testing. *Clinical Chemistry*, 65(1), 45–47.

Takano, T. (2019). How safe is GEDmatch? https://blog.genomelink.io/posts/how-safe-is-gedmatch

Tandy-Connor, S., Guiltinan, J., Krempely, K. LaDuca, H., Reineke, P., Gutierrez, S., Gray, P., & Davis, B. T. (2018). False-positive results released by direct-to-consumer genetic tests highlight the importance of clinical confirmation testing for appropriate patient care. *Genetics in Medicine*, 20, 1515–1521.

United States Census. (2020). U.S. and world population clock. www.census.gov/popclock

Update to "Direct-to-Consumer genetic testing: An examination of privacy and security concerns". (2015). *Penn Bioethics Journal*, 11(2), 9.

US Courts. (n.d.) What does the Fourth Amendment mean? https://www.uscourts.gov/about-federal-courts/educational-resources/about-educational-outreach/activity-resources/what-does-0

US Department of Education. (2006). The health literacy of America's adults: Results from the 2003 national assessment of adult literacy (NAAL). *Institute of Education Sciences: National Center for Education Statistics*. https://nces.ed.gov/pubs2006/2006483.pdf

van Dijk, J.A.G.M. (2006). Digital divide research, achievements and shortcomings. *Poetics*, 34(4–5): 221–235.

Wiggins, S., Whyte, P., Huggins, M., Aedam, S., Theilmann, J. Bloch, M., Sheps, S.B., Schechter, M., & Hayden, M.R. (1992). The psychological consequences of predictive testing for Huntington's Disease. *New England Journal of Medicine*, 327(20): 1401–1405.

Winston, J. (2017, May 17). Ancestry.com takes DNA ownership rights from customers and their relatives. https://thinkprogress.org/ancestry-com-takes-dna-ownership-rights-from-customers-and-their-relatives-dbafeed02b9e/

Wojcicki, A. (2019, Feb. 5). 23andMe responds: Empowering consumers. [Letter to the editor]. *New York Times*. https://www.nytimes.com/2019/02/05/opinion/letters/23andme-genetic-test.html

Index

Page numbers in *italics* refer to content in *figures*; page numbers in **bold** refer to content in **tables**.

A

AARP, 95, 98
Abdel-Wahab, N., 81
Academic Search, 62
activities of daily living (ADLs), **28**, 95, 105, 108, 159, 166, 167, 175, 183, 186
   definition, 167
   user engagement, 167
activity trackers, 28, 227
adolescents, 102–103, 123
   chronic illnesses, 102–103
adult literacy, 34–36
Advancing Care Information, 119
advertising, 74, 80, **85**, 149, 193, 206, 219
advertising policy, 49, 80
advocacy organizations, 9, 11, 85, **86**, 152
African Americans, 126, 182, 217
AfterTheInjury website, 101
age, 50, 94
Agency for Healthcare Research and Quality (AHRQ), 26, 86
Aitken, M., 150
alcoholism, 184, 222
algorithms, 49, 50, 58, 168, 172
All of Us (NIH), 7, 21
Allam, A., 74
Allan, R., 191
Alnasser, A.A., 145, 146
ALS Digest (weekly magazine), 183
alternative medicine, 59, 64; *see also* complementary and alternative medicine
Alzheimer's disease, 99, 105, 149, 163, 172, 205, 207, 209, 217, 221
   testing, 209
Amazon, 168, 169, 206, 207
   Amazon Echo, 169
ambient sensors, 159, 226, 227
ambulatory activities (Ni *et al.*), 166

American Academy of Otolaryngology, **86**
American Cancer Society, 9, **86**
American Civil Liberties Union, 169
American College Health Association, 103
American Diabetes Association, 52
American Health Information Management Association, 203
American Heart Association, 9, **83**
American Journal of Bioethics, 219
American Library Association, 203
   Presidential Committee on Information Literacy, 41
American Medical Association, 42, 75, 203
American Medical Informatics Association, 27, 29, 66
   AMIA Dental Informatics Working Group, 25
   code of ethics, 202
American Nurses Association, 25, 203
American Psychological Association, 63
American Public Health Association, 203
American Recovery and Reinvestment Act (ARRA, 2009), 119
American Syringomelia and Chiari Alliance Project, 183
Amyotrophic Lateral Sclerosis (ALS), 7, 12–13, 183, 185, 189
Ancestry.com, 204, 208, 218, 224
Ancker, J. S., 46–48
Anderson, M., 212
Android apps, 108
Android Google Play Store, 141
Annas, G. J., 210
ANSI (American National Standards Institute), 124
anxiety, 103, 150
aorta, 15
APOE e4 allele, 209
Apostilidis, K., 9
app, definition, 134

Printed in the United States
By Bookmasters